MOHR

Color Atlas
of Diagnostic Endoscopy
in Otorhinolaryngology

COLOR ATLAS OF DIAGNOSTIC ENDOSCOPY IN OTORHINOLARYNGOLOGY

Eiji Yanagisawa, M.D.
Clinical Professor of Otolaryngology
Yale University School of Medicine
Attending Otolaryngologist, Yale–New Haven Hospital
Attending Otolaryngologist, Hospital of St. Raphael
New Haven, Connecticut

Graphics by
Ray Yanagisawa, B.A.
New Haven, Connecticut

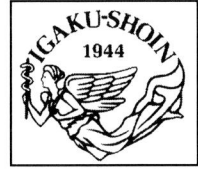

IGAKU-SHOIN   New York • Tokyo

Published and distributed by

IGAKU-SHOIN Medical Publishers, Inc.
One Madison Avenue, New York, New York 10010

IGAKU-SHOIN Ltd.,
5-24-3 Hongo, Bunkyo-ku, Tokyo 113-91.

Copyright © 1997 by IGAKU-SHOIN Medical Publishers, Inc.
All rights reserved. No part of this book may be translated or
reproduced in any form by print, photo-print, microfilm or any
other means without written permission from the publisher.

Library of Congress Cataloging-in-Publication Data

Yanagisawa, Eiji.
    Color atlas of diagnostic endoscopy in otorhinolaryngology / Eiji
Yanagisawa; graphics by Ray Yanagisawa.
       p.   cm.
    Includes bibliographical references and index.
    1. Otolaryngologic examination—Atlases. 2. Video endoscopy—
Atlases. 3. Otolaryngology—Diagnosis—Atlases. I. Title.
    [DNLM: 1. Otorhinolaryngologic Diseases—diagnosis—atlases.
2. Endoscopy—atlases.   WV 17 Y21c 1996]
RF48.5.E53Y36 1996
617.5' 107545—dc20
DNLM/DLC
for Library of Congress   96-15369
                                                                  CIP

ISBN: 0-89640-316-5 (New York)
ISBN: 4-260-14316-6 (Tokyo)

Printed in Hong Kong
10 9 8 7 6 5 4 3 2 1

Preface

When I was an ENT resident at Yale 40 years ago, Dr. John A. Kirchner, then Chief of Otolaryngology, showed me his collection of Dr. Paul Holinger's most beautiful photographs of the larynx. How I wished that some day I could take laryngeal pictures like Dr. Holinger. I have since tried numerous methods of still photography, cinematography, and videography to document the anatomy and pathology of otorhinolaryngological structures.

My interest in videography began in 1975 when I purchased my first home video color camera (Magnavox CV440) to take pictures of my children. I soon realized that the same video camera could be used for videography of the microsurgery of the larynx. Using a C-mount adapter, I was able to connect it to the Zeiss operating microscope and perform my first successful videography of the larynx on a patient with an obstructive verrucous carcinoma. I then decided to apply this technique of videographic documentation to other areas of otorhinolaryngology and have subsequently published early works in videolaryngoscopy (1981, 1984, 1985, 1991), videorhinoscopy (1986), video-otoscopy (1987), stroboscopic videolaryngoscopy (1987, 1993), videonasopharyngoscopy (1989), simultaneous velolaryngeal videoendoscopy (1990, 1991), videopharyngoscopy, and other videoendoscopic techniques.

In the course of my endeavor to obtain the best possible images of the ear, nose, and throat, I was inspired by the works of many otorhinolaryngologists around the world. Drs. Bruce Benjamin, Paul Holinger, Oscar Kleinsasser, Richard Buckingham, Paul Ward, Minoru Hirano, Koichi Yamashita, and Heinz Stammberger all had a major influence on my work.

This atlas of diagnostic endoscopy in otorhinolaryngology is the culmination of my 20 years of personal experience of videographic documentation in otorhinolaryngology. I selected and compiled these images from over 10,000 cases of ENT endoscopy. Because of the limited scope of my practice, I could not cover all diseases of the otorhinolaryngologic field. However, this book shows useful anatomy and pathology of commonly encountered ear, nose, and throat disorders.

The unique feature of this atlas is that almost all of the pictures shown in this book were taken from video images reproduced either by color video printers or by a computer. I believe that videographic documentation is the most practical and effective means for a precise ENT diagnosis today. It is my sincere hope that this book will be of practical value for otolaryngologists and serve as a useful guide to the understanding of anatomy and pathology of otorhinolaryngological structures.

Eiji Yanagisawa, M.D.

This book is dedicated to my wife June
and my children, Ken, Kay, Amy, and Ray.

Foreword

Throughout my 40-year association with Dr. Yanagisawa, I have marveled at his penetrating power of observation, particularly for the kind of minute detail that might escape a less attentive witness. Unlike most of us who simply store away our observations in a mental file box, Dr. Yanagisawa captures them with his camera, always near at hand to record the usual and the unusual, such as the wisp of hair in contact with the tympanic membrane. In the early years of this project, Dr. Yanagisawa's photographs became an important part of the residents' training at the Yale–New Haven program, and they continue to be. As the collection grew, its teaching value to the profession at large was recognized by national organizations in this country and across the world. His meticulous attention to detail provides the reader of this volume with key landmarks that guide him through a safe but thorough examination of the nasal chamber and paranasal sinuses. His success in photographing structures in areas ordinarily hidden from casual inspection such as the sphenoid ostium in the sphenoethmoidal recess reflects a dogged determination to demonstrate what he sees. Important structures within the sphenoid sinus—the carotid artery and optic nerve ridges—are displayed with unmistakable clarity. Seeing the fenestra in the horizontal semicircular canal under the skin flap photographed in living color would have delighted Julius Lempert.

The author has not restricted the atlas to normal anatomy, its variations, and its abnormalities, but has included short, concise comments on the clinical significance of the structure or condition being displayed in the photograph. The reader will find these comments useful in practice. The 90-degree telescopic view into the ventricle, for example, solves the problem of assessing the lateral extent of a glottic carcinoma and its suitability for hemilaryngectomy.

Dr. Yanagisawa's extensive collection of endoscopic photographs has outgrown its original storage area on the ground floor of his home. How such a wealth of material could be organized for presentation appeared to be an almost insurmountable task, but he has indeed succeeded. In presenting to us these unique and comprehensive photographic views of the upper aerodigestive tract, Dr. Yanagisawa has rendered an incomparable service to every practicing otolaryngologist.

John A. Kirchner, M.D.
Professor Emeritus of Otolaryngology
Yale University School of Medicine
New Haven, Connecticut

Acknowledgments

I acknowledge the valuable contributions of the following individuals: Drs. Mario Andrea and Oscar Diaz, Lisbon, Portugal (Chapter 12); Dr. Dennis Poe, Boston, Massachusetts (Chapter 13); Dr. Edward M. Weaver, New Haven, Connecticut (Chapters 8 and 10); and Dr. Ken Yanagisawa, New Haven, Connecticut (Chapter 10). I also extend my appreciation to Dr. John A. Kirchner, New Haven, Connecticut, for providing me with his valuable histopathology photographs of the larynx.

I thank Dr. Valerie Asher for proofreading the manuscript and thank Dr. Edward M. Weaver for his assistance in writing, editing, and proofreading the manuscript. My special thanks go to my son Ray Yanagisawa for his tireless efforts and perseverance to attain the superb graphics, and I am grateful to Melissa Pisani for carrying out the extensive work of retrieving the video images from my large collection.

I would like to express my deep appreciation to Mr. Gene Kearn of Igaku-Shoin Publishers for the conception of this book and for his encouragement, guidance, patience, and understanding during its preparation.

Contributors

Mario Andrea, M.D., Ph.D.
Professor and Chairman
Department of Otolaryngology
Faculty of Medicine of Lisbon
Lisbon, Portugal

Oscar Dias, M.D., Ph.D.
Assistant Professor
Department of Otolaryngology
Faculty of Medicine of Lisbon
Lisbon, Portugal

Dennis S. Poe, M.D.
Associate Professor of Otolaryngology
Tufts University School of Medicine
Boston, Massachusetts

Edward M. Weaver, M.D.
Senior Resident in Otolaryngology
Yale–New Haven Hospital
New Haven, Connecticut

Eiji Yanagisawa, M.D.
Clinical Professor of Otolaryngology
Yale University School of Medicine
Attending Otolaryngologist, Yale–New Haven Hospital
Attending Otolaryngologist, Hospital of St. Raphael
New Haven, Connecticut

Ken Yanagisawa, M.D.
Clinical Instructor of Otolaryngology
Yale University School of Medicine
New Haven, Connecticut

Key to Figure Abbreviations

A	Arytenoid		MMA	Middle meatal antrostomy
AC	Anterior commissure, Anterior crus of stapes		MO	Maxillary sinus ostium
AEA	Anterior ethmoidal artery		MS	Maxillary sinus
AF	Anterior fontanelle		MSO	Maxillary sinus ostium
AMO	Accessory maxillary sinus ostium		MT	Middle turbinate
AN	Agger Nasi		NL	Nasolacrimal duct
AO	Accessory ostium		NP	Nasopharynx, Neopharynx
AP	Anterior pillar (palatoglossal arch), Atretic plate		NS	Nasal septum
BA	Body of arytenoid cartilage		ON	Optic nerve
BE	Ethmoid bulla (bulla ethmoidalis)		OP	Oropharynx
BL	Basal lamella (ground lamella)		P	Polyp
C	Choana		PD	Pseudodiverticulum
CA	Cancer		PE	Posterior ethmoid sinus, Pyramidal eminence, Pressure equalizing (tube)
CB	Concha bullosa			
CCD	Charge-coupled device		PEO	Posterior ethmoid sinus ostium
CE	Conus elasticus		PF	Posterior fontanelle
CEMS	Contact endoscopy in microlaryngeal surgery		PG	Pseudoglottis
CP	Cribriform plate		PM	Promontory
CR	Cricoid cartilage		PP	Posterior pillar (palatopharyngeal arch)
CT	Corniculate tubercule		PPW	Posterior pharyngeal wall
D	Dissector		PR	Pterygoid recess (inferolateral recess)
E	Epiglottis		PS	Pyriform sinus
EI	Ethmoidal infundibulum		PT	Palatine tonsil
ES	Ethmoid sinus		PW	Pharyngeal wall
ET	Eustachian tube orifice		RBR	Retrobullar recess (lateral sinus)
ETT	Endotracheal tube		REMS	Rigid endoscopy in microlaryngeal surgery
F	Facial nerve		RMT	Retromolar trigone
FE	Fovea ethmoidalis		RNC	Roof of nasal cavity
FF	False vocal fold		RW	Round window
FMI	Fused malleus and incus		S	Stapes
FN	Facial nerve		SBR	Suprabullar recess (lateral sinus)
FR	Frontal recess		SER	Sphenoethmoidal recess
FSS	Floor of sphenoid sinus		SF	Stapes footplate
GT	Glomus Tumor		SG	Subglottis
HS	Head of stapes		SIT	Sinus tympani
HSL	Hiatus semilunaris		SM	Superior meatus, Squamous matrix
HSLI	Hiatus semilunaris inferior		SO	Sphenoid sinus ostium
HSLS	Hiatus semilunaris superior		SP	Soft palate, Stapes prosthesis
HT	Hypotympanum		SS	Sphenoid sinus, Sigmoid sinus
I	Incus		SSO	Sphenoid sinus ostium
ICA	Internal carotid artery		ST	Superior turbinate
IM	Inferior meatus		STF	Superior tonsillar fossa
IMA	Inferior meatal antrostomy		SVHS	Super VHS
IOR	Infraoptic recess		T	Tumor, Tongue, Trachea
IT	Inferior turbinate		TAM	Thyroarytenoid muscle
ITF	Inferior tonsillar fossa		TC	Thyroid cartilage
KR	Kirchner's ridge		TF	True vocal cord
KS	Karl Storz		TT	Torus tubarius
L	Lacrimal bone		U	Uvula, Umbo
LNW	Lateral nasal wall		UP	Uncinate process
LP	Lamina papyracea		V	Vallecula, Ventricle
LS	Lateral sinus		VHS	Video home system
M	Malleus		VL	Vocal ligament
MA	Mastoid antrum		VM	Vascular mass
ME	Middle ear		VP	Vocal process of arytenoid cartilage
MM	Middle meatus, Malleus manubrium			

Contents

Key to Figure Abbreviations   x

Part I. General Considerations

Chapter 1.   Introduction and Historical Background   3

Chapter 2.   Equipment   7

Chapter 3.   Documentation   13

Part II. Endoscopy in Otorhinolaryngology

Chapter 4.   Endoscopy of the External Ear and Tympanic Membrane (Video-otoscopy)   19

Chapter 5.   Endoscopy of the Nose (Video Nasal Endoscopy, Videorhinoscopy)   41

Chapter 6.   Endoscopy of the Paranasal Sinuses (Videosinoscopy)   67

Chapter 7.   Endoscopy of the Nasopharynx (Videonasopharyngoscopy)   86

Chapter 8.   Endoscopy of the Oropharynx (Videopharyngoscopy)   102

Chapter 9.   Endoscopy of the Larynx (Videolaryngoscopy)   114

Chapter 10.   Stroboscopy of the Larynx (Stroboscopic Videolaryngoscopy, Strobovideolaryngoscopy)   145

Chapter 11.   Simultaneous Velolaryngeal Videoendoscopy   158

Chapter 12.   Rigid and Contact Endoscopy in Microlaryngeal Surgery   168

Chapter 13.   Endoscopy of the Middle Ear (Middle Ear Videoendoscopy)   180

Bibliography   179

Index   185

Color Atlas
of Diagnostic Endoscopy
in Otorhinolaryngology

Part I
General Considerations

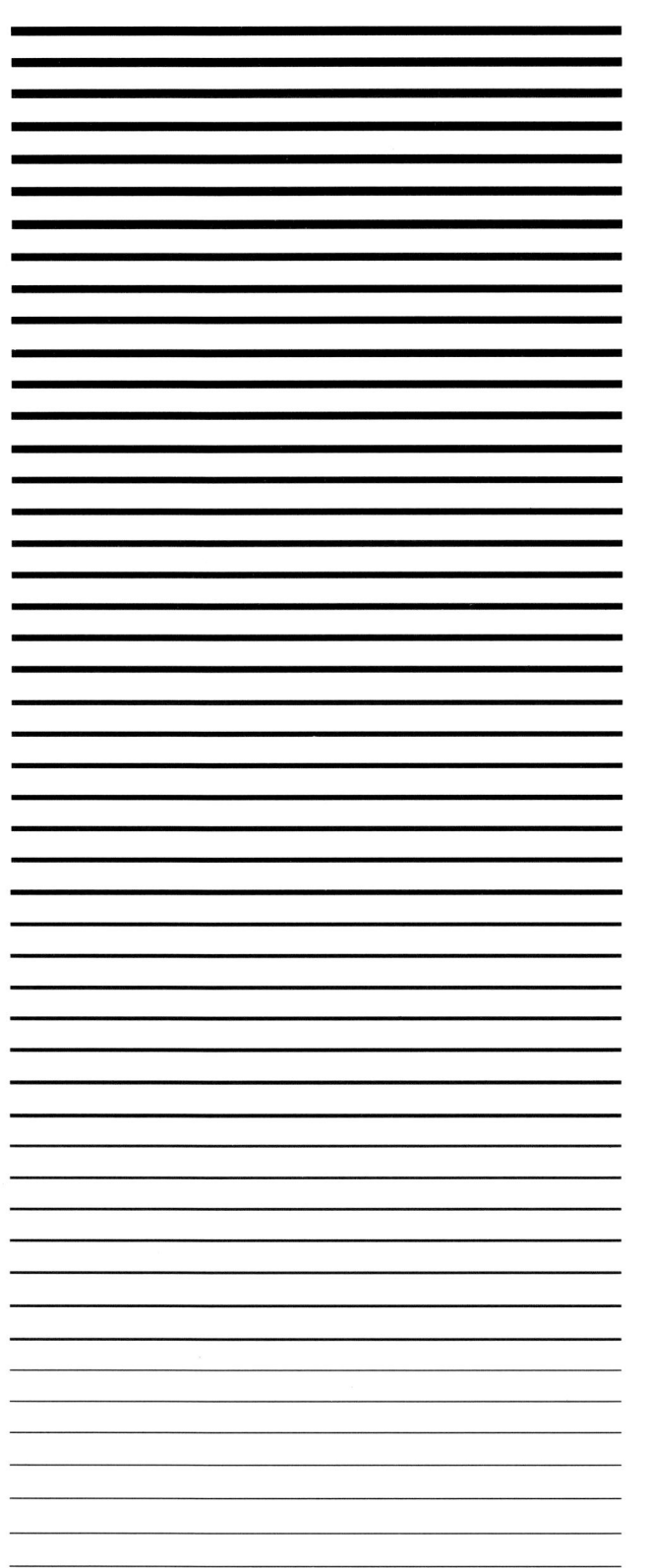

CHAPTER 1
INTRODUCTION AND HISTORICAL BACKGROUND

Videoendoscopy in otorhinolaryngology now includes a wide variety of techniques using an array of rigid and flexible endoscopes with video cameras, monitors, recorders, and printers. The various techniques provide access to the different structures and movements of the ear, nose, and throat and are the focus of the following chapters. Most of these techniques can be performed in the office.

Video-otoscopy uses a rigid telescope to view the tympanic membrane (Figure 1-1A). Pneumatic video-otoscopy records the tympanic membrane movement in real time (Figure 1-1B). Videorhinoscopy provides a complete view of the nasal cavities through rigid telescopes (Figure 1-1C). Videosinoscopy reveals intra-antral anatomy with rigid telescopes introduced directly into the maxillary sinus through a trocar (Figure 1-1D). Videonasopharyngoscopy uses angled telescopes to view the nasopharynx and posterior nasal cavity from below (Figure 1-1E). Videopharyngoscopy displays close-up views of the oropharynx with various transoral rigid telescopes (Figure 1-1F). Fiberscopic videolaryngoscopy is a common and relatively easy technique of examining the larynx (Figure 1-1G). Telescopic videolaryngoscopy yields a clearer image of the larynx than does the fiberscopic technique (Fig. 1-1H). Stroboscopic videolaryngoscopy (strobovideolaryngoscopy) provides a unique examination of the vocal fold movements (Figure 1.1I).

Videography allows immediate viewing of ear, nose, and throat (ENT) pathology by the examiner and patient and instantaneous production of video prints for the permanent record. Almost all of the color images shown in this atlas were taken with a video camera and reproduced by either a color video printer or a computer.

The purpose of this book is to (1) describe various techniques of diagnostic endoscopy in otorhinolaryngology, (2) show clear color pictures of detailed endoscopic anatomy and pathology (many common pathological states, as well as some rare but clinically important conditions, were selected from the author's collection), and (3) illustrate the value of many different forms of videoendoscopy in otorhinolaryngology.

Each clinical chapter consists of (1) brief introduction, (2) overview, (3) techniques, (4) endoscopic anatomy, and (5) common disorders. In some chapters, special newer endoscopic techniques, such as simultaneous velolaryngeal videoendoscopy, stroboscopic videolaryngoscopy, rigid and contact endoscopy in microlaryngeal surgery, and middle ear videoendoscopy, are described.

HISTORICAL BACKGROUND OF ENDOSCOPIC DOCUMENTATION IN OTORHINOLARYNGOLOGY

Otology

The critical milestones in otologic photography included the development of otoscopic photography in the late

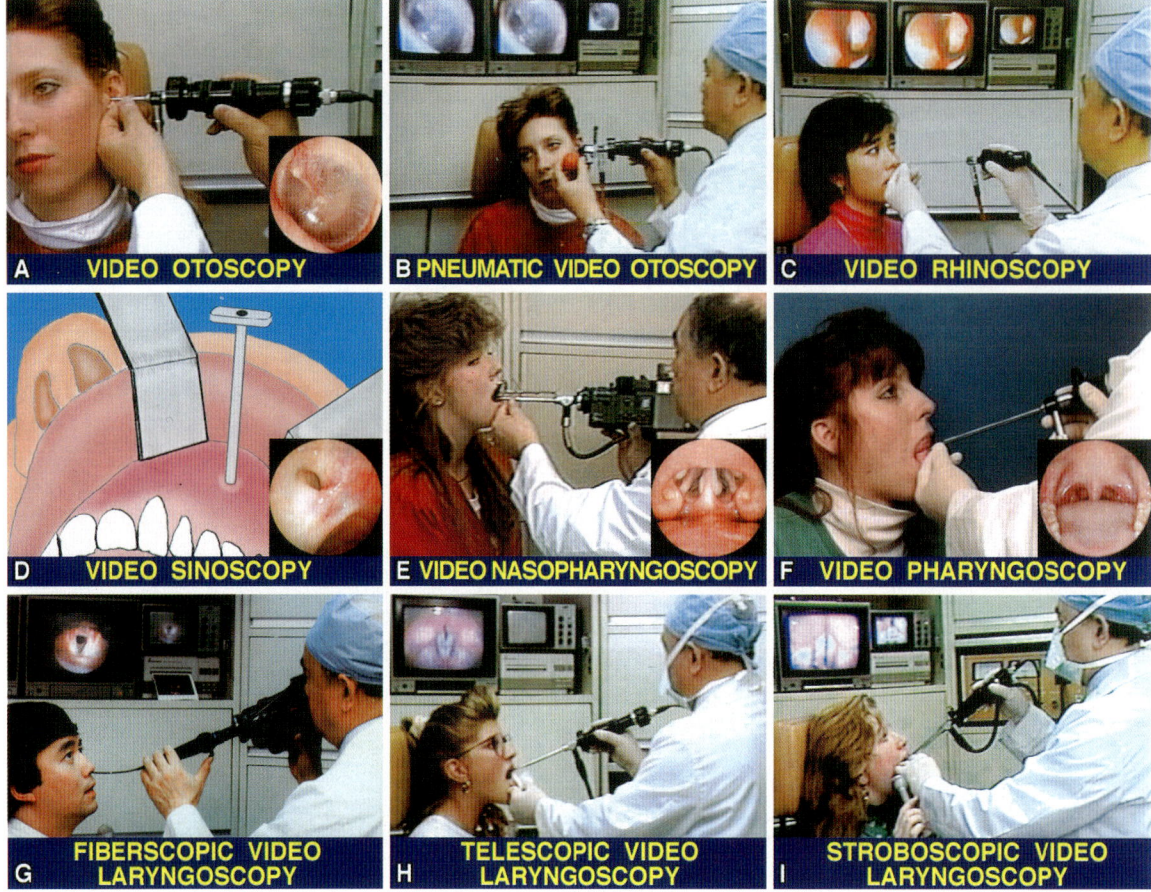

Figure 1-1. Overview of videoendoscopy in otorhinolaryngology. (A) Video-otoscopy (Chapter 4). (B) Pneumatic video-otoscopy (Chapter 4). (C) Videorhinoscopy (Chapter 5). (D) Videosinoscopy (Chapter 6). (E) Videonasopharyngoscopy (Chapter 7). (F) Videopharyngoscopy (Chapter 8). (G) Fiberscopic videolaryngoscopy (Chapter 9). (H) Telescopic videolaryngoscopy (Chapter 9). (I) Stroboscopic videolaryngoscopy (Chapter 10).

1800s, microscopic photograhy in the 1950s, and telescopic photography in the 1970s. The advent of motion picture photography and later videography greatly enhanced visual documentation of ear anatomy and pathology.

In 1865, Adam Politzer published a remarkable chromolithographic illustration of the tympanic membrane in health and disease. The first photographic reproductions of the tympanic membrane appeared in 1866 in Rudinger's *Atlas des Menschlichen Gehororganes*. S. T. Stein of Frankfurt illustrated a technique for the reproduction of the *in vivo* tympanic membrane image in the *Archiv für Ohrenheilkunde* in 1873 (Figure 1-2A). In 1938, Schultz van Treek introduced an optical lens system to which a camera and a speculum were fitted. He obtained good field visualization and produced black-and-white photographs of exceptionally high quality. I. Hantman, using a camera designed by the Cameron Surgical Specialty Company of Chicago, was the first to publish color photographs of the tympanic membrane.

In 1940, J. D. Brubaker first developed an endoscopic camera for proctoscopic photography. It was adapted by P. Holinger, J. D. Brubaker, and J. E. Brubaker for open-tube endoscopic photography of the larynx, bronchi, and esophagus. R. A. Buckingham of Chicago was the first to adapt the Brubaker–Holinger camera for ear photography (Figure 1-2B). He produced color photographs of superior quality.

In the late 1950s, the Carl Zeiss operating microscope—a milestone in optics—came into use. Shortly after the introduction of the microscope to otologic surgery, the House–Urban observation tube, 35-mm still (Figure 1-2C) and 16-mm motion picture cameras, and later color video cameras were added. These additions enhanced the teaching and documentation of microsurgery of the ear.

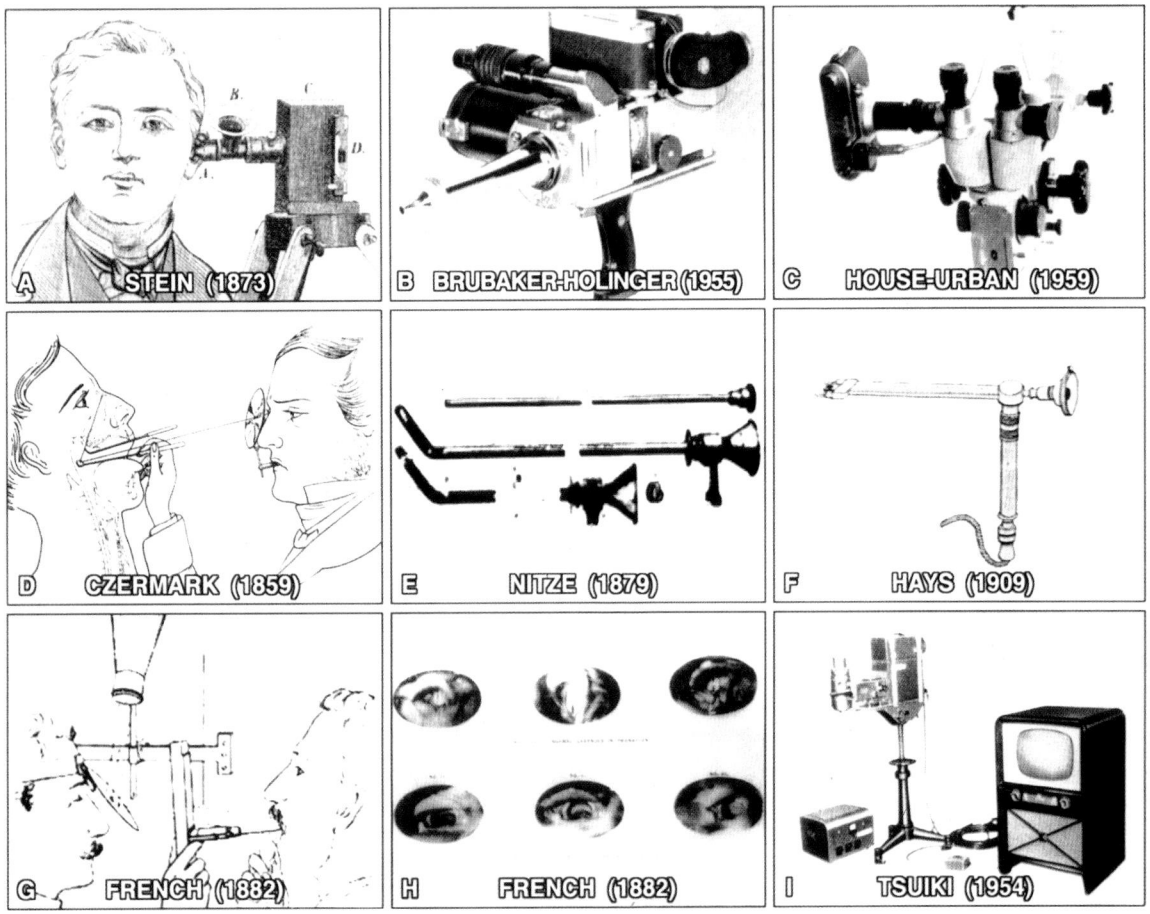

Figure 1-2. Historical milestones. (A) Stein's photographic otoscope. (B) Buckingham's modified Brubaker–Holinger camera. (C) Zeiss operating microscope with a House–Urban 35-mm camera. (D) Czermark's nasopharyngeal mirror. (E) Nitze's cystoscope. (F) Hays' transoral nasopharyngoscope. (G) French's indirect laryngoscope. (H) Larynx photographs by French. (I) Tsuiki (1954) laryngeal "tele-endoscope." (Figs. A, B, C from Pensak ML, Yanagisawa E. Tympanic membrane photography, historical perspective. *Am J Otol* 5:324–332, 1984. Figs. D, E, F from Yamashita K. Diagnostic and therapeutic ENT endoscopy. Tokyo, Medical View, 1988. Figs. G, H from French TR. On a perfected method of photographing the larynx. *New York Med J* 4:655–656, 1984. All figures used with permission.)

One of the most significant advances in endoscopic photography is the development by H. H. Hopkins of the telescope with the new rod lens system. The air-containing spaces between the conventional series of lenses have been replaced with glass rods, with polished ends separated by small "air lenses." The optics of this new invention are such that light transmission and magnification are significantly increased. The wide-angle view of the Hopkins telescopes provides an almost infinite depth of field so that the entire tympanic membrane is in focus. Perhaps the most attractive feature of this new telescopic system is the ease with which still, video, or movie cameras and teaching attachments can be coupled to the new telescopes.

At the American Academy of Otolaryngology Meeting in 1979, Yanagisawa et al. presented a comparison of techniques for tympanic membrane and middle ear photography. Subsequently reporting to the 1981 annual meeting of the Academy, Yanagisawa concluded that telescopic photography was the most effective method of tympanic membrane photography.

The disadvantages of telescopic otoscopy include (1) lens fogging, (2) distortion due to the wide-angle lens, and (3) risk of tympanic membrane or ossicular chain injury. In spite of these shortcomings, with the high-quality video printers available today, video-otoscopy now is the most effective and reliable method of tympanic membrane photography. Excellent full-view detailed color images of the tympanic membrane can be recorded on video and printed.

This immediate hard copy is useful for teaching and records, and it allows for a 100% successful image capture rate.

Rhinology

In 1806, Bozzini published the first description of a nasopharyngeal endoscope. He called his primitive endoscope a "light conductor" and described its use in a number of body cavities, including the nasopharynx. In 1838, Baumes described his technique using a mirror to examine the larynx and choanae. Czermark in Vienna also described nasopharyngeal mirror exams, including a posterior nasal exam in 1859 (Figure 1-2D). Anterior rhinoscopy with a nasal speculum received renewed interest in 1860 when Markusowsky had a nasal speculum made. He did not realize that others had used similar devices centuries earlier. Wertheim was able to examine the anterior and middle thirds of the nasal cavity with his conchoscope in 1869.

In 1879, Nitze invented his cystoscope, used for examining the bladder and other anatomical spaces (Figure 1-2E). Leiter adapted the Nitze cytoscope for nasal and nasopharyngeal examinations. Zaufal used this scope in 1880 to view the eustachian tube orifice. This device was infrequently used because the hot platinum wire light source required a bulky built-in water cooling system.

Even the cooler electric light was slow to catch on until 1903 when Valentin developed a 4.5-mm endoscope with a small electric light source not requiring a coolant system. This scope could pass easily through most noses even allowing consistent exams of the eustachian tube orifices. The year before, in 1902, Hirschman and Valentin viewed the maxillary sinus with a modified cystoscope through an enlarged dental alveolus. Throughout that decade various people used the endoscopes to perform primitive endoscopic sinus surgery for chronic empyema or foreign body removals. Independently in 1909–1910 Flatau and Hays described transnasal salpingoscopy and transoral nasopharyngoscopy with similar endoscopes (Figure 1-2F).

Nevertheless, nasal and nasopharyngeal endoscopy remained unpopular until after World War II because it was considered unnecessary. In the 1950s, microscopic endonasal surgery was initiated by Heermann. By 1956, Hopkins introduced his new rigid rod endoscope with glass rods separated by "air lenses." His endoscopes used a separate light source and provided excellent resolution with high contrast, large field of vision despite slim scope diameter, and true fidelity of color. Messerklinger initiated modern endoscopic sinus surgery in the late 1960s, and his techniques have advanced since then through the work of many endoscopists including Hellmich and Herberholdt, Draf, Wigand, Yamashita, Friedrich, Stammberger, and Kennedy.

Laryngology

The Spanish-born singing teacher Manuel Garcia was the first to visualize the intact larynx. In 1854, he observed the movements of his own vocal folds using a dental mirror, with a hand-held mirror for reflecting sunlight. Thomas French of New York in 1882 was the first to photograph the larynx successfully. Using a box camera with an attached laryngeal mirror and a device to concentrate sunlight (Figure 1-2G), he was able to produce remarkably clear black-and-white photographs (Figure 1-2H).

Since the early photographs of the larynx by French, other methods of laryngeal documentation have been developed. These techniques include (1) indirect laryngoscopic photography, (2) direct laryngoscopic photography, (3) fiberscopic photography, (4) telescopic photography, and (5) microscopic photography.

In 1941, P. Holinger, J. D. Brubaker, and J. E. Brubaker introduced the Holinger and Brubaker 35-mm camera. This camera set a new standard for laryngeal photography. The clarity, color, and brilliance of these photographs have not been surpassed even by today's standards. This system, however, was expensive and bulky; it is no longer used.

In 1954, Yutaka Tsuiki of Tohoku University, Japan, was the first to "televise" the larynx. He used his "tele-endoscope" attached to a large television camera (Figure 1-2I). He predicted the importance of video recording the larynx as a method of documentation and teaching.

In 1963, Oscar Kleinsasser of Cologne used a 400-mm objective lens to adapt the Zeiss otological microscope for laryngoscopic use. Later he used a photoadapter, beam splitter, and single-lens reflex (SLR) camera to produce outstanding pictures of the larynx.

In 1968, Sawashima and Hirose of Japan introduced the flexible laryngoscope, which is now standard equipment for the practicing otolaryngologist. While this instrument is easy to use and produces acceptable pictures, modern telescopes such as the Hopkins rod lens (Karl Storz), the Lumina optic system (Richard Wolf), and the full Lumen system (Nagashima) produce superior images. These telescopes provide brilliant, high-resolution, magnified images with a significant depth of field. The use of these instruments by Paul Ward, George Berci, and Bruce Benjamin has set a high standard for laryngeal photography. Video recording, as pioneered by Koichi Yamashita, has become the standard technique of the serious endoscopist who requires high-quality documentation of laryngeal form and function. He called the procedure "VTR endoscopy" (1977). Yanagisawa in 1981 named video recording of the larynx as "videolaryngoscopy" and popularized this technique.

CHAPTER 2
EQUIPMENT

Equipment used for endoscopic otorhinolaryngological procedures consists of (1) endoscopes (fiberscopes and telescopes), (2) video cameras, (3) video adapters, (4) light sources, (5) video recorders, (6) video monitors, (7) video printers, and (8) video enhancers.

ENDOSCOPES

Most diagnostic endoscopy in otorhinolaryngology can be accomplished with either a flexible fiberscope or a rigid telescope. The advantages of the flexible fiberscopes are as follows: (1) The flexible nasopharyngolaryngoscope allows the examination of the entire upper respiratory tract (nasal cavity, nasopharynx, oropharynx, hypopharynx, larynx, and subglottis) with only one pass; (2) the procedure is relatively simple and well tolerated by children and adults and is particularly useful for laryngoscopy in a patient with a hypersensitive gag reflex; and (3) nasal endoscopy can be performed even on a patient with a septal deviation, and laryngoscopy can be done in a patient with an anomalous epiglottis or obstructive supraglottic lesion. The subglottis and the ventricle can often be examined well.

Disadvantages of fiberscopic endoscopy are as follows: (1) The image on the monitor is small and of rather limited resolution; (2) the wide-angle lens distorts the image; (3) the disturbing moiré effect (unwanted color stripes) is peculiar to fiberscopic video documentation (it can often be eliminated by turning the head of the fiberscope); and (4) the fiberscope provides poor illumination for video documentation.

Telescopic endoscopy has many advantages over fiberscopic endoscopy: (1) Telescopic images are larger and brighter with excellent color and resolution; (2) fine vocal fold vibration can be assessed more easily and accurately, particularly with stroboscopy; (3) little optical distortion is noted in the periphery; and (4) video documentation is easier and clearer.

The main disadvantage of telescopic endoscopy is that the rigid telescopes are poorly tolerated by children and by adults who have a hypersensitive gag reflex or obstructed passages. Because of the consistently superior images obtained by rigid telescopy, the author primarily uses these telescopes in otorhinolaryngological endoscopy unless the patient cannot tolerate it.

The telescopes are available with a variety of viewing angles: (1) straight forward (0 degrees), (2) forward oblique (30 degrees), (3) lateral (70 and 90 degrees), and (4) retrospective (120 degrees) (Figure 2-1A). The telescopes are also available in different lengths (typically 3–20 cm) and diameters (typically 2.7 or 4.0 mm) depending on the use. Most of the telescopes described here are Karl Storz telescopes using the Hopkins rod lens system. A few Richard Wolf (Lumina optic system) and Nagashima (full Lumen optic system) telescopes were used.

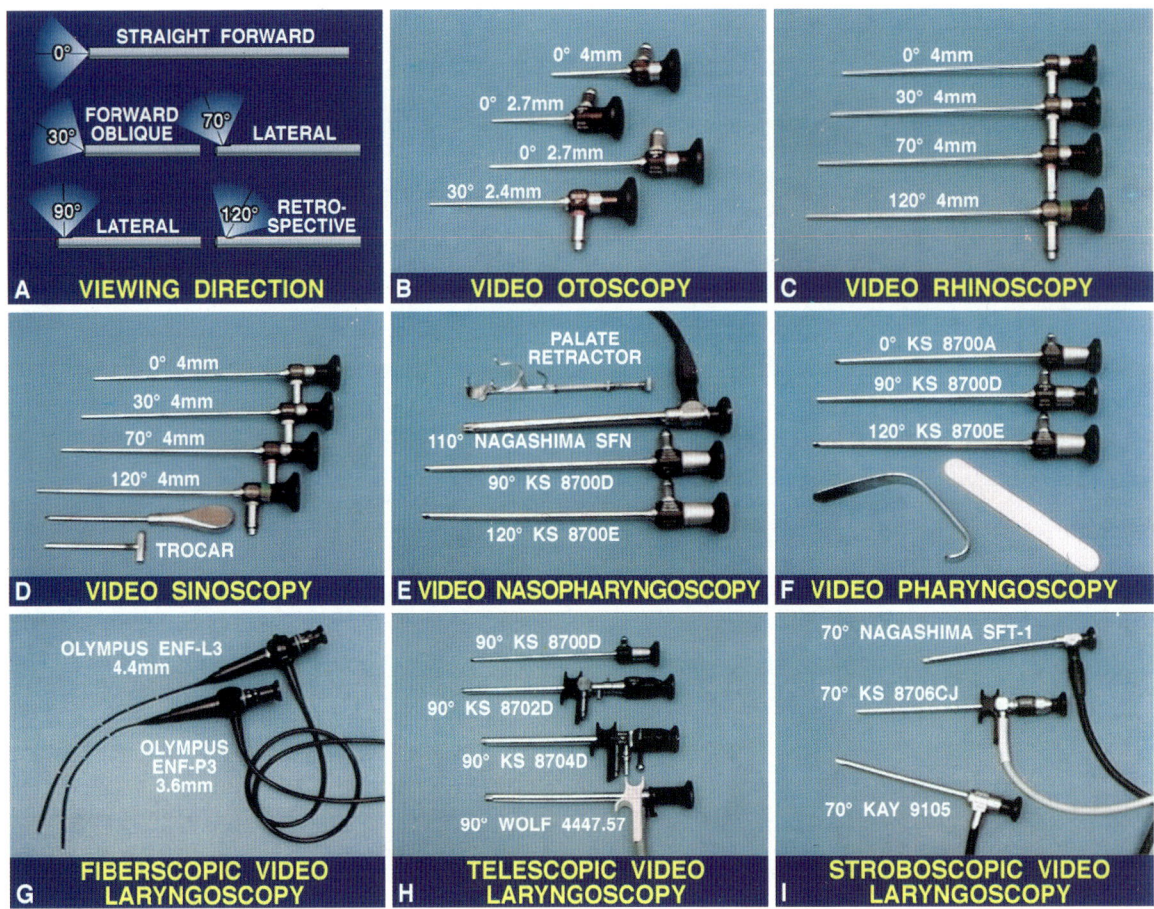

Figure 2-1. Endoscopes. (A) Viewing directions. (B) Ototelescopes. (C) Nasal telescopes. (D) Sinus telescopes and trocar. (E) Nasopharyngeal telescopes and palate retractor. (F) Pharyngeal telescopes and tongue depressors. (G) Fiberscopes. (H) Laryngeal telescopes. (I) Stroboscopic telescopes.

For video-otoscopy (viewing the external auditory canal and tympanic membrane) (Chapter 4) (Figure 2-1B), the 4.0-mm 6-cm-long 0-degree ototelescope (KS 1215A) is used for adults and older children, and the 2.7-mm 6-cm-long 0-degree ototelescope (KS 1218A) is used for younger children, infants, and very narrow ear canals. The 2.7-mm 11-cm-long 0-degree telescope (KS 1230A) can also be used. For transtympanic membrane telescopy (Chapter 13), one can use the 1.9-mm 12-cm-long 5 and 25-degree ototelescopes (Richard Wolf) or the 1.9-mm 0 and 30-degree ototelescopes (KS 28-301A and D, respectively). The 1.0-mm 5-cm-long flexible fiberscope (Machida MES-10) can also be used for eustachian tube and middle ear endoscopy in some cases. For otosurgical endoscopy (transtympanotomy or transmastoid telescopy) (Chapter 13), one can use the 2.7-mm 11-cm-long 0- and 30-degree telescopes (KS 1230 A and B, respectively) or the 4.0-mm 6-cm-long 0- and 30-degree ototelescopes (KS 1218A and B, respectively).

For videorhinoscopy (Chapter 5) (Figure 2-1C), the 4.0-mm 18-cm-long 0-, 30-, 70-, and 120-degree nasal telescopes (KS 7200A, B, C, and E, respectively) are used for adults; and the 2.7-mm 18-cm-long 0-, 30-, and 70-degree nasal telescopes (KS 27018A, B, and C, respectively) are used for children or adults with stenotic nasal passages. For videosinoscopy (Chapter 6) (Figure 2-1D), the same telescopes are used through external and transnasal approaches to the sinuses.

Videonasopharyngoscopy (Chapter 7) (Figure 2-1E) can be approached transnasally with the 0-, 30-, and 70-degree nasal telescopes (see above) or with the 3.6-mm fiberscope (Olympus ENF-P3). For transoral videonasopharyngoscopy the author uses the 4.0-mm 18-cm-long 90- and 120-degree telescopes (KS 7200D and E, respectively), the 5.8-mm 20-cm-long 90- and 120-degree telescopes (KS 8700D and E, respectively), and the 110-degree retrospective telescope (Nagashima SFN).

For videopharyngoscopy (Chapter 8) (Figure 2-1F), the

Equipment

0-, 90-, and 120-degree nasal telescopes (see above) are used in conjunction with a tongue depressor. For larger, clearer images, however, one uses the 10-mm 20-cm-long 0-degree telescope (KS 8700A) and the 5.8-mm 20-cm-long 90- and 120-degree telescopes (KS 8700D and E, respectively).

For fiberscopic videolaryngoscopy (Chapter 9) (Figure 2-1G), the author uses 3.6-mm and 4.4-mm flexible fiberscopes (Olympus ENF-P3 and -L3, respectively). The former is used for most fiberscopic exams (nose, nasopharynx, oropharynx, hypopharynx, larynx, and subglottis), while the latter is used for fiberscopic strobovideolaryngoscopy because it provides a much larger, clearer fiberscopic image.

For telescopic videolaryngoscopy (Chapter 9) (Figure 2-1H), the author uses a variety of 90-degree telescopes, including (1) a 5.8-mm 20-cm-long 90-degree telescope (KS 8700D), (2) a Berci–Ward 14-cm-long 90-degree laryngopharyngoscope (KS 8702D), (3) a 15-cm-long 90-degree telelaryngopharyngoscope with 4× magnification (KS 8704D), and (4) a 90-degree Wolf telescope (Wolf 4447.57). These 90-degree telescopes produce excellent images, but the view is from the oropharynx. It tends to show the larynx in the posterior portion of the telescopic image with the base of the tongue in the anterior portion of the view. In order to position the 90-degree telescope lens closer to the larynx and enlarge the view, the whole telescope must be pushed down on the tongue. For those patients who tolerate it, the 70-degree telescope is used instead. It can be angled downward, bringing the lens closer to the larynx, enlarging the image, and displaying both the anterior and posterior commissures. This superior image is necessary for stroboscopic videolaryngoscopy (Chapter 10) (Figure 2-1I), where the author uses a variety of 70-degree telescopes (Nagashima SFT-1, Karl Storz 8706CJ, and Kay 9105). The light cords are integrated into the body of the telescopes, thus providing brighter images.

VIDEO CAMERAS

Color video cameras have evolved remarkably in the last 20 years. The development of solid-state image pickup devices, increased light sensitivity, and miniaturization were all important improvements.

The image pickup device is a critical component to any video camera. The conventional pickup vacuum tubes create video images with electron beam scanning, which horizontally scans a photoconductive surface to convert light intensity to an electrical signal. It is effectively a cathode ray tube in reverse. The advantages of this system are good resolution and light sensitivity. The newer solid-state pickup devices (charge-coupled devices or CCD) use integrated circuits (chips) and form video images by simultaneously accumulating light intensity from all of the picture elements (pixels) that cover the pickup surface. This system is analogous to the method of storing pictures on movie film. The advantages of this system are size and durability. The chips are small, lightweight, and shock-resistant.

In order to improve color sensitivity, brightness, and resolution, a three-pickup system was developed where the incoming light is divided into primary colors, each focused on a separate pickup device. The three-tube cameras were expensive, awkward, and fragile but did produce superior images. The newer three-chip cameras are very expensive but represent the gold standard for video cameras. They are compact and durable, and they produce the highest-quality images.

Illumination is often the limiting factor in producing an acceptable video image, especially with the fiberscope. Therefore, high light sensitivity is an important parameter in a video camera used for videoendoscopy. Video cameras each have a minimum required illumination (lux) to produce adequate images. A camera with a low lux produces a brighter image with better color saturation.

Figure 2-2 displays some of the video cameras used by the author over the last 20 years. The Magnavox CV440 (Figure 2-2A) was the author's first color video camera. It was a cumbersome single-tube camera, but it produced decent videoendoscopic images. Other home video cameras included the JVC GXN8U (1/2-inch single tube, 10 lux), Olympus Movie 8 VX801 (single chip CCD, 7 lux), and Ricoh R620 (4 lux) (Figure 2-2C). Early miniaturized cameras included the Stryker single chip CCD and Circon single-tube compact cameras from the early 1980s (Figure 2-2B). The Hitachi DK5050 three-tube camera (Figure 2-2D) produced excellent images but was awkward to use. Various miniaturized single-chip cameras were used by the author, including the Karl Storz 9000 (17 lux), 9050B, 9080 (10 lux), Supercam 9000B (7 lux) (Figure 2-2E), Telecam (3 lux) (Figure 2-2F), DX-cam (3 lux), and ENT 62 (7 lux); Toshiba N-3 (10 lux) (Figure 2-2E,F); Elmo EC 202 (10 lux) (Figure 2-2C,F), EC 102 (15 lux) (Figure 2-2E), and MN401 (10 lux); Wolf Endocam (10 lux) (Figure 2-2F); Panasonic GP KS152 (5 lux); Videomedics Phase 4 (10 lux); and Aztec VID1 The best video image quality is produced with the three-chip CCD cameras, such as the Stryker 782 (Figure 2-2G) and the Karl Storz Triacam 9070N (Figure 2-2H).

Most endoscopic cameras today are equipped with a built-in adapter including (a) single-chip cameras such as Supercam (Karl Storz), Telecam (Karl Storz), DX-cam (Karl Storz), and Wolf Endocam and (b) three-chip CCD cameras such as Stryker 782 and Tricam (Karl Storz). An endoscope can be directly connected to the built-in adapter of these cameras.

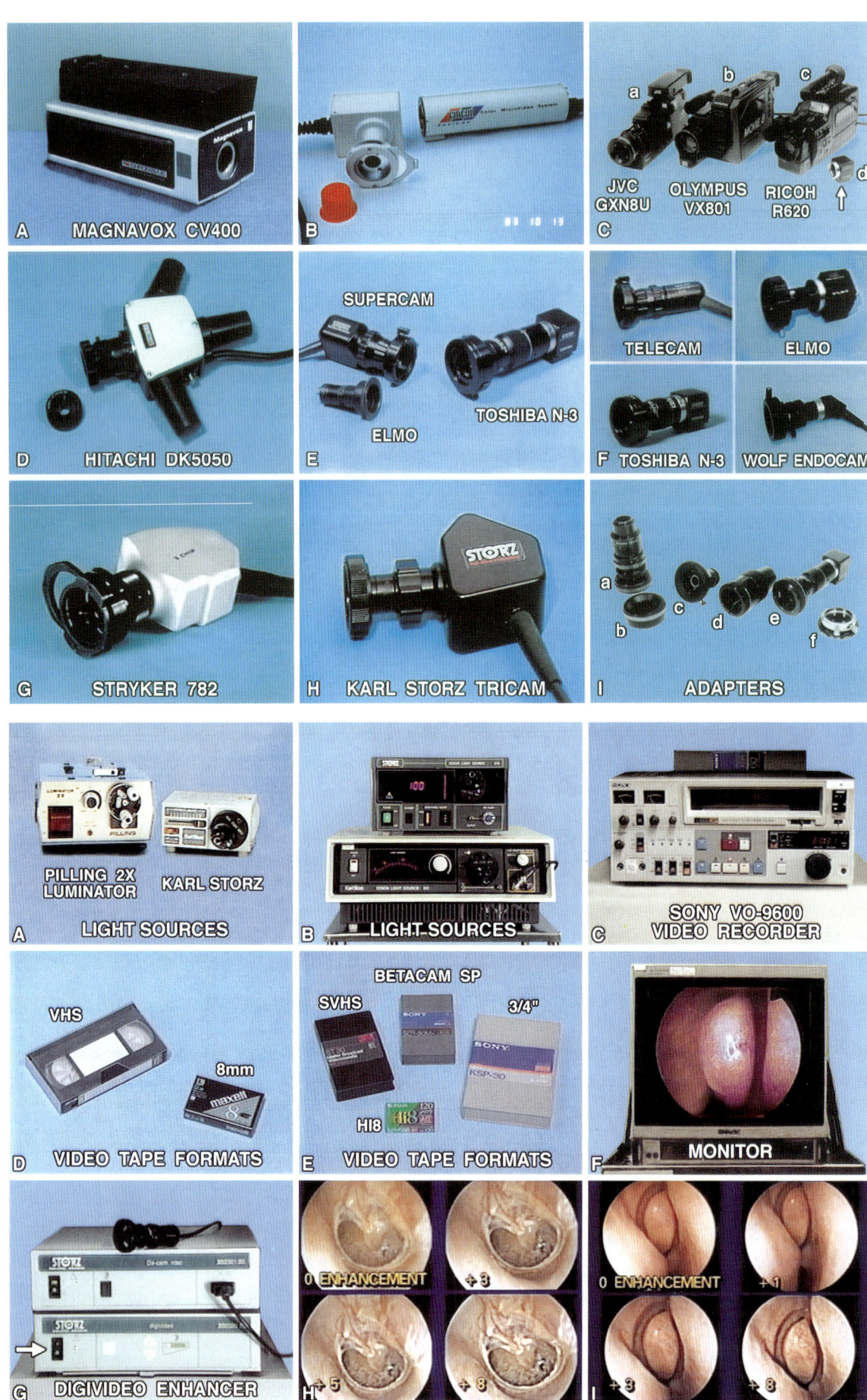

Equipment

Figure 2-2. Video cameras. (A) Magnavox CV440, single tube (1975). (B) Early compact cameras (1983). *Left:* Stryker single chip. *Right:* Circon single tube. (C) Home video cameras versus a miniature single-chip camera. (a) JVC GXN8U (10 lux), (b) Olympus Movie 8 VX801 (7 lux), (c) Ricoh R620 (4 lux), and (d) Elmo EC-202 (10 lux). (D) Hitachi DK5050 three-tube camera. (E) Single-chip CCD cameras: Karl Storz Supercam (7 lux), Elmo EC 102 (15 lux), and Toshiba N-3 with a Nagashima zoom lens adapter. (F) Single-chip CCD cameras: Karl Storz Telecam (3 lux), Elmo 202 (10 lux) with Olympus adapter, Toshiba N-3 (10 lux) with a Nagashima zoom lens adapter, and Wolf Endocam (10 lux). (G) Stryker 782 three-chip CCD. (H) Karl Storz Tricam 9070N three-chip CCD. (I) Endoscope adapters: (a) Karl Storz zoom, (b) Karl Storz quick connect adapter, (c) Olympus, (d) Nagashima, (e) Nagashima zoom lens adapter with Elmo EC 202 camera, and (f) Machida.

Figure 2-3. Equipment. (A) Light sources: *Left:* Pilling 2X Luminator. *Right:* Karl Storz 481C miniature light source. (B) Xenon light sources: *Top:* Karl Storz 615. *Bottom:* Karl Storz 610. (C) Sony VO-9600 video cassette recorder. (D) Videotape formats: VHS and 8 mm. (E) Videotape formats: SVHS, Betacam SP, 3/4-inch, and Hi8. (F) Monitor. (G) *Top:* DX-cam single-chip CCD video camera. *Bottom:* Digivideo enhancer. (H) Tympanic membrane perforation with different levels of enhancement (0 to +8). (I) Middle turbinate with different levels of enhancement (0 to +8).

A miniature camera with a c-mount aperture can be used for endoscopic videography using an appropriate adapter such as the zoom lens adapters (Karl Storz and Nagashima) or a fixed focus endoscopic adapter recommended by each camera company (Figure 2-2I). For home video cameras, a quick-connect camera adapter by Karl Storz can be attached to the front of the video camera lens to which an endoscope is connected.

LIGHT SOURCES

Light sources used were: Karl Storz Xenon light source 487C, 610, or 615 (Figure 2-3B). Standard illuminators such as the Pilling 2X Luminator and Karl Storz Miniature light source 481 (Figure 2-3A) were also used and found to be quite satisfactory. However, xenon light sources are recommended to obtain consistently satisfactory video images of high quality.

VIDEO RECORDERS

The primary recorders used in the office were the Sony 3/4-inch videocassette recorder VO-5600 and the Sony 3/4-inch SP videocassette recorder VO-9600 (Figure 2-3C). The Sony Video 8 EV DT-1 (8 mm) was also used in some cases.

There are multiple formats for video recording, namely 3/4-inch (U-matic), 1/2-inch (VHS, SVHS, Betacam SP), and 8-mm (Hi8) (Figures 2-3D and E). The equipment is not always compatible. The author started with and continues to use the 3/4-inch format. For those people setting up new systems, however, he recommends either the 1/2-inch SVHS or the 8-mm Hi8 format. These newer formats produce excellent images and are more compact than the 3/4-inch format. For those who wish to obtain consistently high quality images, Betacam SP system is recommended, but it is costly. Videotapes have a limited life span. It is advisable to make a copy of tapes every 10 years, particularly of unusual cases of teaching and publication value. Make sure that you make color videoprints or slides of those important images or transfer them to a computer file.

Also available are digital recorders that record still images directly to a floppy disk without motion video. The Panasonic Video Floppy Recorder AG810 stores up to 25 images on each disk, and the Sony Still Video Recorder MVR5300 saves up to 50 images on its floppy disk (Sony Mavipak MP50). The images can be printed with a video printer or transferred to slides or prints as described in Chapter 3 for digitized images. The advantages of this image recording technique are (1) permanent image storage (digitized images will not degrade) and (2) ease of labeling images and making composite images. The main disadvantage of digital recorders is that no motion is recorded (still images only).

VIDEO MONITORS

The monitors that the author has used are: Panasonic BTS 1900, Panasonic CT 110, CT 1030, Sony Video 8 EV DT-1, and Sony Trinitron PVM 1343 MD.

VIDEO ENHANCER

Digivideo (digital video enhancer) is a new piece of equipment (Figure 2-3G) that allows contrast enhancement of video images on the screen. This unit can be used with any video camera system, as long as there is "S-video" output in the processor of the video camera. The amount of the contrast enhancement is measured on a 0–10 scale. In Figure 2-3G, a single-chip CCD camera and its processor are shown, connected to the enhancer below. Shown in Figure 2-3H is a composite picture of a large TM perforation, with different degrees of digital contrast enhancement: 0, +3, +5, and +8. Also shown is a composite picture of a right middle turbinate taken with enhancement of 0, +1, +3, and +8 (Figure 2-3I). This system is relatively new and expensive. It appears that the best images can be obtained with +2 or +3 enhancement. Digital video enhancement was not used for any of the images in this atlas.

CHAPTER 3
DOCUMENTATION

The importance of medical documentation cannot be overemphasized. Among its many important functions, communication of physical findings is particularly important in otorhinolaryngology, where the visual examination often determines the diagnosis and the success of treatment. The clearest and most concise way to document a physical finding is to record an image: a drawing, photograph, or video image. A drawing is better than words, but better yet is an objective image by still photography, cinematography, or videography.

Still photography produces the highest-quality images but does not record movement of otorhinolaryngological structures and has a significant time delay during film development. One cannot confirm successful capture at the time of the exam. Cinematography can record movement, but equipment is bulky and costly and the film is voluminous and not reusable. Again, there is a delay before one sees the images. Videography now is the method of choice for imaging otorhinolaryngological endoscopic examinations. Videography provides a real-time record of the examination. Thus one records anatomical structures and their movements (e.g., pneumatic otoscopy, mucus flow in the sinuses, soft palate movements, and true vocal fold postural movements and mucosal waves). The video image can be projected on a video monitor for group and patient viewing. Instantaneous review confirms adequate image capture and allows for patient and student teaching. Instantaneous videoprints provide objective images for medical records, referring physicians, students, and patients. Excellent still images can be produced from video either with a video printer or by photographing the still from a monitor. The author uses videography almost exclusively for medical imaging. Most of the images in this atlas are prints from video records.

TRANSFER OF VIDEO IMAGES TO SLIDES AND PRINT

Video-to-Slide Transfer

Video images can be transferred to slides for presentation in several ways. The first method is to photograph the desired image on the video monitor using daylight Ektachrome ASA 400 color film in a standard 35-mm SLR camera equipped with a 50-mm macrolens and an orange-colored filter (Kodak CC40R or Tiffen CC40) (Figure 3-1A–C). The camera is placed on the tripod. The image on the video monitor is focused through the eyepiece of the camera. The room is darkened to prevent reflection on the surface of the monitor and in the finished picture. The photographs are taken with a shutter speed of one-half second or slower (otherwise, there will be streaks across the picture). The exposure is bracketed using the f stops. The second method to produce color slides for pre-

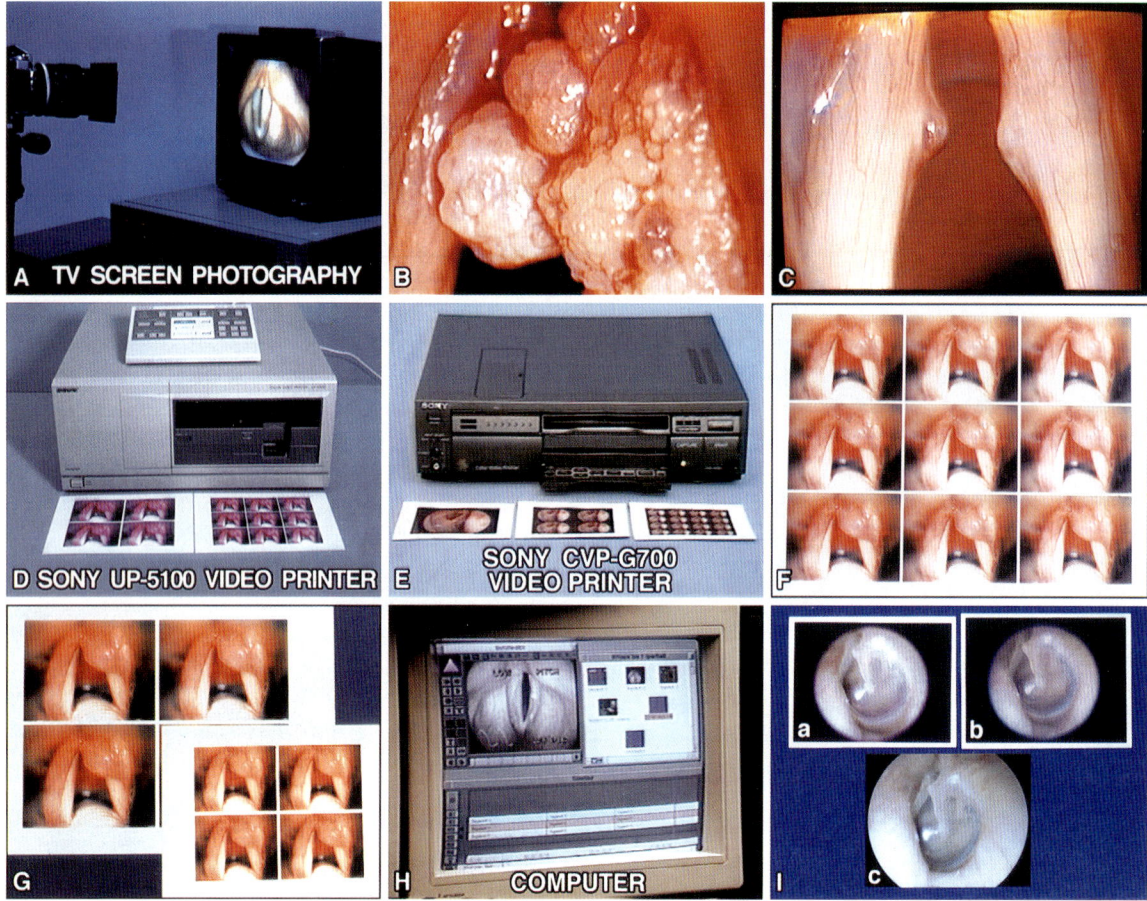

Figure 3-1. Video transfer to slides and prints. (A) TV screen photography, showing the use of a single-lens reflex camera to capture the TV screen image to produce a 35-mm slide. (B) Image of extensive squamous carcinoma of the larynx produced by a TV screen photography. (C) Image of large laryngeal nodules produced by TV screen photography. (D) Sony Color Video Printer (UP-5100). (E) Sony CVP-G700 Color Video Printer showing a single and multiple images on a color print. (F) Multiple images (9-in-1) of a false-fold polyp produced by Sony UP-5100. (G) Comparison of multiple images (4-in-1) of a vocal-fold polyp taken by UP-5100 (*upper left*) and Sony CVP-G700 (*lower right*). (H) Computer image of vocal folds, from which color slides are produced. (I) Comparison of tympanic membrane images produced by UP-5100 (*upper left*), CVP-G700 (*upper right*), and still 35-mm single-lens reflex camera photography.

sentation is to photograph the color video printout using color slide film such as Ektachrome ASA 160 tungsten. The third method is to use a computer to digitize images from the videotape. Software is available which can capture video images either as still frames or as full-motion video. Once the video frame is captured, it is possible to create composite pictures and add text and/or arrows to the image, which can then be saved as a computer file. This file can then be taken to a computer service bureau (usually via high-capacity removable storage devices such as SyQuest or optical drives), which can output the image to a 35-mm slide.

Video-to-Print Transfer

The first method of video-to-print transfer is by the use of a video printer. Newer color video printers allow one to obtain unexpectedly high-quality pictures from video images instantaneously. The color and contrast of the picture can be adjusted before the print is made, and the printer gives the option of single or multiple images on one print (Figure 3-1D–G). The color quality and resolution of videoprints are so good that they are quite adequate for publication. In fact, many color pictures used in this atlas were produced by the Sony UP-5100 color video

Documentation

printer. The more affordable Sony CVP-G700 color video printer made for home camera users can also be used. The second method to produce prints from video is to photograph the images on a video monitor as described for video-to-slide transfer. Print film can be used instead of slide film. The third method to produce prints is to take the computer file (as described in video-to-slide transfer) and output the image to a computer printer. Many of the images in this atlas were printed by a dye sublimation printer (Nikon CP-3000 full color digital printer), which produces high-quality photo-realistic prints. However, since the cost of dye sublimation printers is prohibitive, it is more cost effective to have a computer service bureau make the prints. If a photo-realistic print is not required, the images can be printed on any printer connected to the computer, including black-and-white laser and ink jet printers.

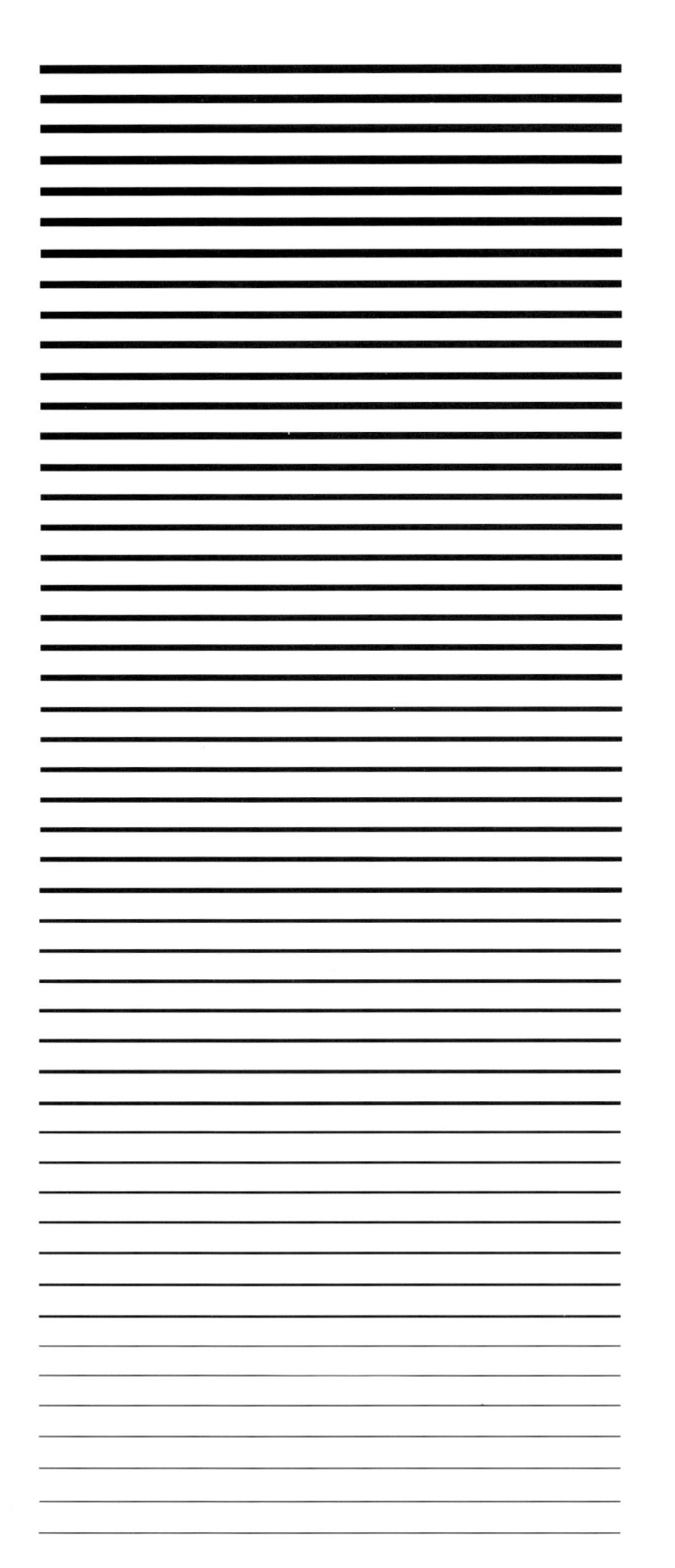

Part II
Endoscopy in Otorhinolaryngology

Chapter 4
Endoscopy of the External Ear and Tympanic Membrane (Video-otoscopy)

Otoscopy is the examination of the external ear and tympanic membrane using a rigid telescope or a standard otoscope (ear speculum, magnifying glass, and light source). When otoscopic findings are documented with a video camera, the procedure is called *video-otoscopy.*

Video-otoscopy is the most practical and effective method of documenting and teaching the anatomy and pathology of the external auditory canal and the tympanic membrane.

The ear canal is first examined with a standard otoscope and cleaned of any wax interfering with visualization of the tympanic membrane. Then, a clear view of the ear canal and the tympanic membrane can be obtained with an ototelescope. With only one or two passes of a telescope, to which a video camera is attached, the anatomy and pathology of the ear canal and the tympanic membrane can be quickly demonstrated and videotaped. Color videoprints of representative images can be made instantaneously. The procedure can be accomplished within 3 minutes. Mobility of the tympanic membrane, bleeding and purulent discharge from the ear canal and middle ear, pulsation of discharge through a tympanic membrane perforation, and pulsation of vascular tumors in the middle ear can be clearly observed with video-otoscopy.

Mobility of the tympanic membrane can best be demonstrated and documented by pneumatic video-otoscopy (Figure 4-3). While several excellent commercial video-otoscopes are available, pneumatic video-otoscopy can be accomplished simply by using a Welch Allyn otoscope head through which the telescope is passed and sealed with wax (e.g., Mack's ear plug wax). The normal tympanic membrane moves readily with pneumatic otoscopy. Decreased mobility may be observed in patients with serous otitis media and tympanosclerosis. Excessive mobility may be noted with an atrophic tympanic membrane or ossicular discontinuity.

Equipment required for endoscopy of the external ear includes (1) standard otoscope for preliminary examination (Welch Allyn), (2) cerumen removal instruments (ear curettes, ear loops, or suction), (3) Hopkins 4.0-mm 6-cm-long 0-degree ototelescope (Karl Storz 1215A) for adults and older children, (4) Hopkins 2.7-mm 11-cm-long 0-degree ototelescope (Karl Storz 1230A) for infants or very narrow ear canals, (5) pneumatic adaptor (Karl Storz 119500) or Mack's ear plug wax, (6) insufflation bulb, and (7) warm water. Video-otoscopy also requires (1) video camera, (2) video recorder, (3) video monitor, and (4) video printer.

The Hopkins telescope provides an excellent method of examining and carefully documenting external ear and tympanic membrane anatomy and pathology. Video-otoscopy facilitates documentation and teaching.

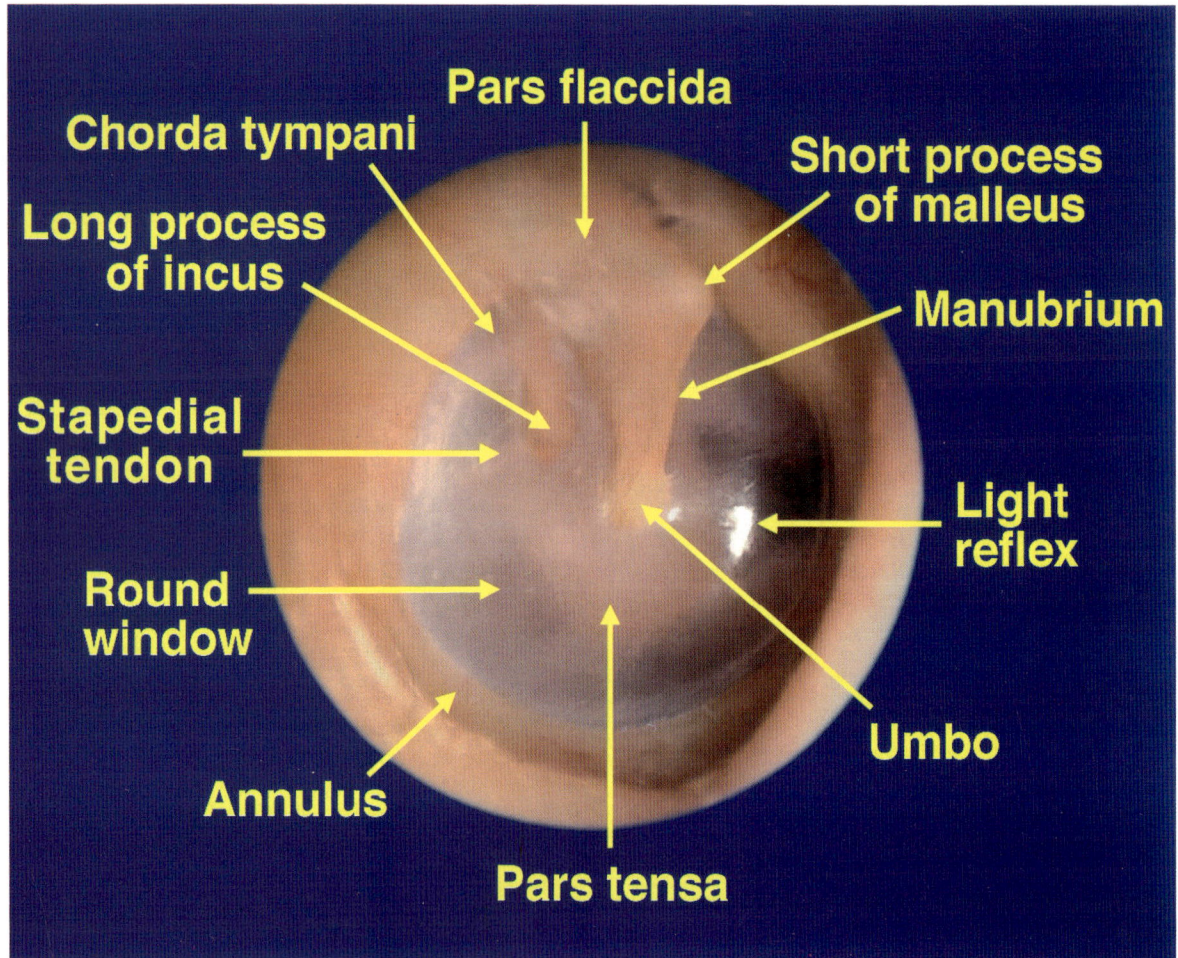

OVERVIEW OF TYMPANIC MEMBRANE ANATOMY

Figure 4-1. Zero-degree ototelescopic view of the normal right tympanic membrane. This wide-angle view of the tympanic membrane demonstrates normal tympanic membrane and middle ear landmarks. The top of this view is superior, and the right-hand side of the view is anterior. The tympanic membrane is attached to the bony canal by the fibrous annulus. The tympanic membrane consists of the pars tensa (five-layered structure making up 80% of the tympanic membrane) and pars flaccida (three-layered structure making up 20% of the tympanic membrane). The light reflex occurs in the anterior inferior quadrant of the normal tympanic membrane and is a good location for a myringotomy. Middle ear structures visible through a clear tympanic membrane include the malleus (umbo, manubrium, and short process), incus (long process), stapedial tendon, chorda tympani nerve, and round window.

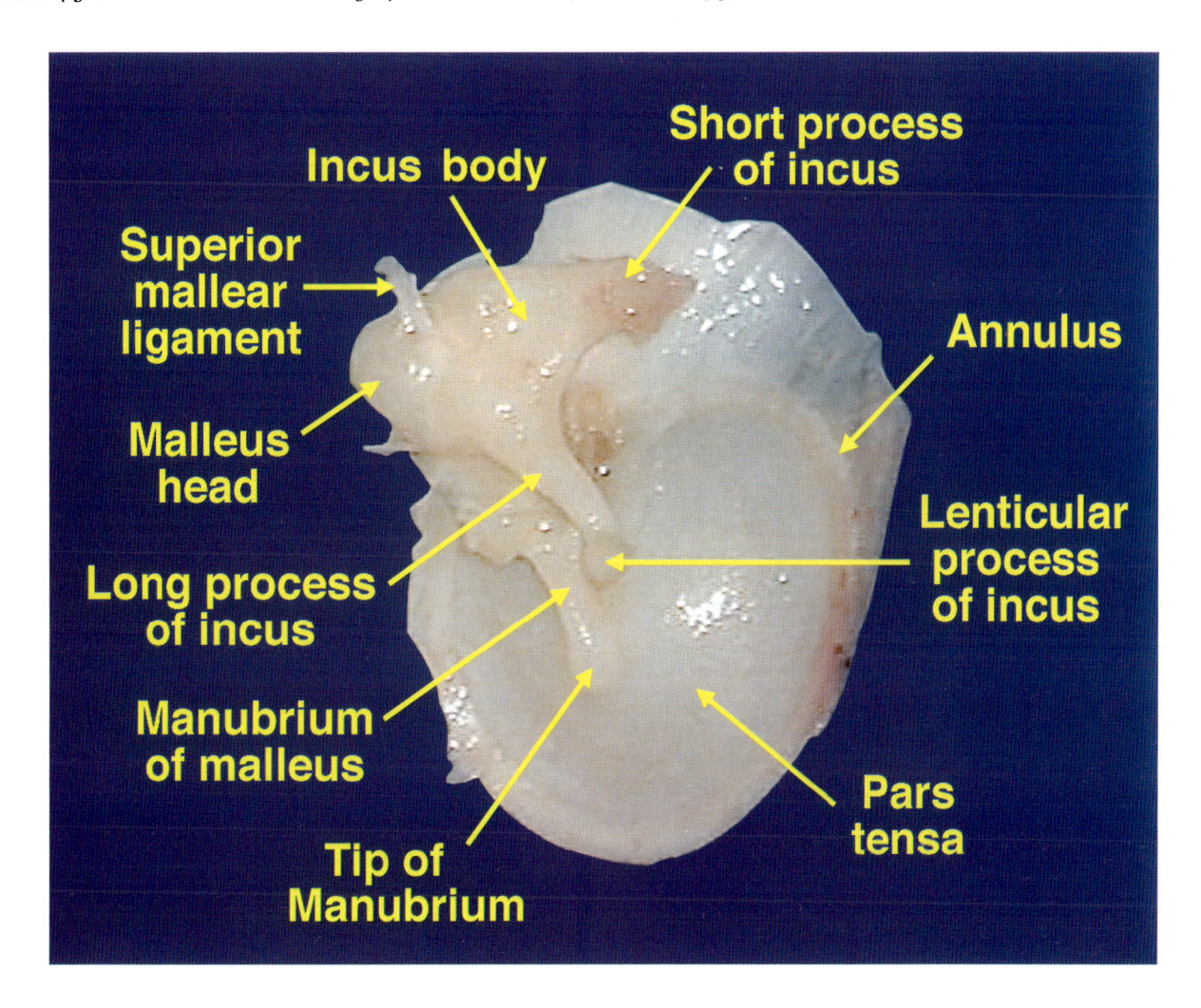

Figure 4-2. Normal anatomy of the medial aspect of the right tympanic membrane in a cadaver. This cadaveric middle ear specimen reveals important middle ear structures adjacent to the tympanic membrane. The ossicles can be seen in detail. Note that the incus head extends superiorly above the level of the tympanic membrane so that it cannot be seen through the tympanic membrane.

TECHNIQUES OF EXTERNAL EAR ENDOSCOPY

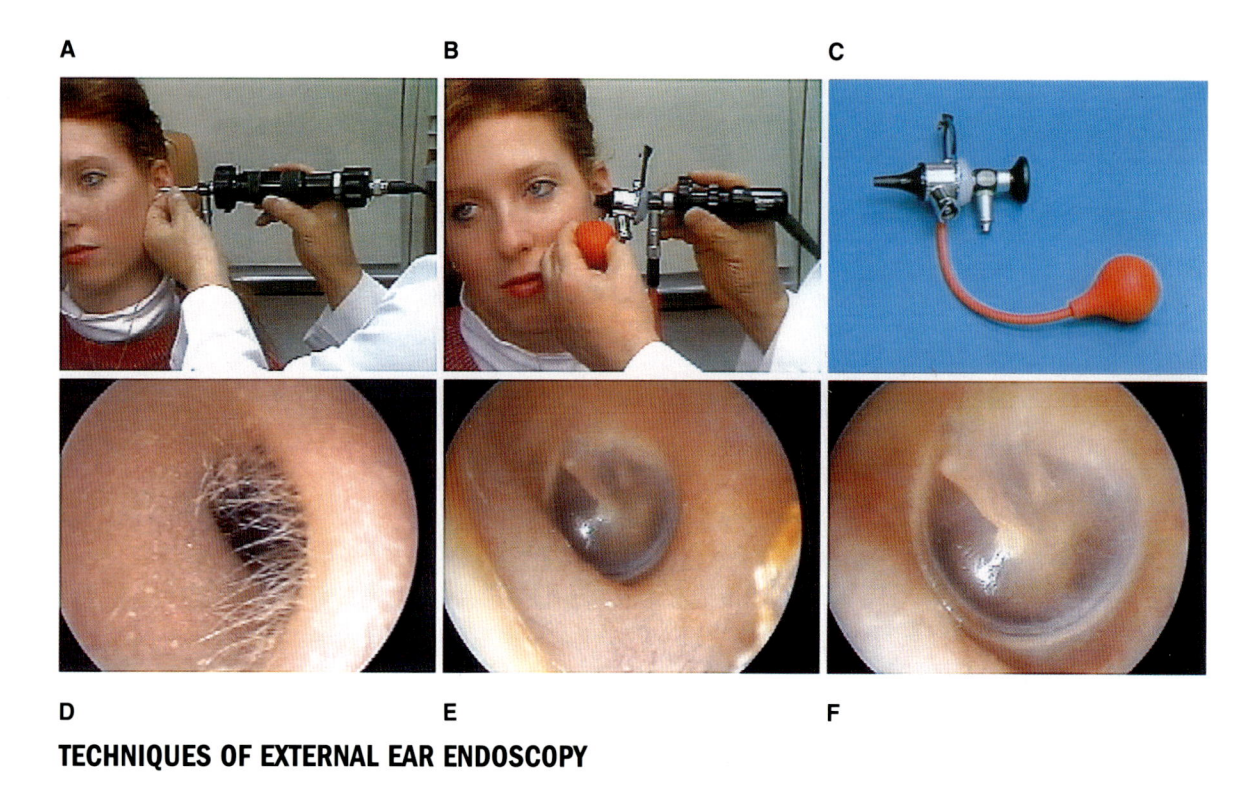

Figure 4-3. *Top row:* Video-otoscopy and pneumatic video-otoscopy. After cerumen removal and reassuring the patient, the telescope is dipped in hot water to prevent fogging and then is carefully advanced through the external ear canal. The endoscope is grasped so that it cannot advance too far into the canal (Figure 4-3A). A pneumatic adaptor allows pneumatic video-otoscopy to be performed (Figure 4-3B). The adaptor can be purchased or else made simply with a standard Welch Allyn otoscope head by passing the endoscope through the open end to the tip of the speculum and sealing the open end with wax (Figure 4-3C). *Bottom row:* Stages of video-otoscopic exam. At the entrance of the external ear canal (cartilaginous portion) (Figure 4-3D) the tympanic membrane is not yet in view and hair is seen. At the cartilaginous–bony junction (Figure 4-3E) the distant tympanic membrane is in full view, and the canal walls are visible through the wide-angle lens. Beyond the isthmus of the ear canal (Figure 4-3F) the tympanic membrane is in full view. This is the best position for the tympanic membrane exam.

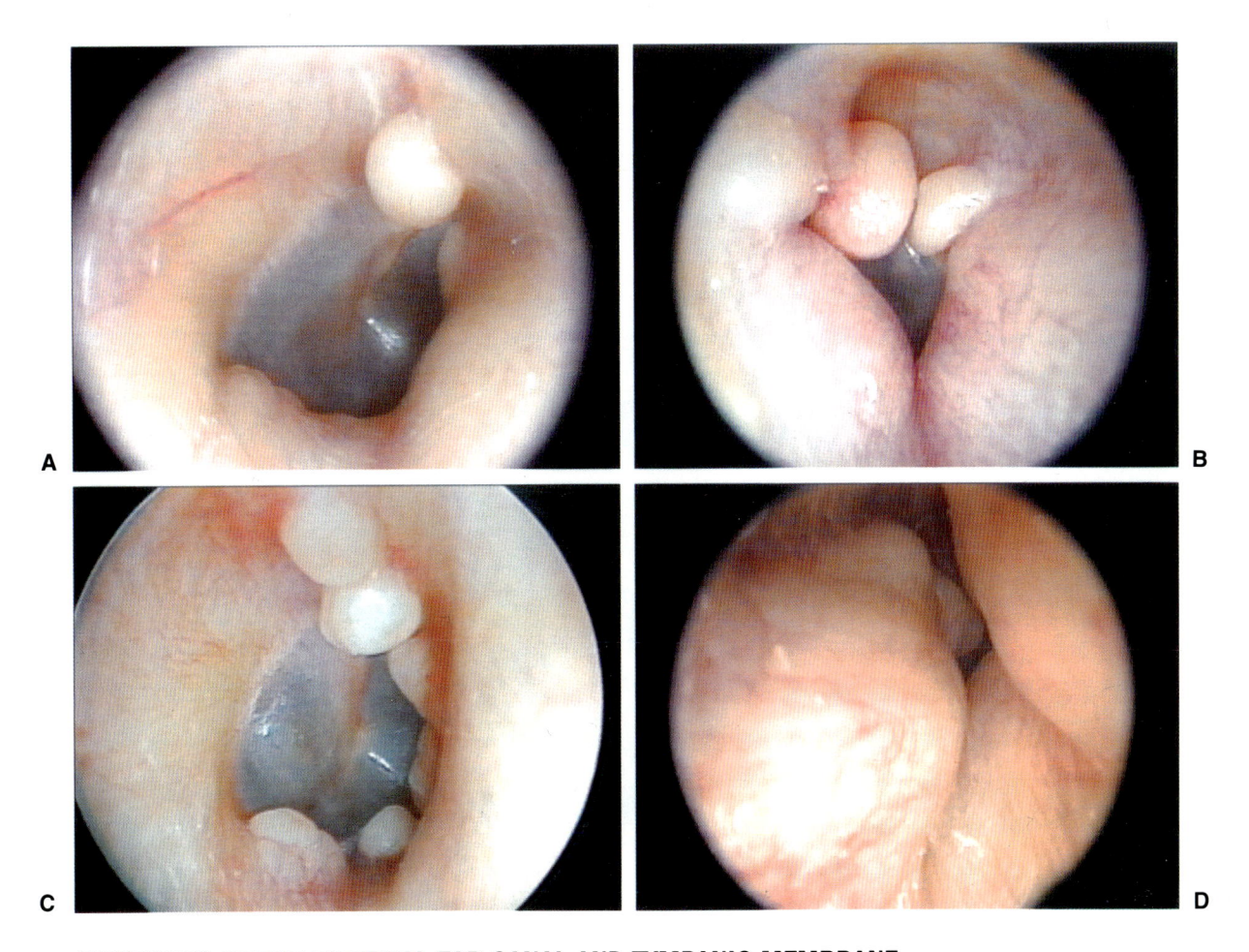

DISORDERS OF THE EXTERNAL EAR CANAL AND TYMPANIC MEMBRANE

Exostoses

Figure 4-4A. Asymptomatic exostoses. One white, rounded bony mass is seen near the right tympanic membrane. Several other diffuse bony protrusions from the walls of the right osseous ear canal are also present.

Figure 4-4B. Multiple exostoses. The external canal is significantly narrowed by multiple exostoses. Only a portion of the left tympanic membrane is visible. Repeated exposure to cold water during swimming and diving has long been regarded as the primary contributing factor in the development of exostoses.

Figure 4-4C. Multiple exostoses. Multiple discrete, rounded, white exostoses are seen to arise from the superior, anterior, and inferior walls of the bony canal near the right tympanic membrane.

Figure 4-4D. Advanced obstructive exostoses. In this patient, multiple exostoses almost totally obstructed the right ear canal. The tympanic membrane was not visible. Because of recurrent retention of epidermal debris and hearing loss, he underwent surgical excision of these exostoses.

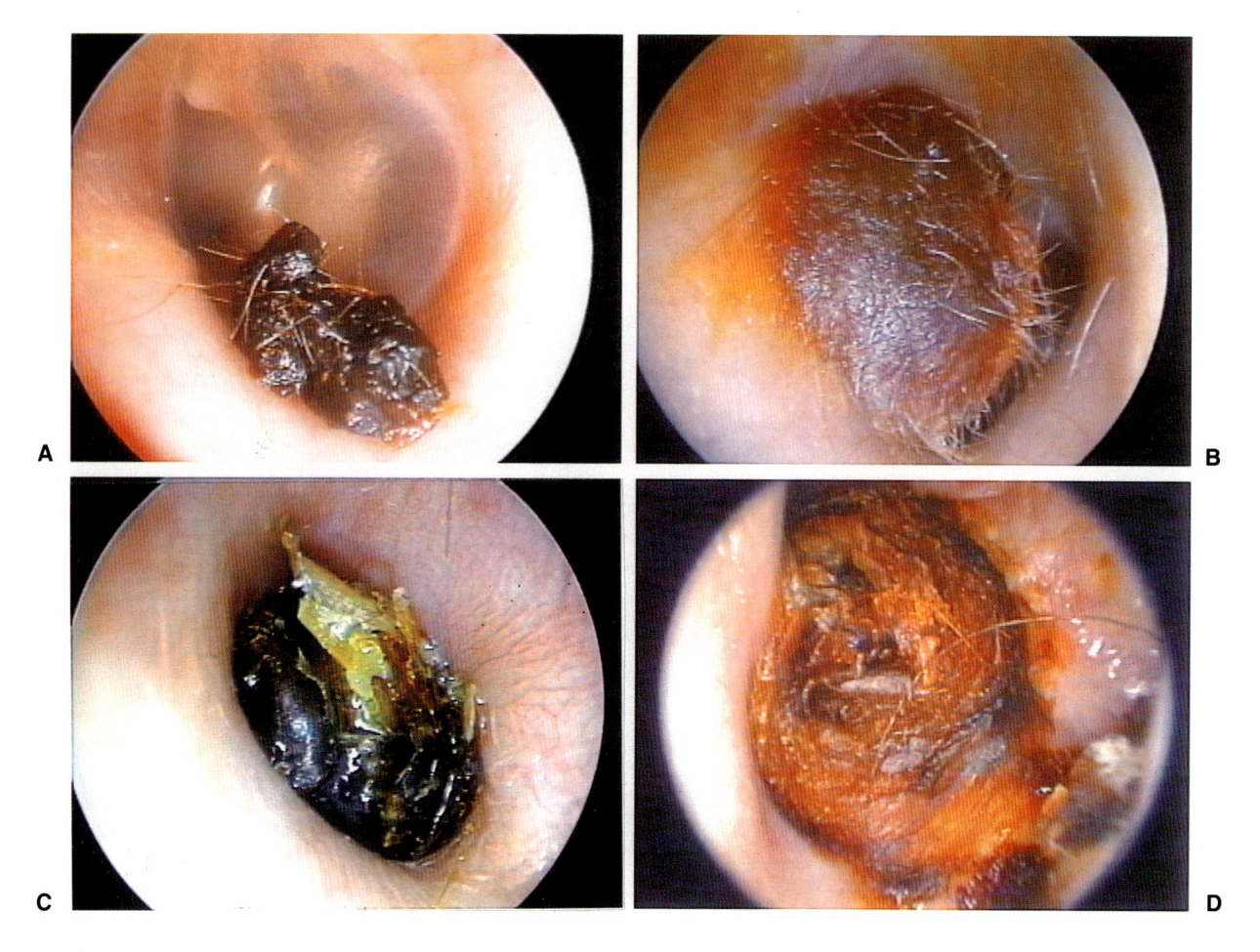

Cerumen

Figure 4-5A. Cerumen. In this patient, asymptomatic cerumen was seen on the floor of the left ear canal.

Figure 4-5B. Large cerumen. This patient complained that his hearing aid function had deteriorated. Removal of a large cerumen plug corrected this problem.

Figure 4-5C. Impacted cerumen. This patient had hard black cerumen impacted in the medial portion of the left ear canal. Often it is necessary to soften the wax with ear drops before removal either by instrumentation or irrigation. Cerumen is the most common cause of conductive hearing loss in adults. It can also cause sudden hearing loss when the cerumen gets wet and expands during showering or swimming.

Figure 4-5D. Impacted cerumen. A large plug of impacted brown cerumen is seen obstructing the entire ear canal. This type of wax can be removed with a wax curette, right-angled hook, or Hartmann's forceps.

Endoscopy of the External Ear and Tympanic Membrane (Video-otoscopy)

A

B

C

D

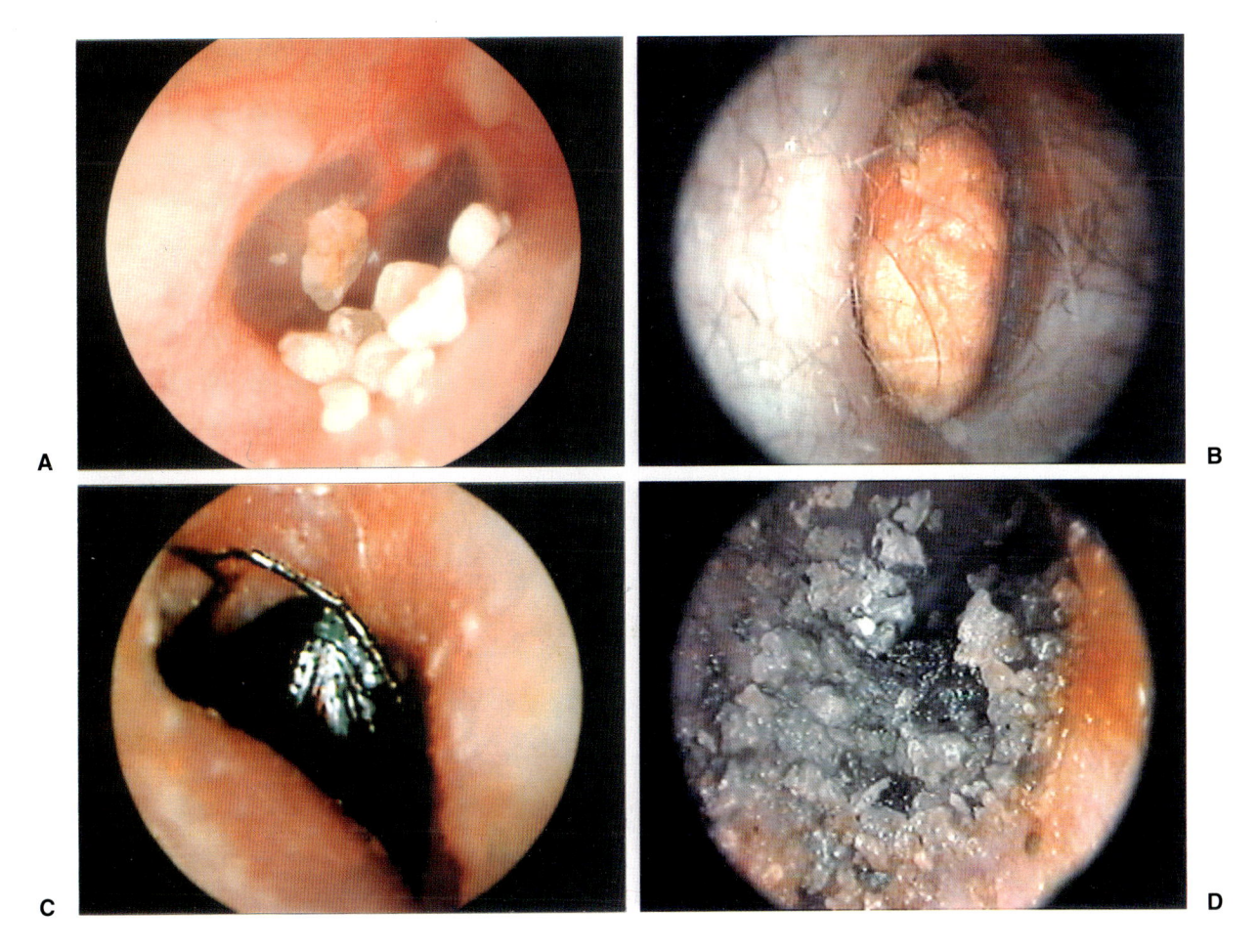

Foreign Bodies

Figure 4-6A. Multiple pebbles. These foreign bodies were found in the medial portion of the ear canal and on the tympanic membrane. They were easily removed with irrigation.

Figure 4-6B. Foreign body. A large cotton ball is shown lodged in the deep portion of the ear canal, causing discomfort.

Figure 4-6C. Live insect. This live beetle took an unwelcome journey into this patient's left ear canal. The two posterior legs were visible. The front legs were probably scratching the tympanic membrane. The patient complained of excruciating ear pain, and it was necessary to remove the beetle under general anesthesia. A smaller insect can be suffocated with mineral oil or lidocaine and removed by irrigation (if the tympanic membrane is intact) or with an operating microscope.

Figure 4-6D. Construction debris. Multiple pieces of construction debris completely filled this patient's left ear canal when he was caught in a large building under construction that collapsed, causing hearing loss. Otoscopy revealed complete obstruction of the ear canal by foreign bodies that were removed with suction and irrigation.

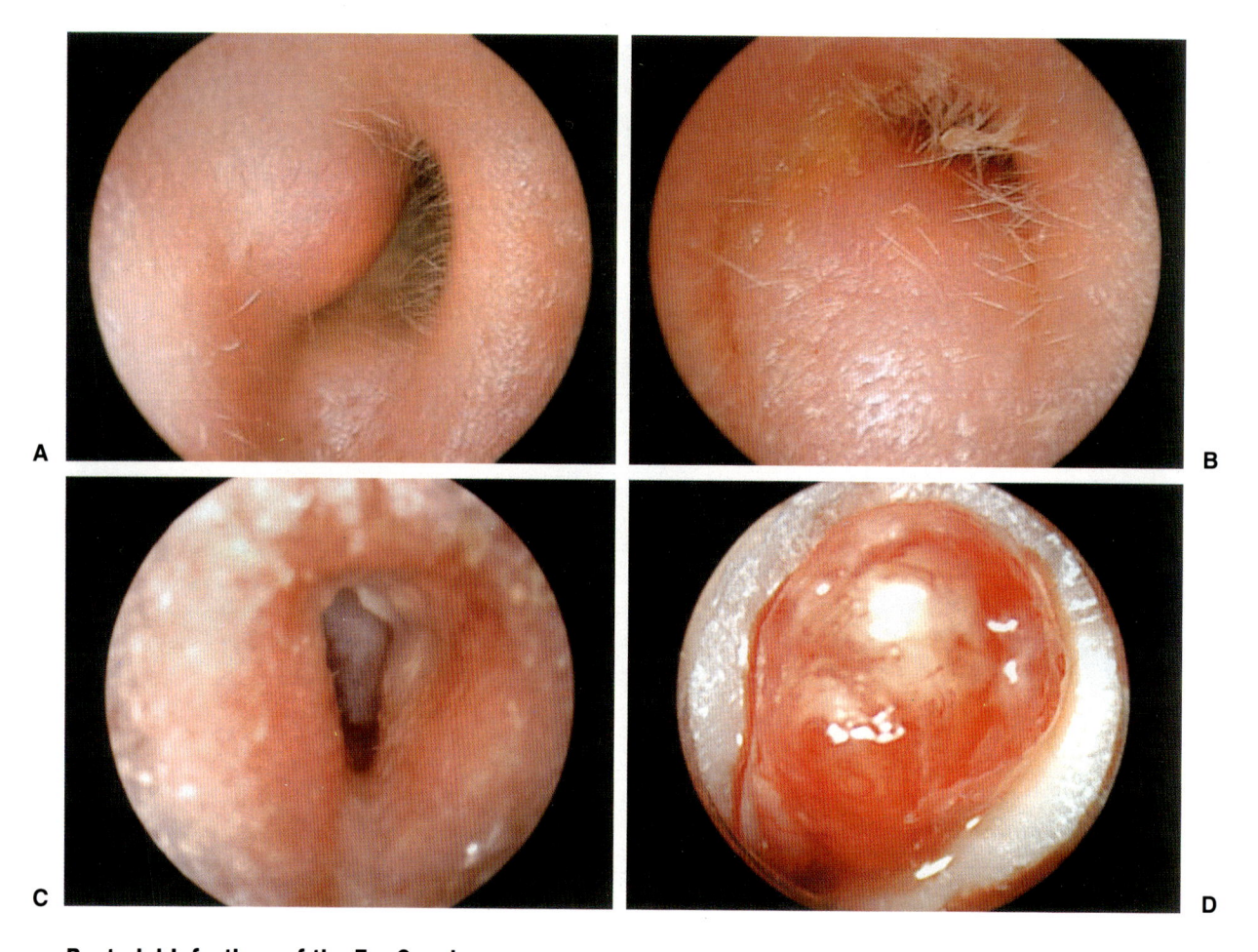

Bacterial Infections of the Ear Canal

Figure 4-7A. Furuncle (acute circumscribed otitis externa). A staphylococcal abscess is shown arising from the base of a hair follicle in the outer cartilaginous portion of the ear canal.

Figure 4-7B. Acute circumscribed otitis externa. In this patient the furuncle originated from the floor of the left ear canal and almost totally occluded the outer canal. The patient complained of excruciating ear pain and hearing loss. The canal was extremely tender. Incision and drainage was necessary to evacuate purulent material and relieve the symptoms.

Figure 4-7C. Acute diffuse otitis externa. The skin of the right external ear canal is diffusely swollen, red, and painful. Note that the lumen of the ear canal is markedly obliterated. A cotton tip or wick is usually required to deliver antibiotic ear drops into the medial portion of the ear canal.

Figure 4-7D. Necrotizing (malignant) otitis externa. In this case a granulomatous mass originated from the floor of the right ear canal at the junction of the bony and cartilaginous portions. Culture grew *Pseudomonas aeruginosa*. This patient was treated with systemic and local anti-Pseudomonal antibiotics in addition to local débridement. Malignant otitis externa is a serious (although not truly malignant) form of infection with high mortality occurring in elderly diabetics or otherwise immunocompromised patients.

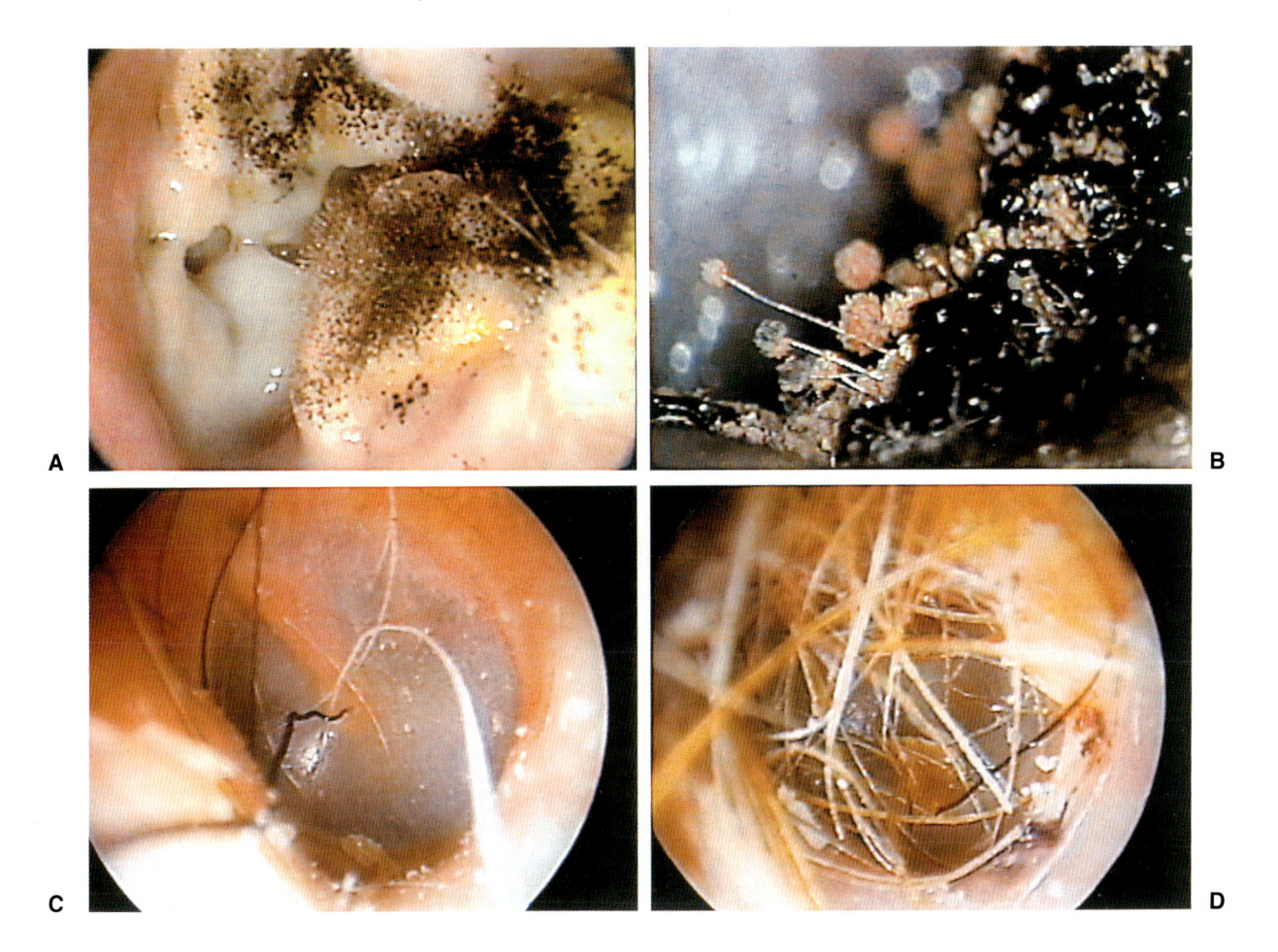

Fungal Infections of the Ear Canal

Figure 4-8A. Otomycosis (fungal otitis externa). Otomycosis is an inflammation of the epidermis of the external auditory canal by fungal invasion. The most common pathogenic fungi are *Aspergillus* and *Candida*. Itching is the most frequent symptom, but otalgia, stuffiness of the ear, and hearing loss may develop with severe infections. Diagnosis is made on the basis of clinical appearance and fungal culture. The left ear canal is completely obstructed by purulent material covered by the brown conidiophores of *Aspergillus*. Treatment of otomycosis includes thorough removal of the fungal material, followed by the application of antimycotic topical agents.

Figure 4-8B. Otomycosis. Microscopic examination (25× magnification, 200-mm objective lens) shows the presence of a fungal mass with multiple light-brownish conidiophores.

Hairs

Figure 4-8C. Hairs contacting the tympanic membrane. This patient complained of scratching noises on swallowing and chewing in his left ear as well as a dry cough. His symptoms disappeared after removal of the hairs. The cough was produced by stimulation of the vagus nerve via Arnold's nerve in the floor of the ear canal.

Figure 4-8D. Excessively hairy ear canal. This patient developed hearing loss due to recurrent impaction of cerumen within the hairs of his external canal. He has required regular "haircuts" for removal of the cerumen.

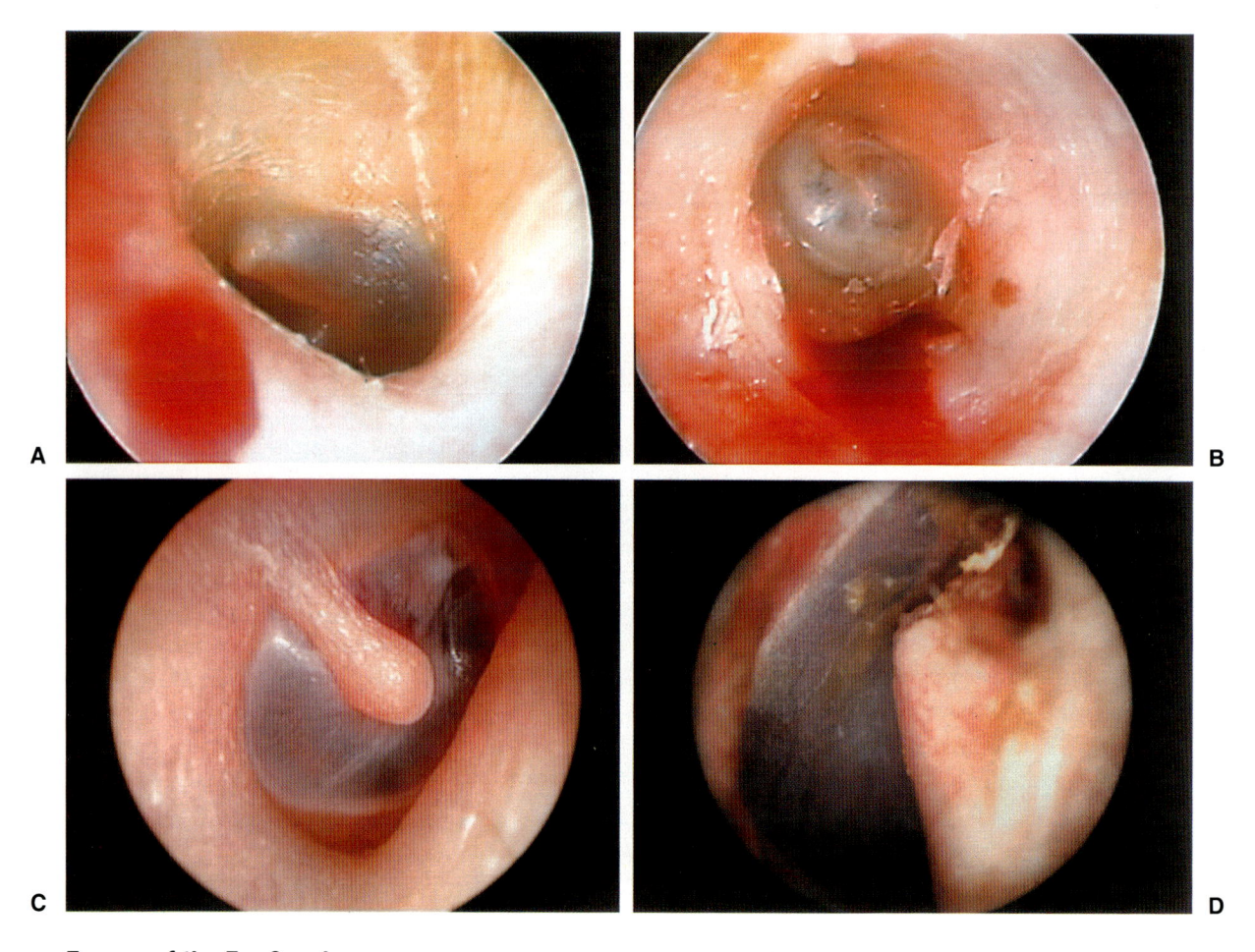

Trauma of the Ear Canal

Figure 4-9A. Hematoma. Subcutaneous hematoma of the anterior wall of the right ear canal is seen caused by a wax curette.

Figure 4-9B. Bleeding from the floor of the ear canal. This bleeding was secondary to cotton swab injury. No treatment was needed.

Figure 4-9C. Traumatic dislocation of incus. This patient developed a profound mixed hearing loss following a fracture of the base of the skull caused by an automobile accident. The incus was found to be dislocated into the posterior–superior and medial portion of the right ear canal.

Figure 4-9D. Fracture of anterior canal wall. In this patient the anterior wall of the right ear canal was fractured due to a mandibular fracture caused by an automobile accident. Note that the anterior bony wall was displaced posteriorly, obscuring the view of the anterior half of the right tympanic membrane. Note also that there was hemotympanum.

Endoscopy of the External Ear and Tympanic Membrane (Video-otoscopy)

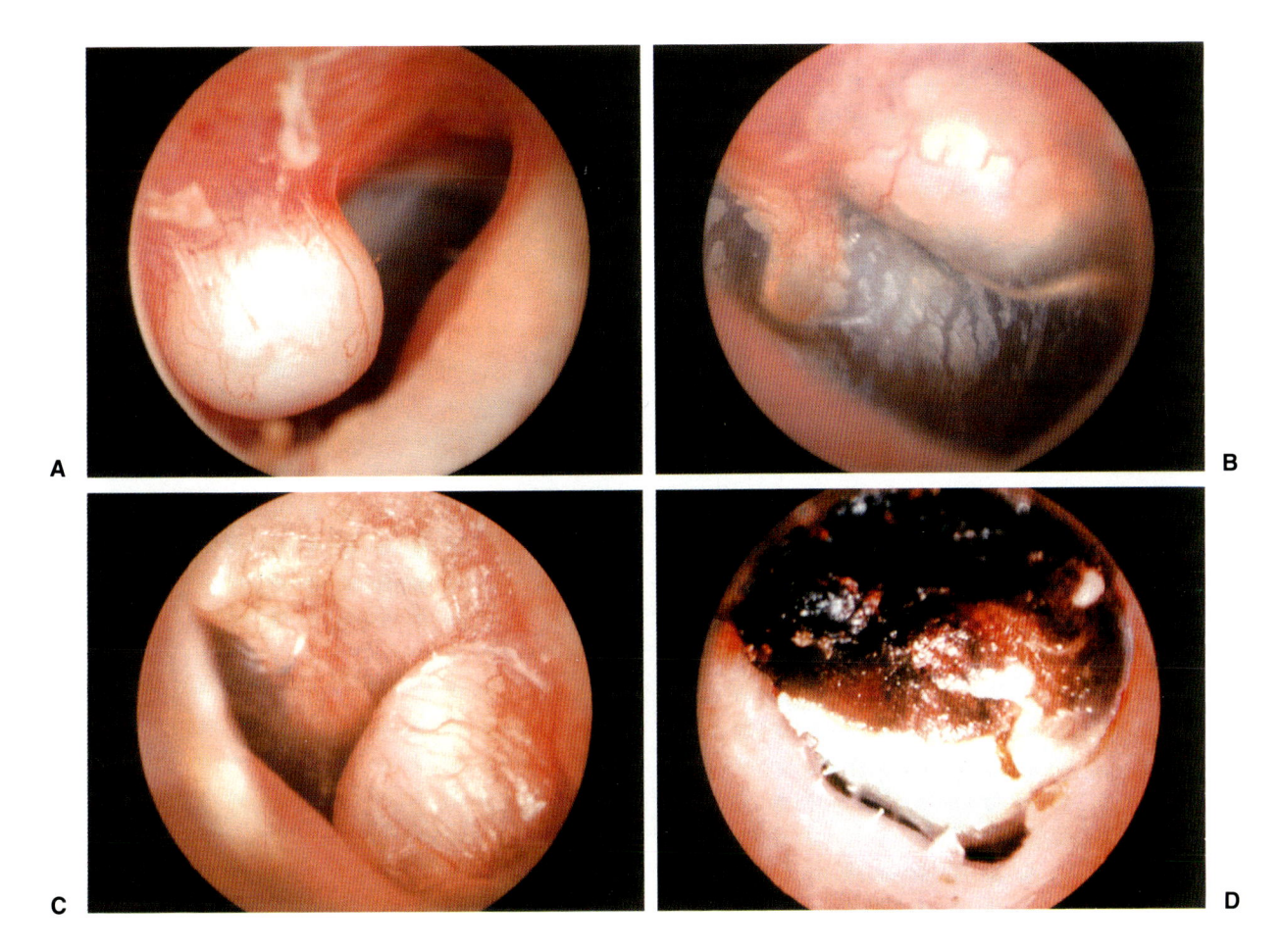

Cholesteatoma of the Ear Canal

Figure 4-10A. Postoperative cholesteatoma of the posterior canal wall. Cholesteatoma of the ear canal may be secondary to chronic infection, trauma, or surgical procedures of the tympanic membrane or the ear canal. In this patient the epidermal cyst developed six months after a medial graft myringoplasty.

Figure 4-10B. Cholesteatoma of the posterior superior canal wall. This bulging of the posterior superior portion of the left ear canal was due to a mastoid and middle ear cholesteatoma eroding into the bony canal. The patient required a canal wall-down tympanomastoidectomy.

Figure 4-10C. Postoperative cholesteatoma. This cholesteatoma involving the floor and posterior canal wall resulted from a lateral graft myringoplasty.

Figure 4-10D. Keratosis obturans. In this patient the medial half of the left ear canal was completely obstructed by a large mass of white keratin debris covered by brownish cerumen. Keratosis obturans (cholesteatoma of the ear canal) exerts pressure on the bony wall of the ear canal and may widen the bony ear canal. Keratosis obturans is often associated with bronchiectasis and chronic sinusitis.

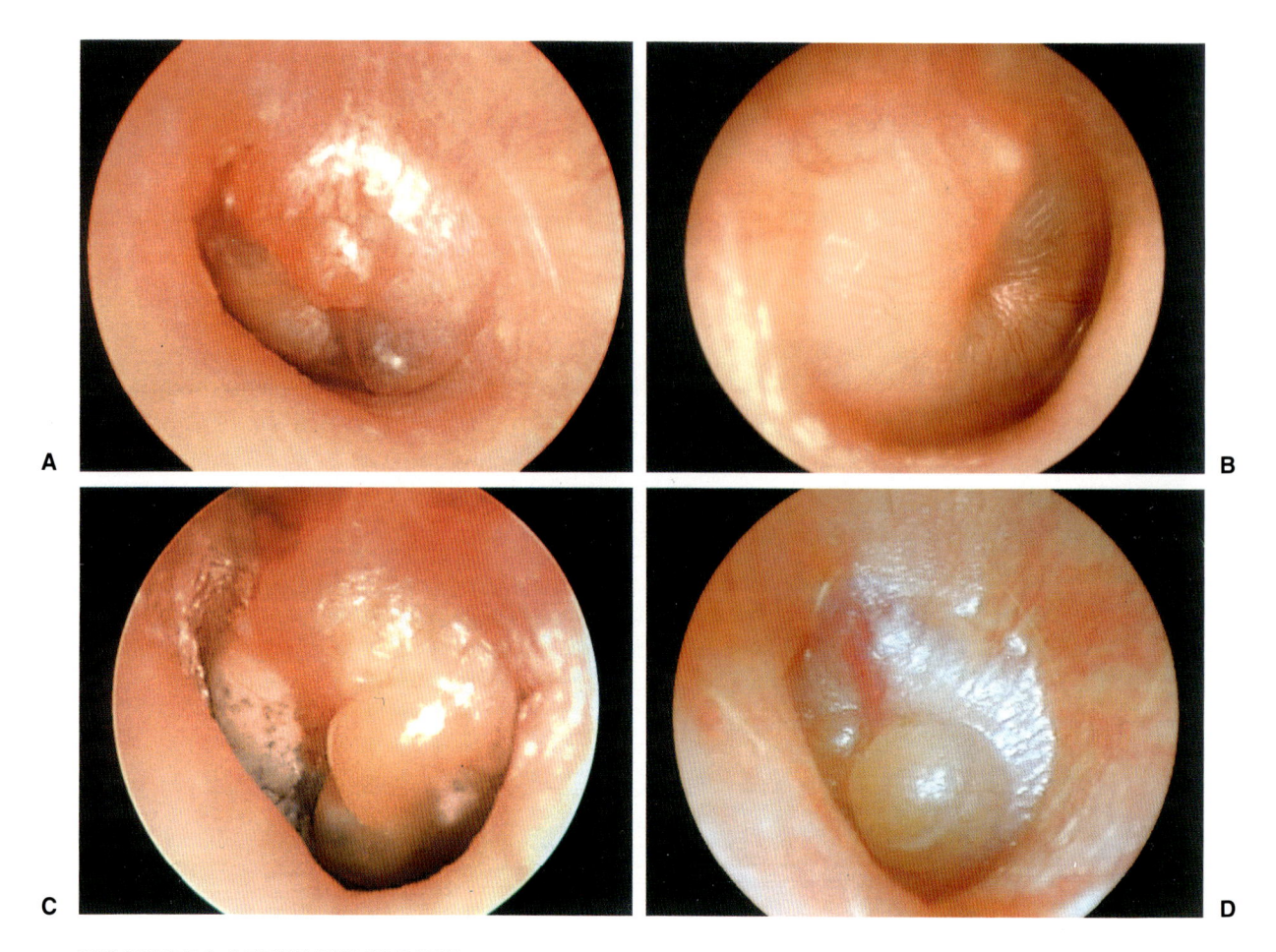

DISORDERS OF THE MIDDLE EAR

Acute Otitis Media

Figure 4-11A. Acute otitis media, suppurative stage. Acute suppurative otitis media is the result of infection of the mucosa of the middle ear caused by pyogenic bacteria. The most common pathogens are *Streptococcus pneumoniae, Hemophilus influenzae,* and *Branhamella catarrhalis.* The clinical course of acute otitis media generally follows four stages: hyperemia, exudation, suppuration, and resolution.

Figure 4-11B. Acute otitis media, exudative stage. Outward bulging of the posterior half of the right tympanic membrane is due to purulent material in the middle ear space.

Figure 4-11C. Acute otitis media, suppurative stage. Note the outward herniation of the posterior superior portion of the left tympanic membrane before its rupture.

Figure 4-11D. Bullous myringitis. A large blister (bulla) is seen arising from the inferior portion of the left tympanic membrane. Bullous myringitis is thought to be caused by an influenza-type virus and is characterized by severe ear pain and bullae. In some cases, it is associated with sensorineural deafness. Mycoplasma pneumonia has also been implicated as a cause.

Endoscopy of the External Ear and Tympanic Membrane (Video-otoscopy) 31

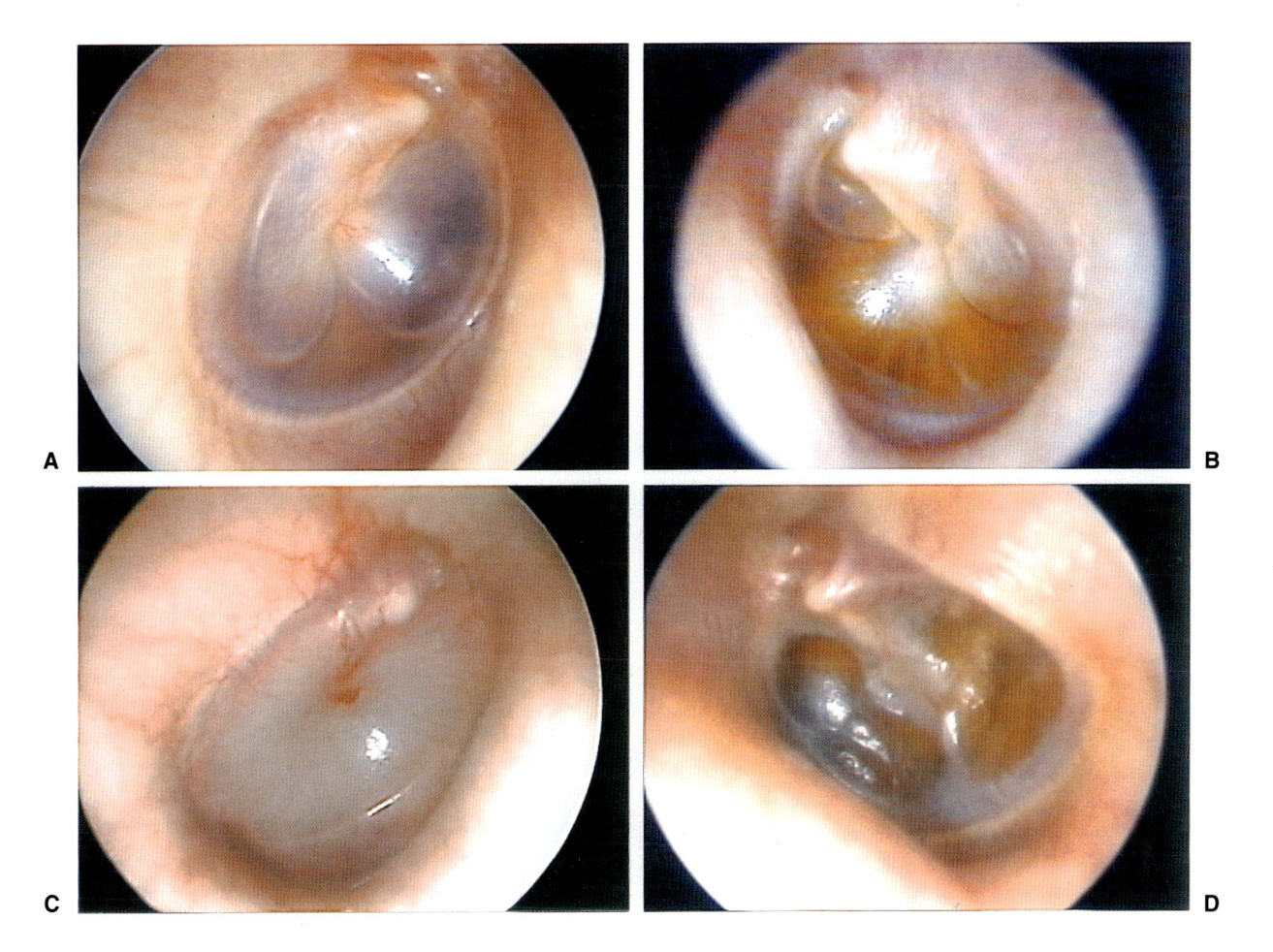

Serous Otitis Media

Figure 4-12A. Serous otitis media with air-fluid level. Serous otitis media is a common disorder characterized by the accumulation of a thin, watery, golden-yellow serous effusion within the middle ear cavity, as seen behind this right tympanic membrane. The fundamental cause of serous otitis media is eustachian tube dysfunction often associated with adenoid hypertrophy.

Figure 4-12B. Serous otitis media with air-fluid level. Serous otitis media is the most common cause of conductive hearing loss in children. It often produces a pressure sensation in the ear and a popping or clicking sound on swallowing.

Figure 4-12C. Mucoid otitis media. Note the gray-white bulging right tympanic membrane indicative of mucoid otitis media. Extremely tenacious, thick creamy-white mucoid secretions were found in the middle ear at the time of myringotomy. A child with mucoid otitis media usually presents with more marked conductive hearing loss than one with serous otitis media.

Figure 4-12D. Mucoid otitis media. This patient who had multiple PE tube insertions in the past was found to have thick mucoid secretions in the middle ear. Note the marked retraction of the entire tympanic membrane including the pars flaccida. Also note the chalky white short process of the malleus and abnormal light reflex.

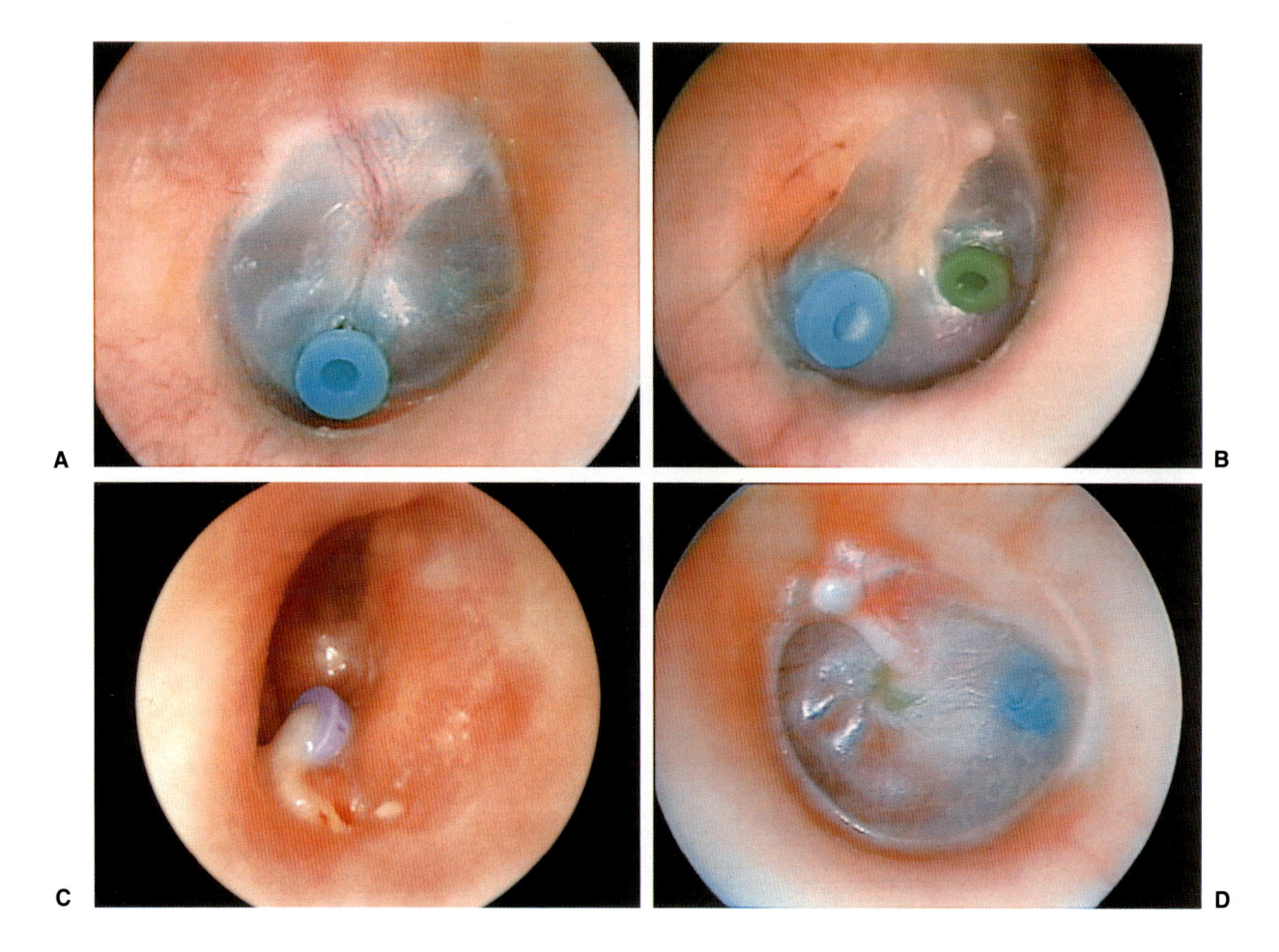

Pressure Equalizing Tubes (PE Tubes)

Figure 4-13A. PE Tube. An Armstrong PE tube is seen in the right tympanic membrane. Indications for myringotomy and insertion of PE tubes include: (1) recurrent or persistent middle ear effusion with hearing loss, (2) recurrent acute otitis media, (3) eustachian tube dysfunction following reconstructive middle ear surgery, and (4) complicated acute suppurative otitis media and mastoiditis in a patient too sick to undergo mastoidectomy. The safe area for incision is the anterior or posterior inferior quadrants of the tympanic membrane. The anterior superior portion is also safe but insertion of the tube may sometimes be difficult due to bulging of the anterior canal wall.

Figure 4-13B. Two PE tubes placed in the same right tympanic membrane. In this patient who had mucoid otitis media, a Donaldson tube is placed in the anterior superior quadrant and an Armstrong tube is placed in the posterior inferior quadrant. Indications to insert two PE tubes are as follows: (1) to decrease frequency of PE tube insertions in a patient who has had multiple PE tube operations in the past, (2) when "unexpected" bleeding from the incision site, canal walls, or from the medial wall of the middle ear obstructs the lumen of the inserted tube, and (3) when tenacious mucoid secretions cannot be evacuated from the middle ear and obstruction of the tube is anticipated postoperatively. These tubes are extruded spontaneously within two years.

Figure 4-13C. Acute otitis media with PE tube. Note the pus coming out of the patent pressure equalizing tube. Evacuation of pus by suctioning (if possible) and use of topical and systemic antibiotics are recommended.

Figure 4-13D. PE tube in the middle ear. Migration of the PE tube into the middle ear may occur spontaneously or at the time of surgery. The tube can be removed through a myringotomy incision and retrieved with a small cup forceps, suction tip, or sharp right-angled hook.

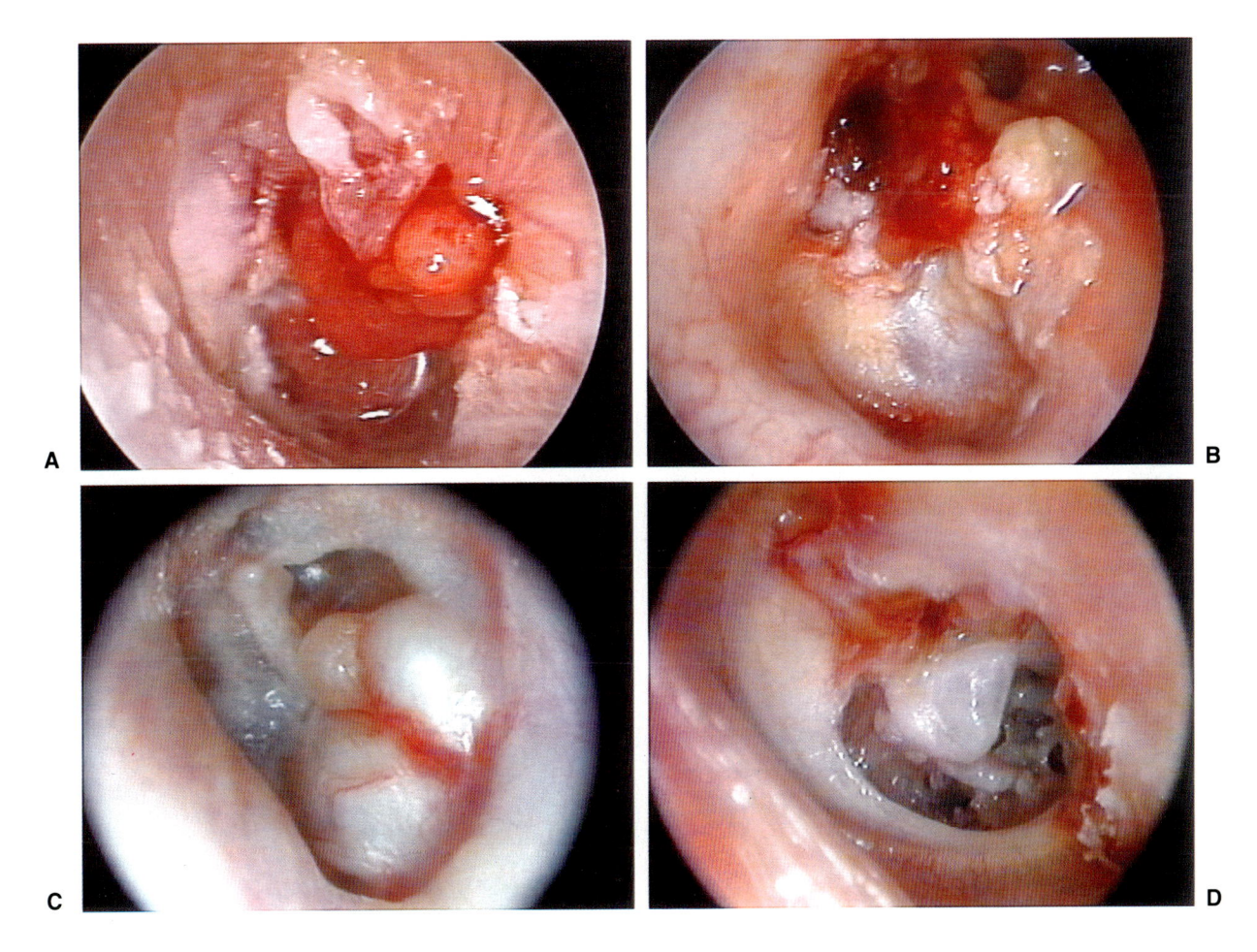

Chronic Otitis Media and Cholesteatoma

Figure 4-14A. Chronic suppurative otitis media with granuloma. Chronic suppurative otitis media is the term used to describe either a recurrent or persistent bacterial infection of the middle ear space typically associated with a tympanic membrane perforation. Note cholesteatoma and bleeding granulomas arising from the posterior superior portion of the left middle ear.

Figure 4-14B. Chronic otitis media with cholesteatoma. Note cholesteatoma and granulomas arising from the attic area and covering the superoposterior portion of the left tympanic membrane. If the patient does not respond to topical and systemic antibiotics, then surgery is indicated, particularly in the presence of persistent otalgia, vertigo, facial paralysis, or impending signs of intracranial spread of infection.

Figure 4-14C. Multiple cholesteatomas. Note cholesteatomas arising from the posterior half of the middle ear space. A retraction pocket is also seen in the posterior superior quadrant of the left tympanic membrane. The treatment is surgical.

Figure 4-14D. Cholesteatoma in the middle ear. In this patient, cholesteatoma in the midportion of the left middle ear was seen through a large tympanic membrane perforation.

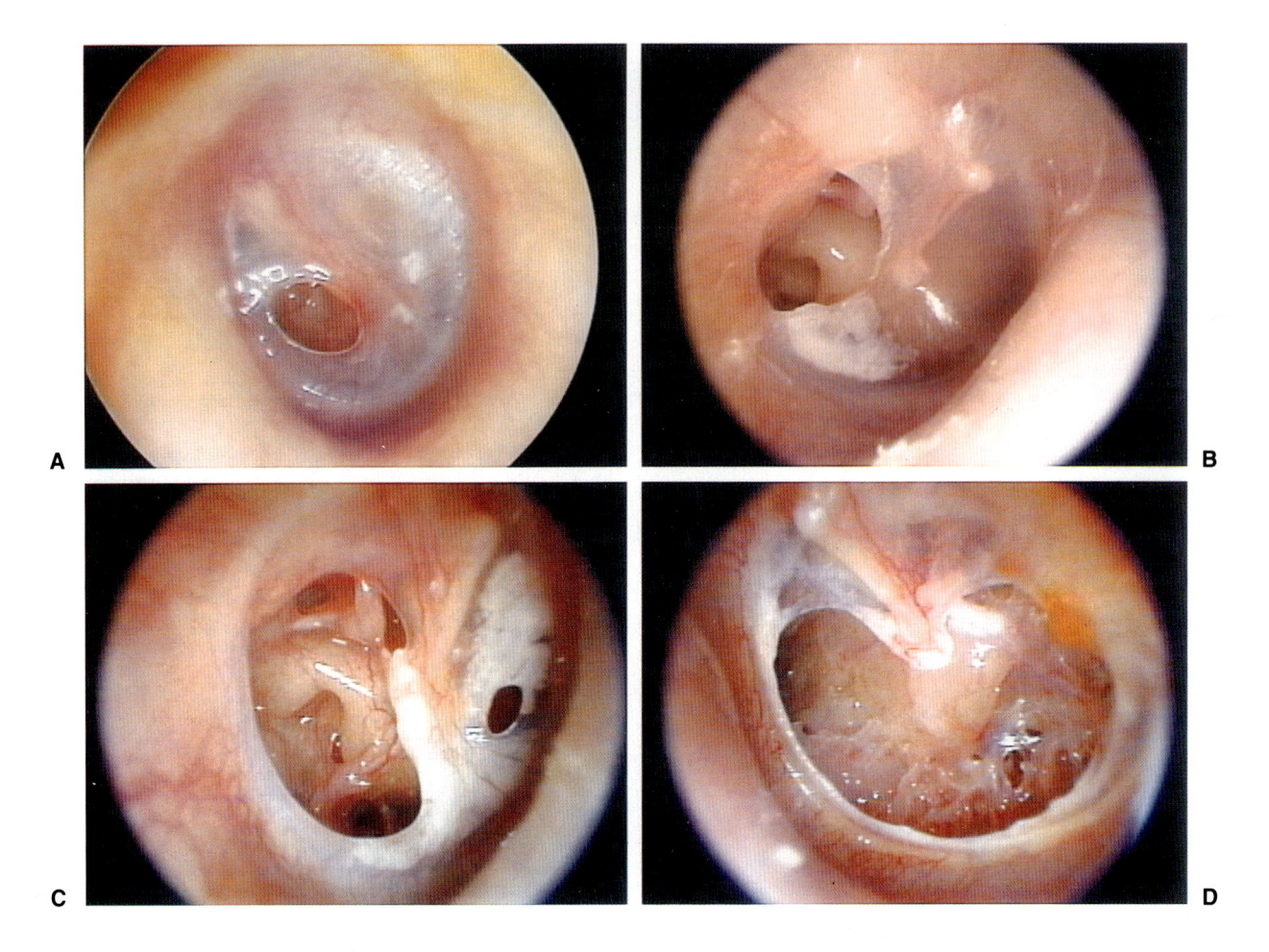

Tympanic Membrane Perforation

Figure 4-15A. Anterior middle tympanic membrane perforation. This post-PE tube perforation can be repaired by medial placement of a graft through the perforation.

Figure 4-15B. Posterior superior tympanic membrane perforation. This type of dry perforation can be successfully repaired by medial placement of a graft inserted through a tympanomeatal flap.

Figure 4-15C. Posterior half tympanic membrane perforation. This postinflammatory perforation may be repaired by medial grafting via the tympanotomy approach or total replacement of the tympanic membrane either by autograft or homograft following removal of the tympanosclerotic plaque.

Figure 4-15D. Near-total tympanic membrane perforation. This type of postinfection perforation can be repaired by medial placement of temporalis fascia with anterior fixation of the temporalis fascia between the tympanic annulus and sulcus or by homograft tympanoplasty.

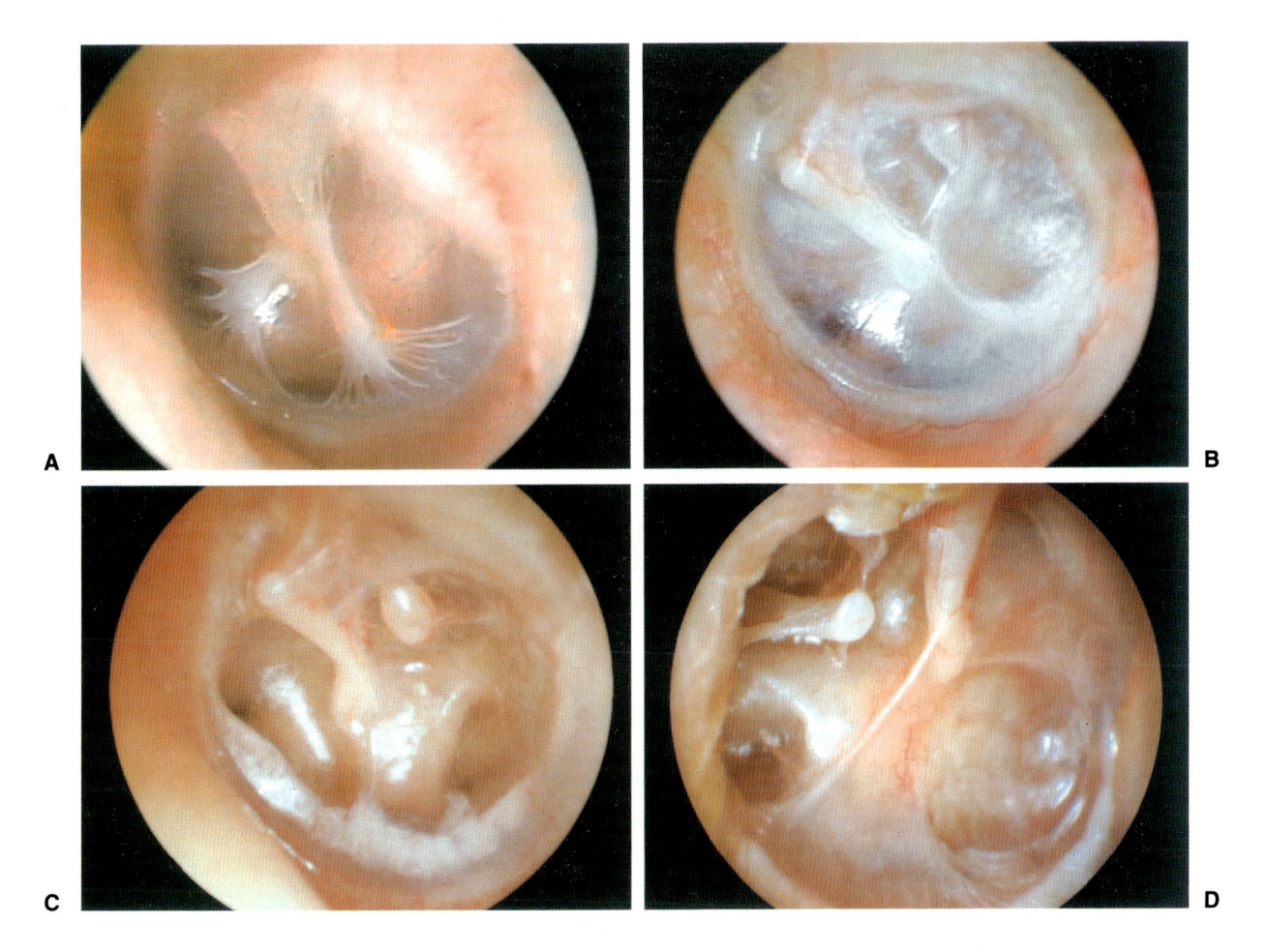

Scarred Tympanic Membrane, Middle Ear Atelectasis, and Adhesive Otitis Media

Figure 4-16A. Scarred tympanic membrane. Scarred tissues are noted in this patient's left tympanic membrane. These scars result from infection, PE tube insertion, or trauma. No treatment is necessary if the patient is asymptomatic.

Figure 4-16B. Attenuated tympanic membrane segment. A medium-sized pulsion hernia is seen in the posterior superior quadrant of the left tympanic membrane. Depending on the middle ear pressure, this dimeric portion of the tympanic membrane may herniate laterally or retract medially against the medial wall of the middle ear.

Figure 4-16C. Adhesive otitis media. In this patient the entire left tympanic membrane is retracted and adherent to the medial wall of the middle ear. Adhesive otitis media, like middle ear atelectasis, is characterized by complete retraction of the thin, atrophic tympanic membrane toward the medial wall of the middle ear. Since the retracted membrane is adherent to the medial wall with fibrous adhesions, reversal of the tympanic membrane retraction by re-aerating the middle ear may not be possible.

Figure 4-16D. Advanced adhesive otitis media. In this patient, almost the entire right tympanic membrane is retracted and adherent to the medial wall of the middle ear. This advanced condition is not reversible. Adhesive otitis media can be differentiated from middle ear atelectasis by pneumatic otoscopy. In adhesive otitis media, there is no motion of the retracted tympanic membrane, while in middle ear atlectasis, there may be motion of a portion of the thin atrophic tympanic membrane.

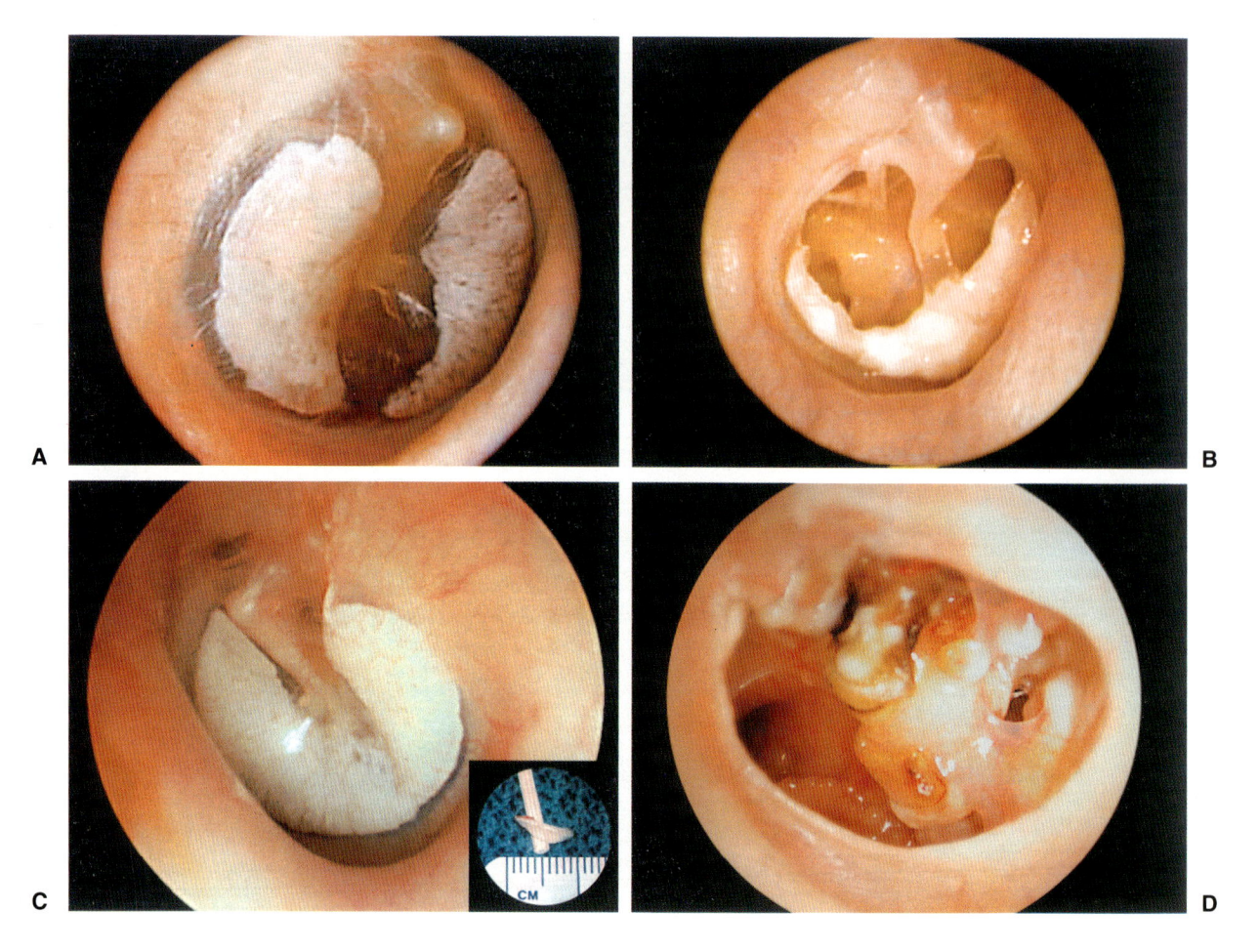

Tympanosclerosis

Figure 4-17A. Tympanosclerosis. Two large discrete plaques are seen in the anterior and posterior halves of the right tympanic membrane. Note that it does not involve the annulus and thus does not affect hearing. Tympanosclerosis is a sclerotic or hyaline change of the submucosal tissue of the middle ear. It appears to be an end product of recurrent acute or chronic ear infections.

Figure 4-17B. Tympanosclerosis with large tympanic membrane perforation. Removal of this plaque may make the right eardrum remnant more receptive to grafting.

Figure 4-17C. Extensive tympanosclerosis. In this patient, tympanosclerosis involved most of the left tympanic membrane. Note that this tympanosclerosis plaque involved the annulus, thus producing a conductive hearing loss. The inset shows the extent of thickness of the tympanosclerosis in this patient's tympanic membrane from a side view.

Figure 4-17D. Middle ear tympanosclerosis. Extensive middle ear tympanosclerosis was seen through a large left tympanic membrane perforation. In this patient, tympanosclerosis involved the promontory, round and oval windows, and stapes.

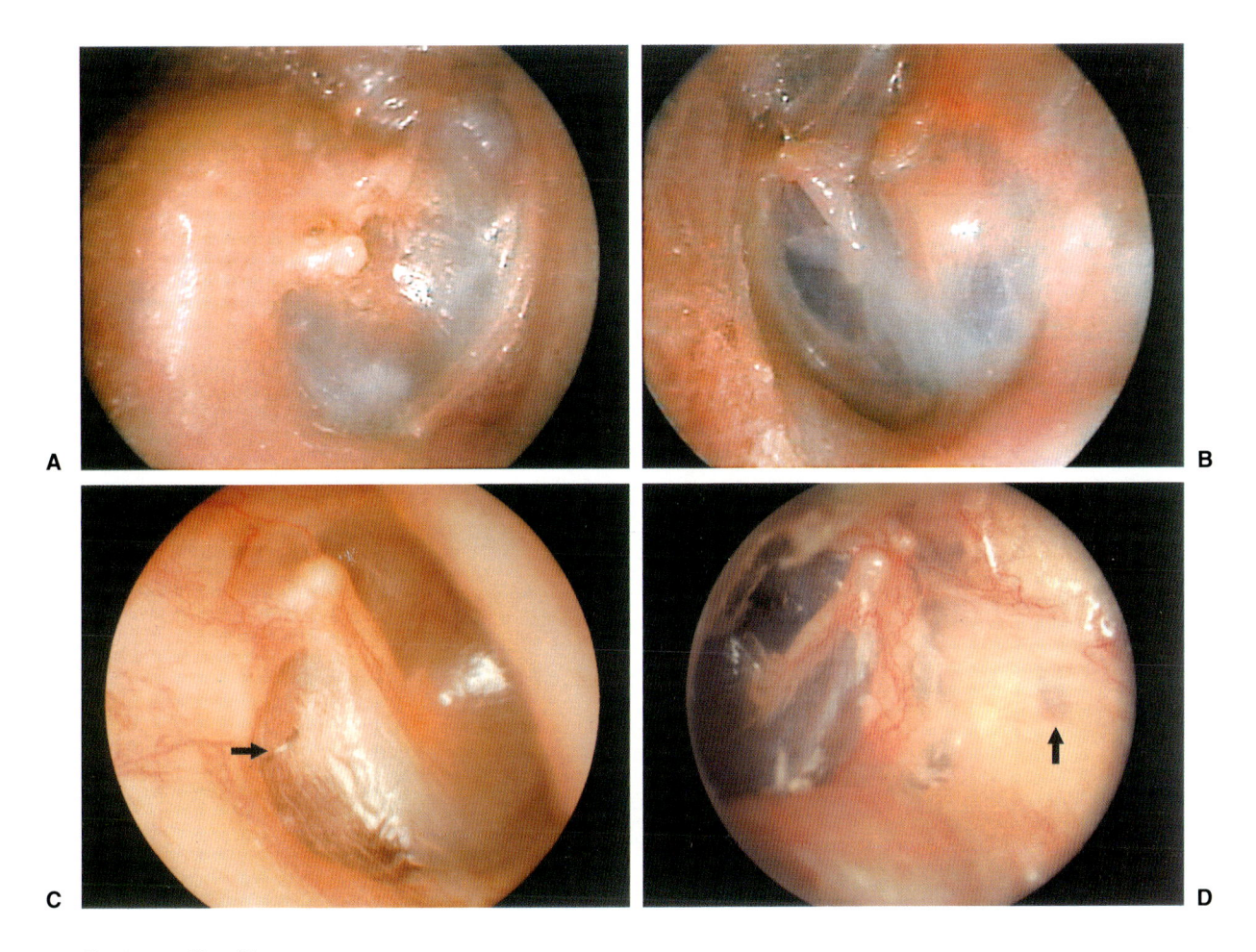

Postoperative Changes

Figure 4-18A. Postoperative Type III tympanoplasty (myringostapediopexy). Note the head of the stapes in the posterior superior quadrant of the right tympanic membrane. Any wax or epithelial debris covering this area must be removed carefully using an operating microscope.

Figure 4-18B. Postoperative tympanoplasty with malleus head ossiculoplasty. Note the absence of the malleus head in the epitympanum in the left ear.

Figure 4-18C. Postoperative stapedectomy. Note the wire prosthesis (*arrow*) placed on the incus as seen through a thin tympanic membrane in the posterior superior quadrant of the right tympanic membrane.

Figure 4-18D. Postoperative fenestration cavity (Lempert). The Lempert fenestration surgery consists of a modified radical mastoidectomy, removal of the head of the malleus and the incus, creation of a window on the lateral aspect of the horizontal semicircular canal, and pedicled skin grafting over the newly created window. Note the window on the horizontal semicircular canal (*arrow*) of the left fenestration cavity. Postoperative hearing loss was 30 dB.

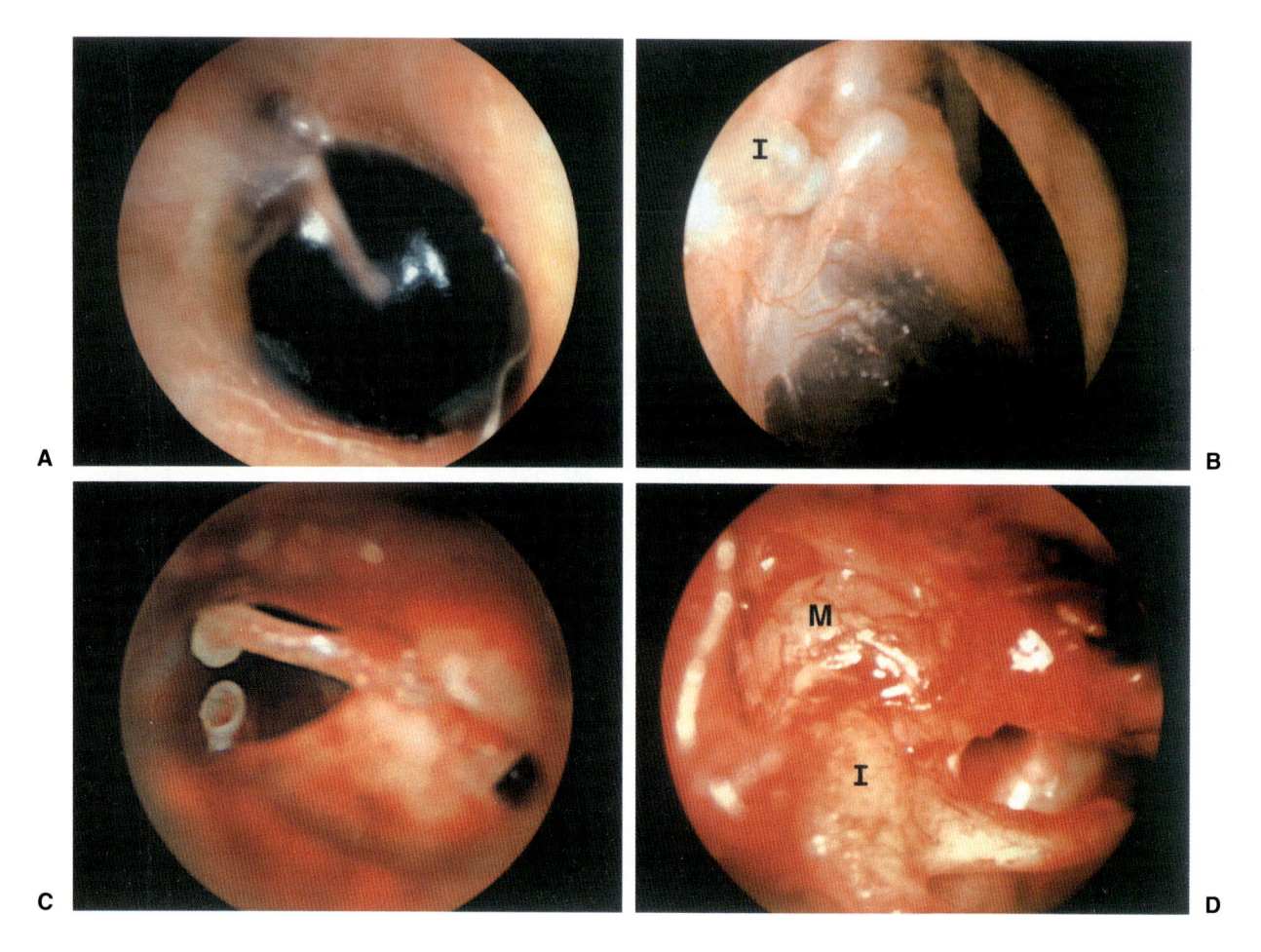

Trauma to the Middle Ear

Figure 4-19A. Hemotympanum. This patient developed hemotympanum as a result of a temporal bone fracture. Note complete filling of the right tympanic cavity by blood. Audiometric testing revealed a 30-dB conductive hearing loss.

Figure 4-19B. Fracture dislocation of the incus. This patient developed a fracture dislocation of the incus (I) as a result of a motor vehicle accident. Note that the distal end of the long process of the right incus including its lenticular process can be seen outside of the tympanic membrane. Audiogram showed a 40-dB conductive hearing loss.

Figure 4-19C. Incudostapedial joint separation. Traumatic dislocation of the ossicular chain produced a 45-dB conductive hearing loss in this patient who had a longitudinal temporal bone fracture due to a motor vehicle accident. The ossicular chain was reestablished by placing a piece of cortical bone between the incus and the stapes. Twenty years later, his hearing remains normal.

Figure 4-19D. Traumatic dislocation of the incudomallear joint. This was repaired by repositioning the incus (I) between the malleus (M) and the mobile stapes head of the right ear, seen on this intraoperative microscopic still photograph.

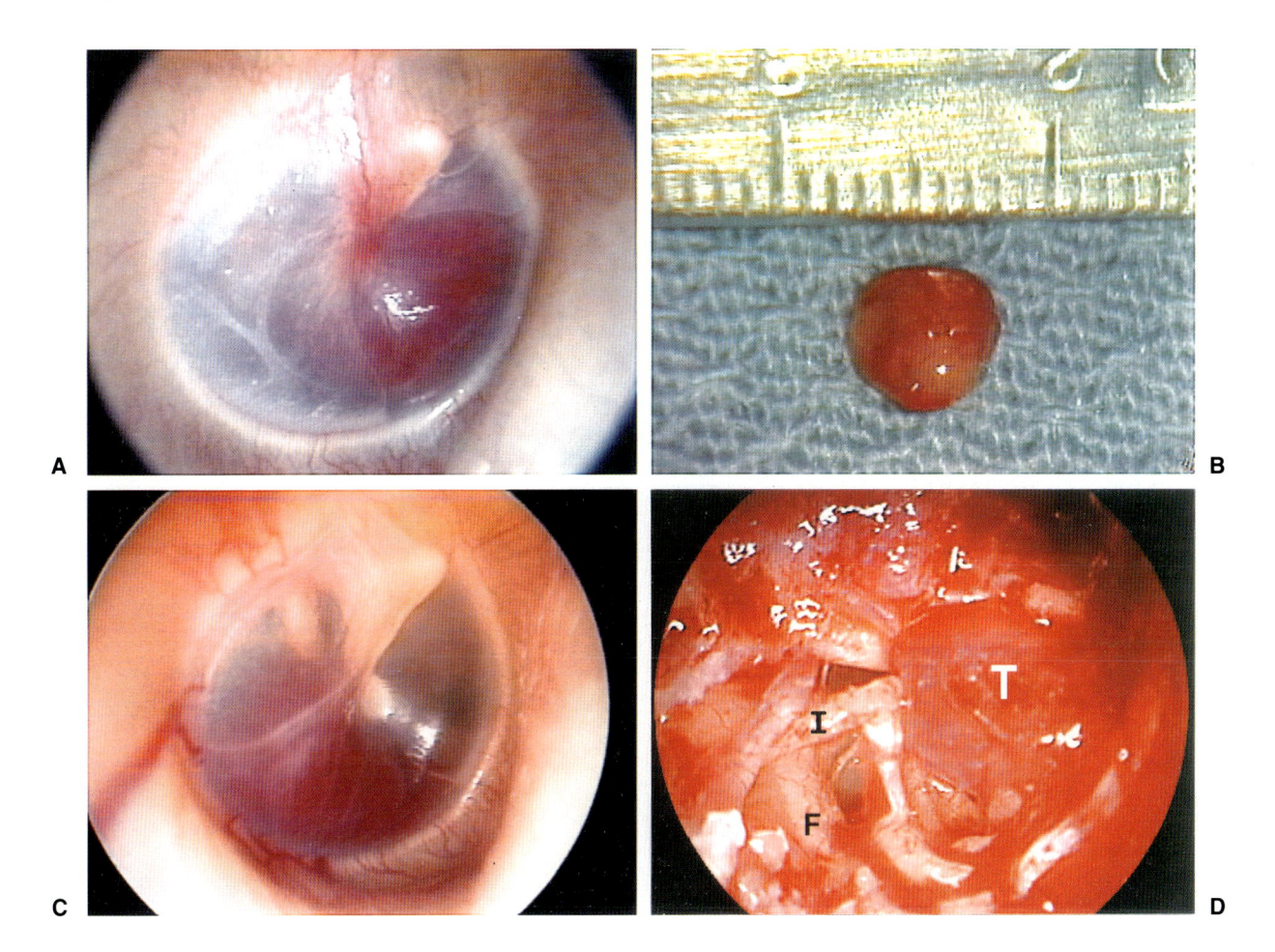

Endoscopy of the External Ear and Tympanic Membrane (Video-otoscopy)

Primary Tumors of the Middle Ear

Figure 4-20A. Glomus tympanicum tumor. The glomus tympanicum is a small and localized vascular tumor (paraganglioma) confined to the middle ear space. This patient had a right glomus tympanicum and presented with unilateral pulsatile tinnitus and conductive hearing loss in that ear. Telescopic examination revealed a red pulsatile mass in the anterior midportion of the right tympanic cavity. The tumor was removed via a transcanal tympanotomy. Bleeding was controlled with bipolar electrocautery.

Figure 4-20B. Glomus tympanicum tumor. This shows the excised glomus tympanicum tumor from the same patient shown in Figure 4-20A.

Figure 4-20C. Glomus jugulare tumor. The glomus jugulare tumor is a large paraganglioma arising from a glomus body located in the jugular bulb that often spreads to the base of the skull affecting cranial nerves VII–XII. This patient complained of constant pulsatile tinnitus in the right ear. Telescopic otoscopy showed a red pulsatile vascular mass involving the inferior two-thirds of the right tympanic cavity. Increased vascularity was noted involving the inferior portion of the tympanic ring extending into the floor of the ear canal. In this patient, Brown's sign (blanching on positive pressure with pneumatic otoscopy) was positive. Audiometric testing showed a 40-dB conductive hearing loss.

Figure 4-20D. Glomus jugulare tumor. This intraoperative 0-degree transmastoid telescopic view (see also Figures 13-2 and 13-3E) of the middle ear of the same patient at surgery shows the large glomus tumor (T) filling the inferior two-thirds of the right middle ear space. The superior portion of the tumor was in direct contact with the incus (I) and stapes as well as the malleus. This explained the patient's 40-dB conductive hearing loss. The glomus jugulare tumor extended inferiorly involving the tympanic bone of the ear canal. Note the middle ear portion of the facial nerve (F).

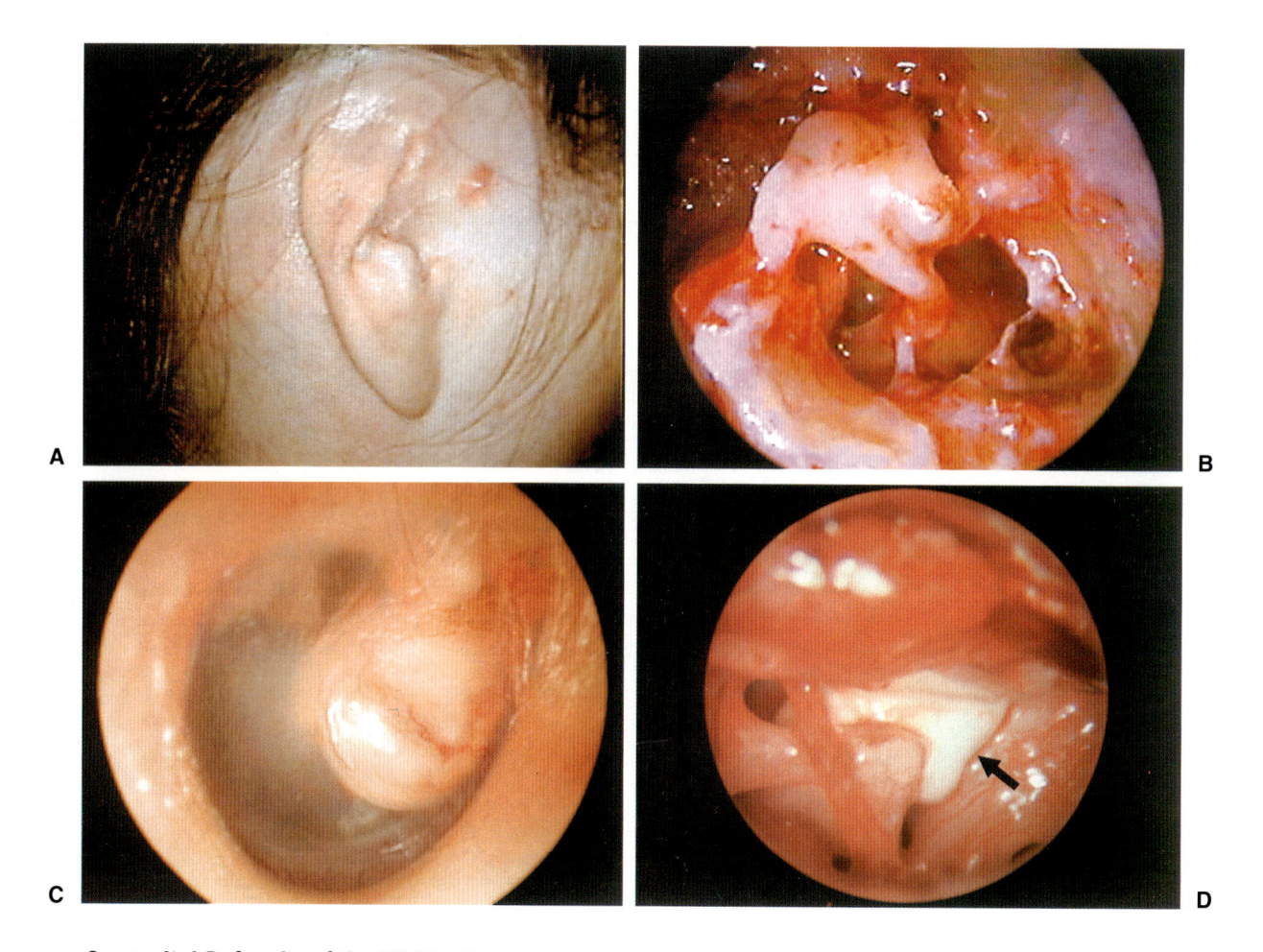

Congenital Deformity of the Middle Ear

Figure 4-21A. Congenital aural atresia. A congenitally deformed auricle is often associated with deformities of the ear canals and middle and inner ears. This patient had an ossicular deformity and presented with a 60% conductive deafness in the right ear.

Figure 4-21B. Congenital anomalies of the middle ear. This is an intraoperative transmastoid telescopic view of the middle ear of the patient shown in Figure 4-21A (see also Figure 13-3H). Fusion of the malleus and incus was found when the atresia plate was removed. Note also the deformed monopod stapes. The patient's hearing improved to 20 dB after tympanoplasty and reconstruction of the ear canal.

Figure 4-21C. Congenital cholesteatoma of the middle ear. In this patient who had no previous history of aural infection or surgery, telescopic otoscopy revealed a white cystic mass behind the anterior superior quadrant of the right intact tympanic membrane.

Figure 4-21D. Congenital cholesteatoma of the middle ear. Middle ear exploration showed congenital cholesteatoma (arrow) in the anterior superior portion of the right middle ear. This type of cholesteatoma can be removed through the transcanal approach by making a wide tympanomeatal flap and separating the superior half of the tympanic membrane from the manubrium of the malleus.

Chapter 5
Endoscopy of the Nose (Video Nasal Endoscopy, Videorhinoscopy)

Nasal endoscopy is the examination of the nasal cavity using a rigid telescope or flexible fiberscope. When nasal endoscopic findings are documented with a video camera, the procedure is called video nasal endoscopy or videorhinoscopy. Videorhinoscopy is the most effective and practical method of demonstrating and documenting the anatomy and pathological conditions of structures within the nasal cavity. Important anatomical structures of the nasal cavities such as turbinates, meatus, nasolacrimal duct openings, natural and accessory ostia of the paranasal sinuses, roof, and septum can be studied in depth, and their findings can be documented.

Equipment required for nasal endoscopy include (1) 4-mm 0-, 30-, 70-, and 120-degree nasal telescopes for adults, (2) 2.7-mm 0-, 30-, and 70-degree nasal telescopes for children, (3) a 4-mm or 2.7-mm short ototelescope for children, (4) a flexible fiberscope such as Olympus ENF P3, (5) a light source, and (6) a topical nasal anesthetic and decongestant. Video nasal endoscopy or videorhinoscopy also requires (1) a video camera, (2) a video recorder, (3) a microphone to record the voice for transnasal observation of velopharyngeal function, (4) a video monitor, and (5) a color video printer.

Videorhinoscopy allows documentation of the anatomy and pathology of intranasal structures for patient counseling, teaching, and permanent records. Videoprints can be made instantaneously and are useful for treatment planning and pre- and postoperative comparison.

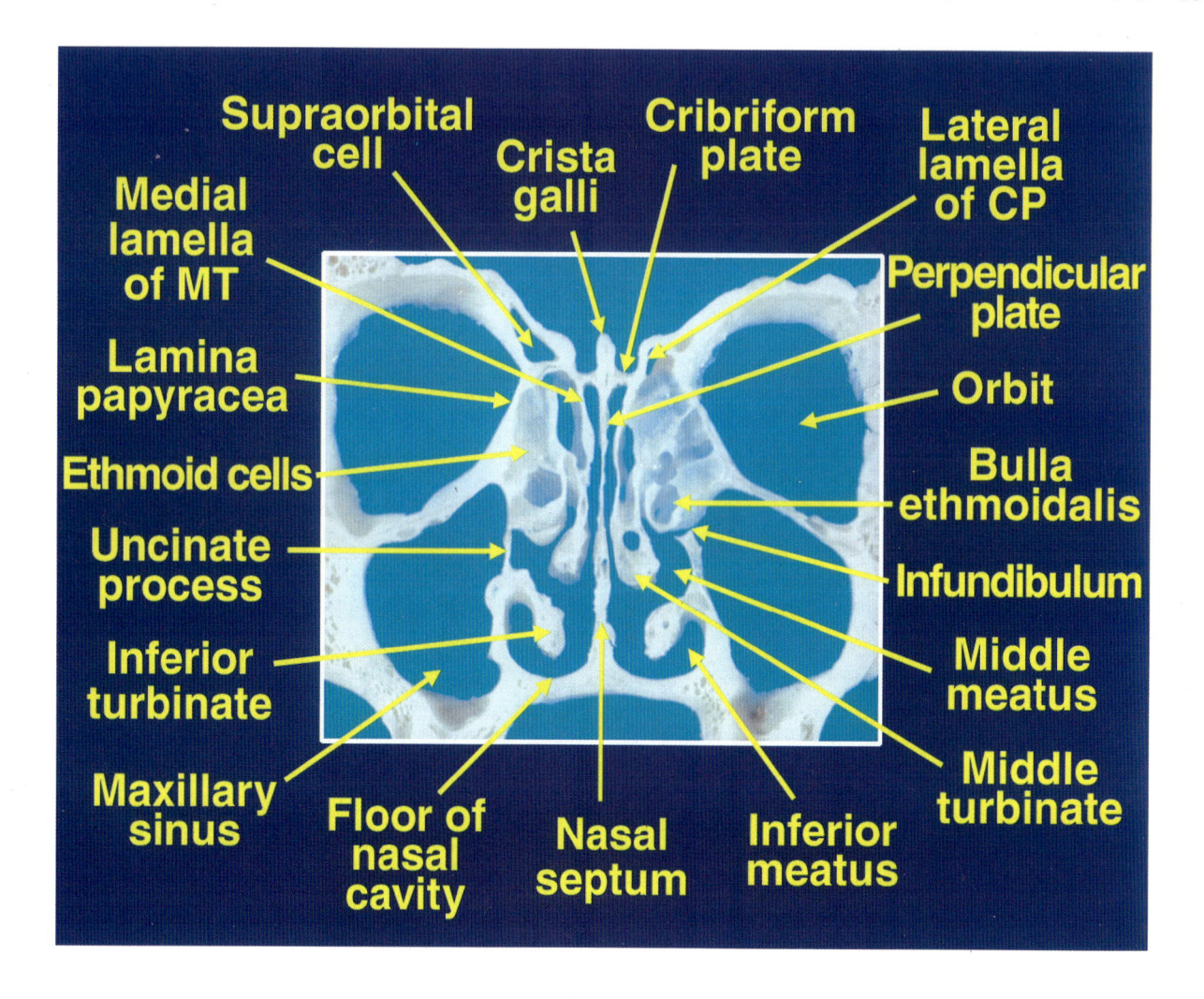

OVERVIEW OF NASAL ANATOMY

Figure 5-1. Anatomical structures of the nasal cavity. This section of a dried skull at the level of the anterior ethmoid shows the anatomical structures of the nasal cavities and paranasal sinuses.

Endoscopy of the Nose (Video Nasal Endoscopy, Videorhinoscopy)

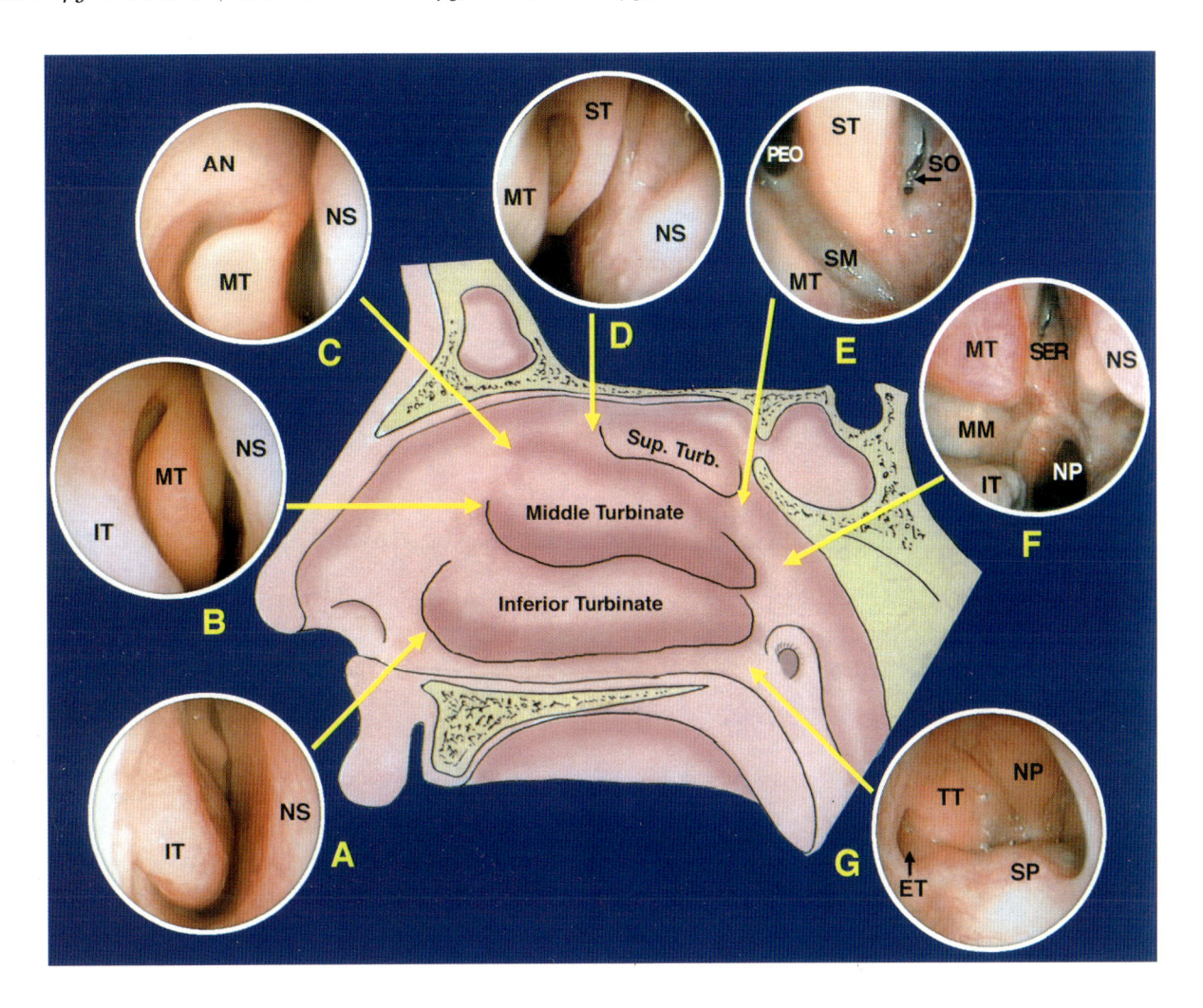

Figure 5-2. Endoscopic anatomy of the nasal cavity. This schematic drawing of the lateral wall of the nasal cavity shows the endoscopic anatomy of pertinent structures (all taken with a 4-mm 0-degree telescope). (A) Inferior turbinate, (B) middle turbinate, (C) agger nasi cell, (D) superior turbinate, (E) superior turbinate and superior meatus (PEO, posterior ethmoid sinus ostium; SO, sphenoid sinus ostium), (F) sphenoethmoidal recess (SER) and related structures (MT, middle turbinate; NS, nasal septum; MM, middle meatus; IT, inferior turbinate; NP, nasopharynx), and (G) posterior nasal cavity and nasopharynx (ET, eustachian tube orifice; TT, torus tubarius; SP, soft palate).

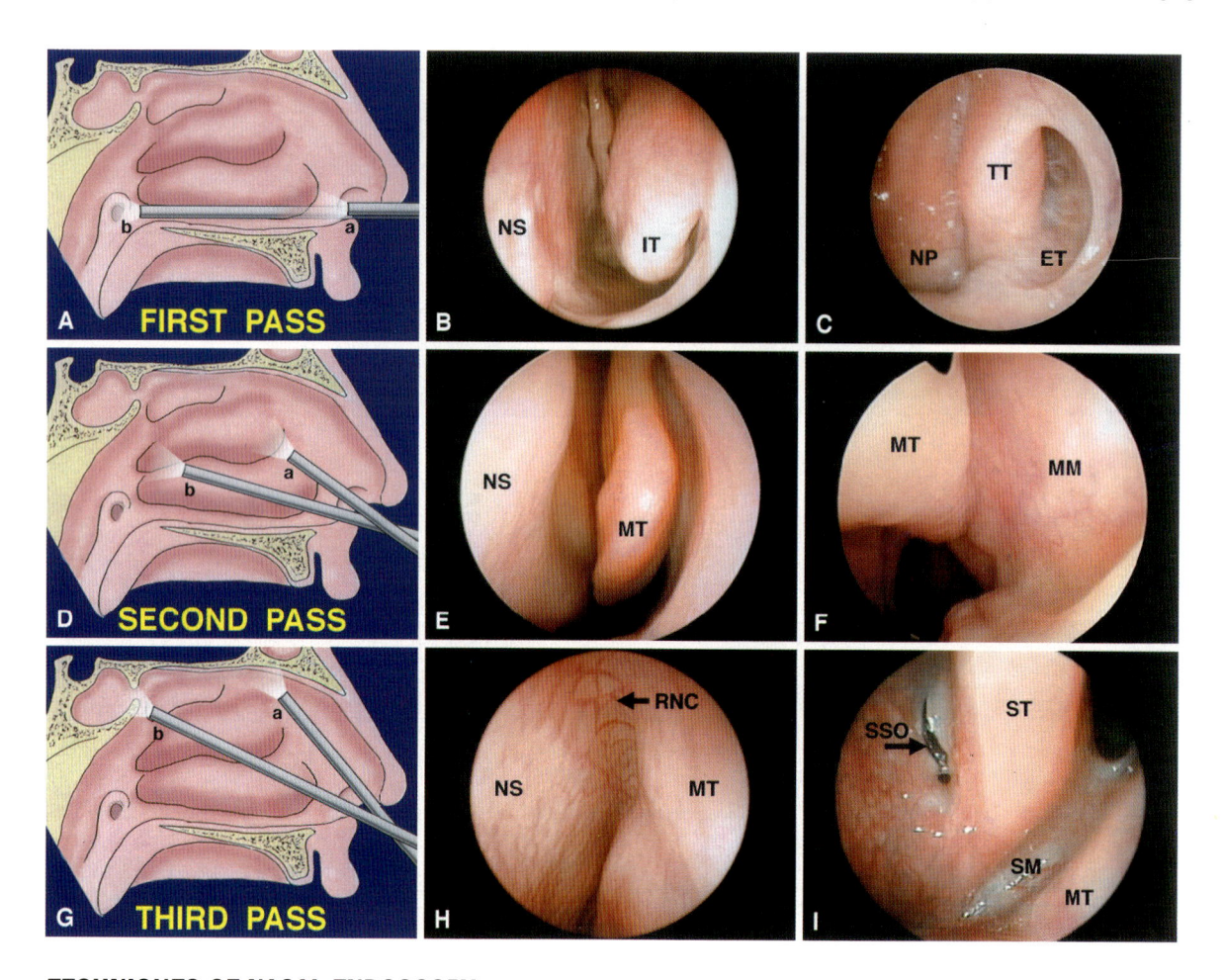

TECHNIQUES OF NASAL ENDOSCOPY

Figure 5-3. Systematic nasal endoscopy. Endoscopic examination of the nasal cavity is carried out in a systematic fashion. *Top row:* The first pass (A–C) is made along the floor of the nose between the nasal septum (NS) and the inferior turbinate (IT) (Figure 5-3B). The anatomical structures to be observed are the inferior turbinate (IT), inferior meatus, floor of the nose, and nasal septum (NS). By advancing the telescope into the posterior nasal cavity, one visualizes the entire nasopharynx (NP), soft palate, eustachian tube orifice (ET), torus tubarius (TT), and the fossa of Rosenmüller (Figure 5-3C). The telescope is slowly withdrawn and the choana and inferior meatus are reexamined. *Middle row:* The second pass (D–F) is made with the patient's head tilted back approximately 45 degrees. The telescope is passed toward the middle turbinate (Figure 5-3Da) and then advanced between the middle turbinate and inferior turbinate (Figure 5-3Db). The structures to be observed are the middle turbinate and the contents of the middle meatus such as the uncinate process, hiatus semilunaris, ethmoid bulla, and accessory ostia of the maxillary sinus. *Bottom row:* The third pass (G–I) is directed toward the roof of the nasal cavity (Figure 5-3Ga) superior and medial to the middle turbinate, and then it is advanced between the middle turbinate and nasal septum toward the sphenoid sinus ostium (SSO) (Figure 5-3Gb). Structures to be recognized include the roof of the nasal cavity (RNC), agger nasi, superior turbinate (ST), and superior meatus (SM).

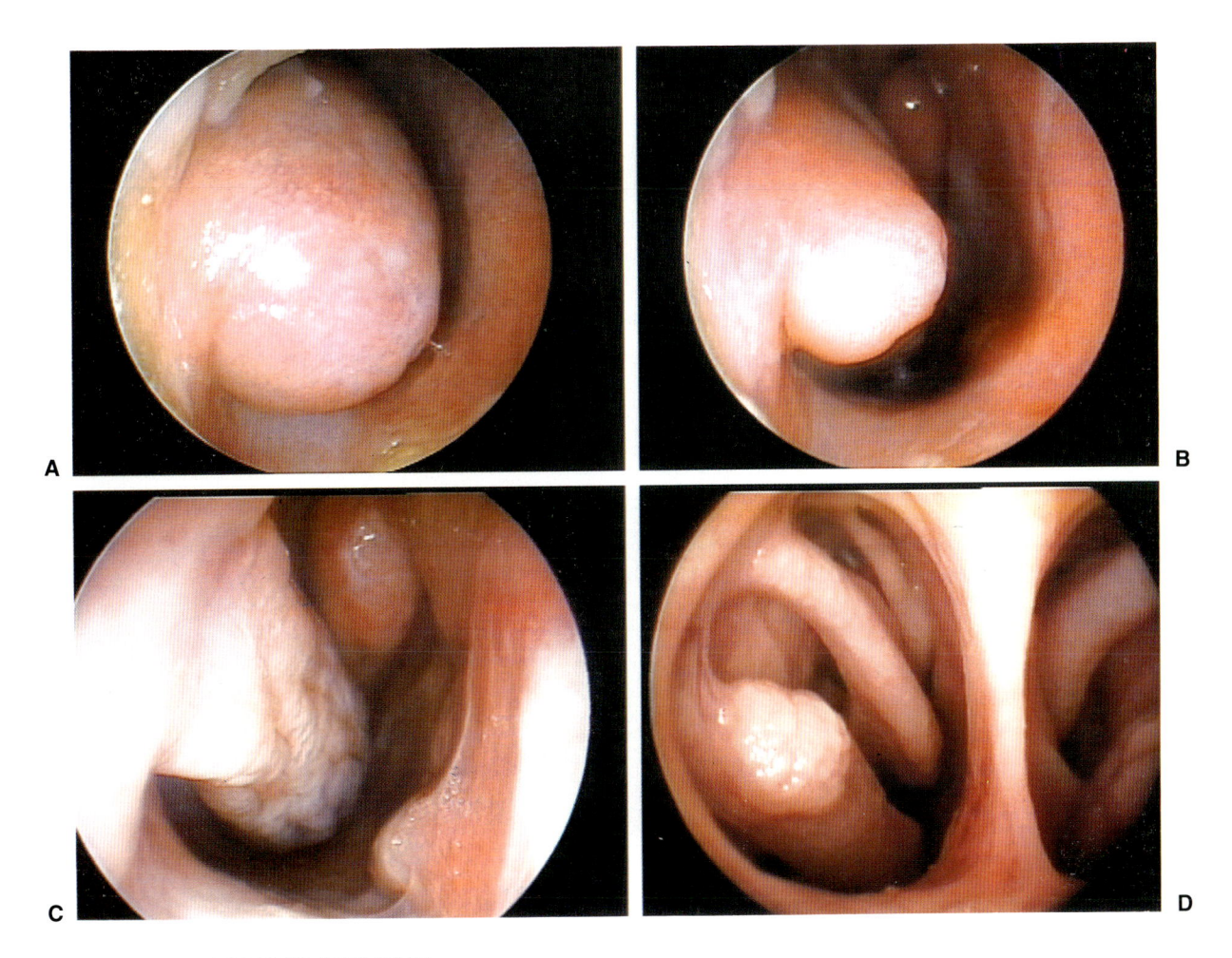

NASAL ENDOSCOPIC ANATOMY

Inferior Turbinate

Figure 5-4A. Hypertrophied inferior turbinate. The 0-degree telescopic view demonstrates the swollen right inferior turbinate.

Figure 5-4B. Decongested inferior turbinate. The same inferior turbinate shown in Figure 5-4A shrinks significantly five minutes after application of 3% ephedrine spray. Note that the air passage has widened, thereby enabling visualization of the middle turbinate and posterior nasal structures. An adequate examination of the nasal cavity cannot be performed until the inferior turbinates have been shrunken with nasal decongestants.

Figure 5-4C. Atrophic inferior turbinate after total laryngectomy. The right inferior turbinate is pale and atrophic.

Figure 5-4D. Posterior end of the inferior turbinate. The mulberry hypertrophy of the posterior end of the right inferior turbinate is seen by transoral retrograde telescopic examination (90-degree). Note that the posterior ends of the superior, middle, and inferior turbinates as well as the superior, middle, and inferior meatus are well shown.

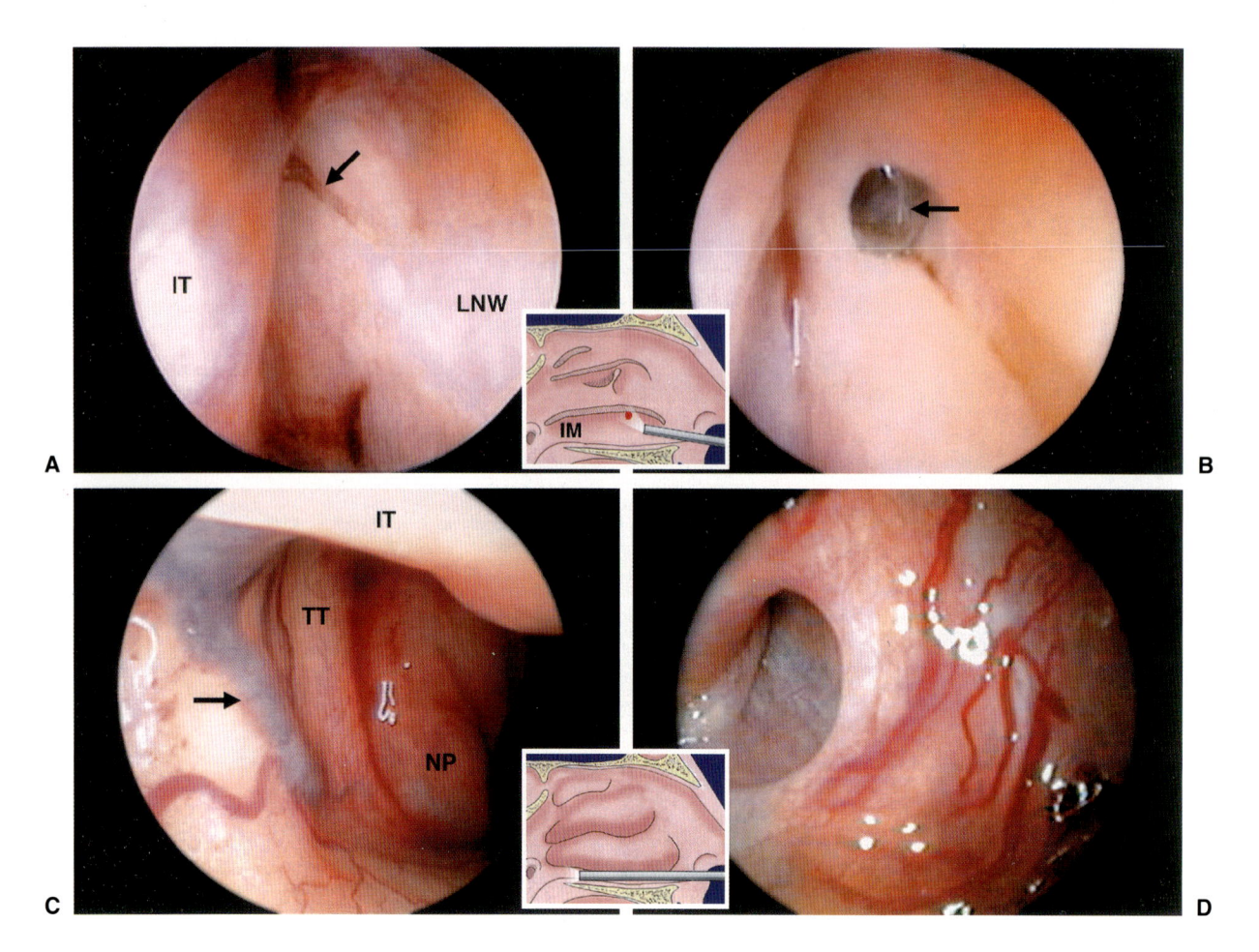

Nasolacrimal Duct Ostium and Nasonasopharyngeal Plexus

Figure 5-5A. Nasolacrimal duct ostium. The lacrimal sac extends downward into the nasolacrimal duct, which travels in a bony canal along the medial wall of the maxillary sinus until it opens into the inferior meatus through the valve of Hasner (*arrow*). The highest portion of the inferior meatus is located at the junction of the anterior and middle thirds of the meatus where the nasolacrimal duct drains into the nasal cavity. In this case, the 4-mm 30-degree telescope is passed into the left inferior meatus (IM) and advanced upward between the inferior turbinate (IT) and the lateral nasal wall (LNW) (see inset). An oblique groove containing the valve of Hasner (*arrow*) is observed.

Figure 5-5B. Nasolacrimal duct ostium. When the telescope is advanced closer toward the opening of the duct, its lumen clearly can be seen in the lateral aspect of the roof of the inferior meatus (*arrow*) A teardrop appears in the rounded opening. The shape of the opening varies considerably from rounded to slit-like. In order to visualize the ostium of the nasolacrimal duct, it may be necessary to displace the anterior portion of the inferior turbinate medially. To avoid injury to this ostium during the inferior meatal antrostomy, the window should be made inferiorly in the middle to posterior portion of the lateral wall of the inferior meatus.

Figure 5-5C. Nasonasopharyngeal plexus (Woodruff's plexus). The nasonasopharyngeal plexus described by Woodruff is usually located along the posterior lateral wall of the inferior meatus. The "Woodruff's plexus" refers to mucosal blood vessels found at the posterior 1 cm of the inferior meatus, inferior turbinate, middle meatus, and nasal floor. Posterior epistaxis usually originates from this region. This transnasal 30-degree telescopic view demonstrates the right nasonasopharyngeal plexus.

Figure 5-5D. Nasonasopharyngeal plexus. In this case the left nasonasopharyngeal vascular network is clearly seen just anterior to the patent eustachian tube orifice on the left side. The inset shows the general location of the plexus as seen with a 4-mm 0-degree telescope.

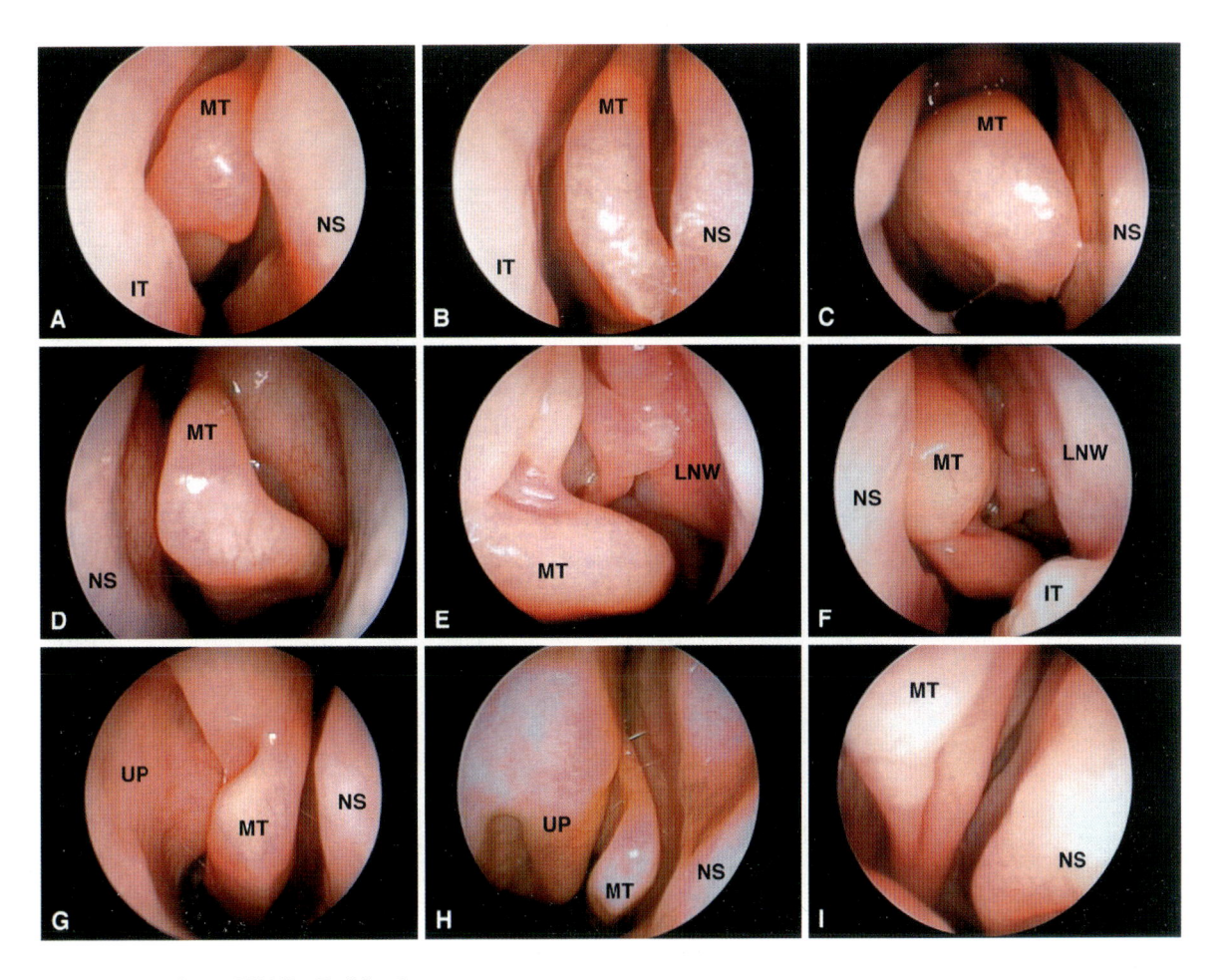

Endoscopy of the Nose (Video Nasal Endoscopy, Videorhinoscopy)

Variations of the Middle Turbinate

Figure 5-6A. Right middle turbinate with anterior polypoid mucosa.

Figure 5-6B. Medially (paradoxically) bent right middle turbinate.

Figure 5-6C. Medially (paradoxically) bent right concha bullosa.

Figure 5-6D. Triangular or L-shaped left middle turbinate.

Figure 5-6E. L-shaped left middle turbinate with a marked horizontal lamella. Note a small polyp in the middle meatus (see also Figure 5-15A).

Figure 5-6F. L-shaped left middle turbinate with a marked horizontal lamella.

Figure 5-6G. Medially displaced right middle turbinate with a well visualized uncinate process (UP) and basal lamella.

Figure 5-6H. Small right middle turbinate between anteriorly and medially bent prominent uncinate process (UP) and nasal septum.

Figure 5-6I. Sagittally clefted middle turbinate. Note the longitudinal cleft along the inferior border of the right middle turbinate.

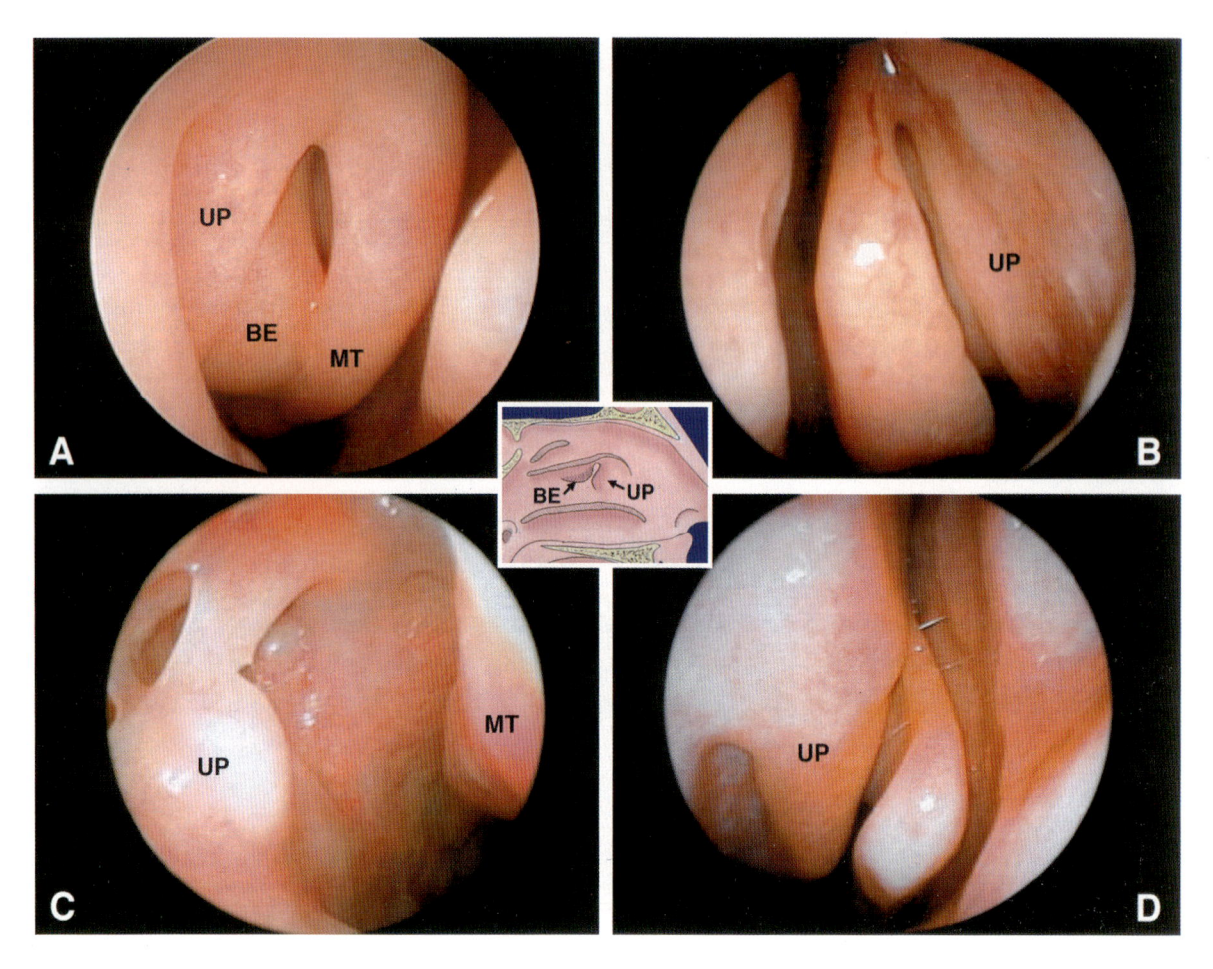

Variations of the Uncinate Process

Figure 5-7A. Uncinate process. The sickle-shaped unicate process normally extends from its anterior superior attachment on the lateral nasal wall down to its posterior inferior attachment on the inferior turbinate. It extends posteromedially to its free margin. In this case the posterior margin of the right uncinate process (UP) extends superiorly and converges with the middle turbinate. Note a prominent ethmoid bulla, also called bulla ethmoidalis (BE), between the uncinate process (UP) and the middle turbinate (MT).

Figure 5-7B. Medially bent uncinate process. In this case, the left uncinate process (UP) is bent medially and anteriorly narrowing the middle meatus.

Figure 5-7C. Unusually shaped uncinate process. The 30-degree telescope reveals an anomalous uncinate process (UP) with a bulbous inferior end and a thin superior bony plate attached to the superior wall of the middle meatus. Note a widely patent middle meatus with the anterior fontanelle anterior to the uncinate process and the posterior fontanelle posterior to the uncinate process. A faint bulging of the ethmoid bulla is seen.

Figure 5-7D. Markedly medially and anteriorly bent uncinate process. Note the small right middle turbinate between the uncinate process (UP) and the nasal septum.

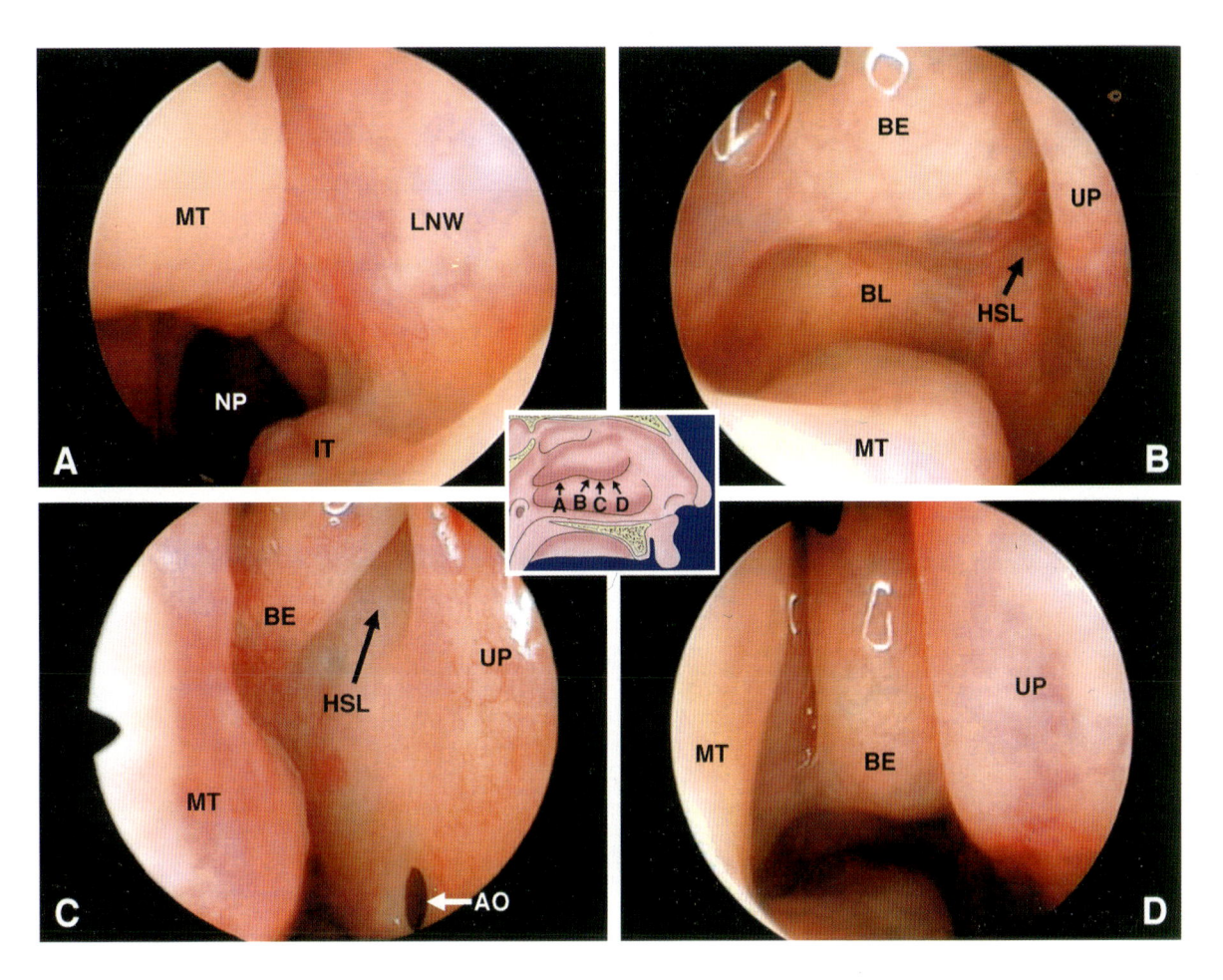

Endoscopy of the Nose (Video Nasal Endoscopy, Videorhinoscopy) 49

The Middle Meatus

Figure 5-8A. Posterior to anterior approach (nasal endoscopy step 2). During the second step of the nasal endoscopic examination, the tip of the telescope (in this case 0-degree) is passed into the posterior portion of the left middle meatus between the middle and inferior turbinates. Note that the posterior portion of the left lateral nasal wall (LNW) is well visualized.

Figure 5-8B. Posterior to anterior approach (nasal endoscopy step 2). As the tip of the 0-degree telescope is drawn anteriorly, the ethmoid bulla (BE) and the upper surface of the laterally bent horizontal lamella of this L-shaped left middle turbinate (MT) come into view. Note the basal lamella (BL) of the middle turbinate is seen posteriorly between the ethmoid bulla (BE) and the middle turbinate (MT). The hiatus semilunaris inferior (HSL) is seen between the inferior portion of the ethmoidal bulla (BE) and the uncinate process (UP).

Figure 5-8C. Posterior to anterior approach (nasal endoscopy step 2). This endoscopic view of the middle meatus shows the hiatus semilunaris inferior (HSL) between the inferior lateral portion of the ethmoid bulla (BE) and the uncinate process (UP). The left middle turbinate (MT) is seen medially, and an accessory maxillary sinus ostium (AO) is seen in the anterior inferior portion of the lateral nasal wall.

Figure 5-8D. Posterior to anterior approach (nasal endoscopy step 2). As the tip of the 0-degree telescope is drawn anteriorly, the anterior face of the left ethmoid bulla (BE) is well visualized. Note the space between the medial aspect of the middle turbinate (MT) and the ethmoidal bulla (BE). This is the beginning of the hiatus semilunaris superior. Note also the laterally bent horizontal lamella of the middle turbinate seen at the bottom of the view.

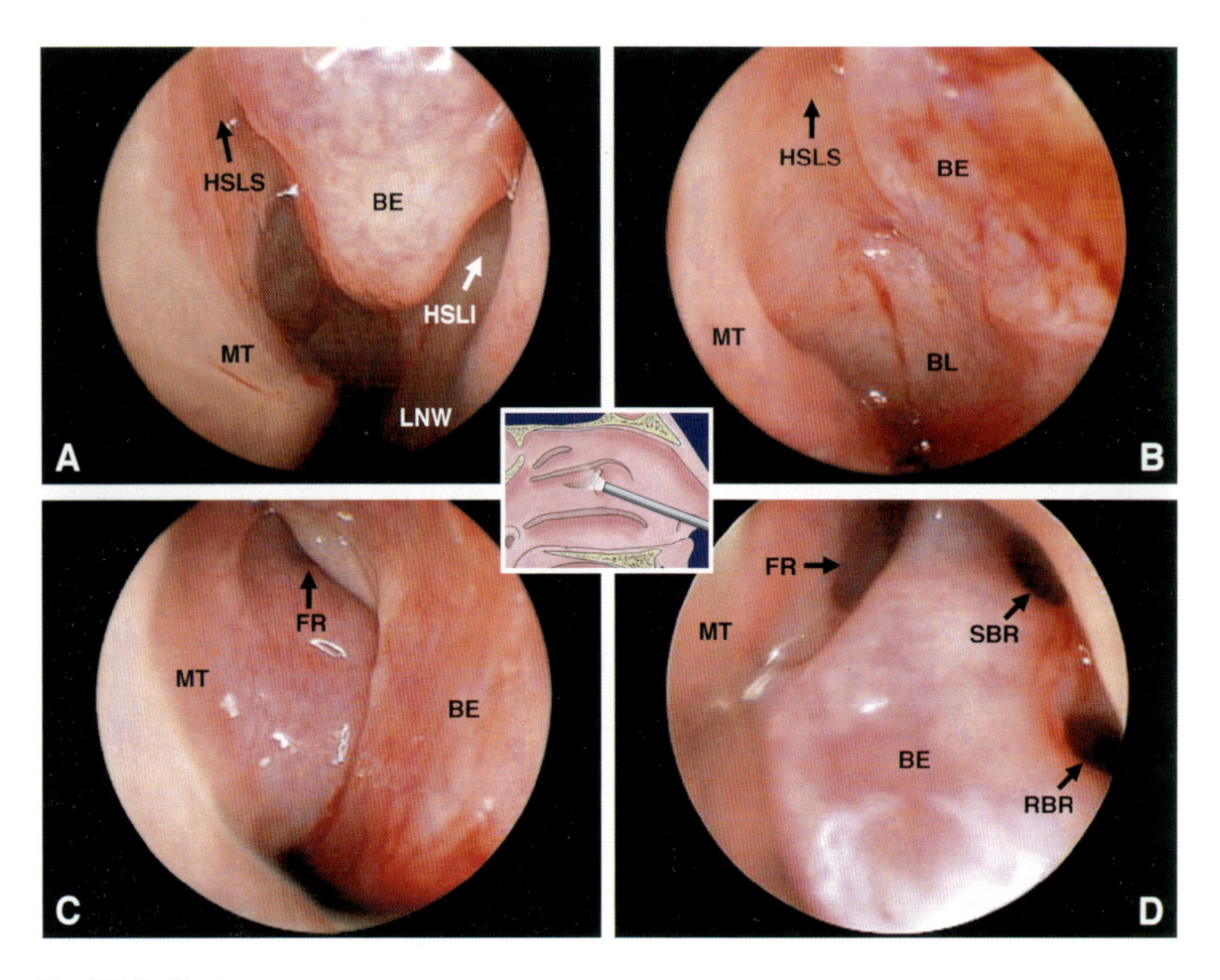

The Middle Meatus

Figure 5-9A. Hiatus semilunaris superior and inferior. This left middle meatal view demonstrates the hiatus semilunaris superior and inferior. The hiatus semilunaris inferior (HSLI) is seen between the inferior portion of the ethmoid bulla (BE) and the uncinate process, leading toward the ethmoid infundibulum. The hiatus semilunaris superior (HSLS) is seen between the lateral surface of the left middle turbinate (MT) and the superior portion of the ethmoid bulla (BE), leading toward the frontal recess. Remember that the hiatus semilunaris inferior is lateral to the ethmoid bulla while the hiatus semilunaris superior is medial to the ethmoid bulla.

Figure 5-9B. Hiatus semilunaris superior (HSLS). This is a vaguely defined crescent-shaped crevice between the ethmoid bulla (BE) and the middle turbinate (MT). Note the basal lamella (BL) of the left middle turbinate posteriorly.

Figure 5-9C. Frontal recess (FR). This is the most anterior and superior portion of the anterior ethmoid complex which leads to and communicates with the frontal sinus. Its medial wall is the lateral surface of the most anterosuperior part of the middle turbinate (MT) as shown in this left middle meatus.

Figure 5-9D. Frontal recess, suprabullar recess, and retrobullar recess. As the tip of the 30-degree telescope is advanced superiorly and medially within the left middle meatus, the frontal recess (FR) is more clearly seen superiorly between the middle turbinate (MT) and the ethmoid bulla (BE). The "sinus lateralis" of Grünwald is more appropriately called the suprabullar recess. Since this space does not have just a single opening for ventilation and drainage and does not satisfy the criteria of a cell, the term *recess* is recommended by Stammberger and by Kennedy et al. The suprabullar recess (SBR) may extend into a retrobullar recess (RBR) when the posterior wall of the bulla lamella does not contact the basal lamella of the middle turbinate. When well pneumatized, this space is bordered superiorly by the ethmoid roof, laterally by the lamina papyracea, inferiorly by the roof of the ethmoid bulla, and posteriorly by the basal lamella of the middle turbinate. It is separated anteriorly from the frontal recess only when the bulla lamella reaches the skull base as shown in this left middle meatal view.

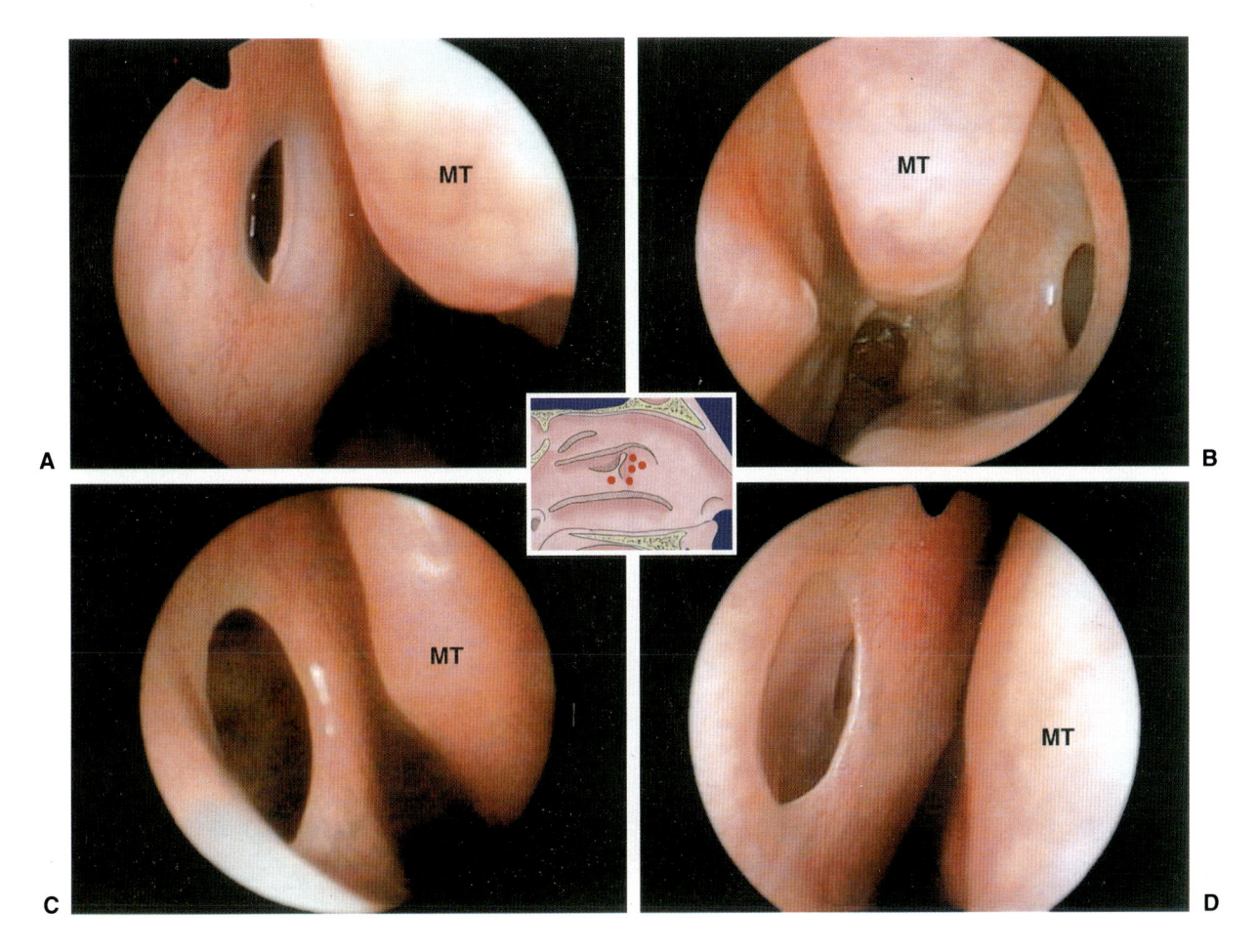

Endoscopy of the Nose (Video Nasal Endoscopy, Videorhinoscopy)

Accessory Maxillary Sinus Ostium

Figure 5-10A. Accessory maxillary sinus ostium. While the natural maxillary sinus ostium is difficult or impossible to visualize during routine nasal endoscopy, an accessory maxillary sinus ostium can often be seen in the lateral wall of the middle meatus. The accessory ostium may be encountered in 25–30% of the population.

Figure 5-10B. Accessory maxillary sinus ostium. The accessory ostium is usually located in the anterior or posterior fontanelle where the medial wall of the maxillary sinus is membranous. In this case, it is located in the left anterior fontanelle.

Figure 5-10C. Accessory maxillary sinus ostium. The size and shape of accessory ostia vary as seen in this right anterior fontanelle. There may be multiple accessory ostia. The accessory ostium allows for the "recirculation" phenomenon whereby maxillary sinus secretions are passed out of the maxillary sinus via ciliary transport through the natural ostium and immediately back into the sinus via an accessory ostium. For this reason, any accessory ostium that is encountered during endoscopic sinus surgery should be connected to the natural ostium to prevent this mucus recirculation problem.

Figure 5-10D. Accessory maxillary sinus ostium. The accessory ostium is usually presented as a hole. However, in this case the accessory ostium is presented as a canal in the lateral wall of the right middle meatus.

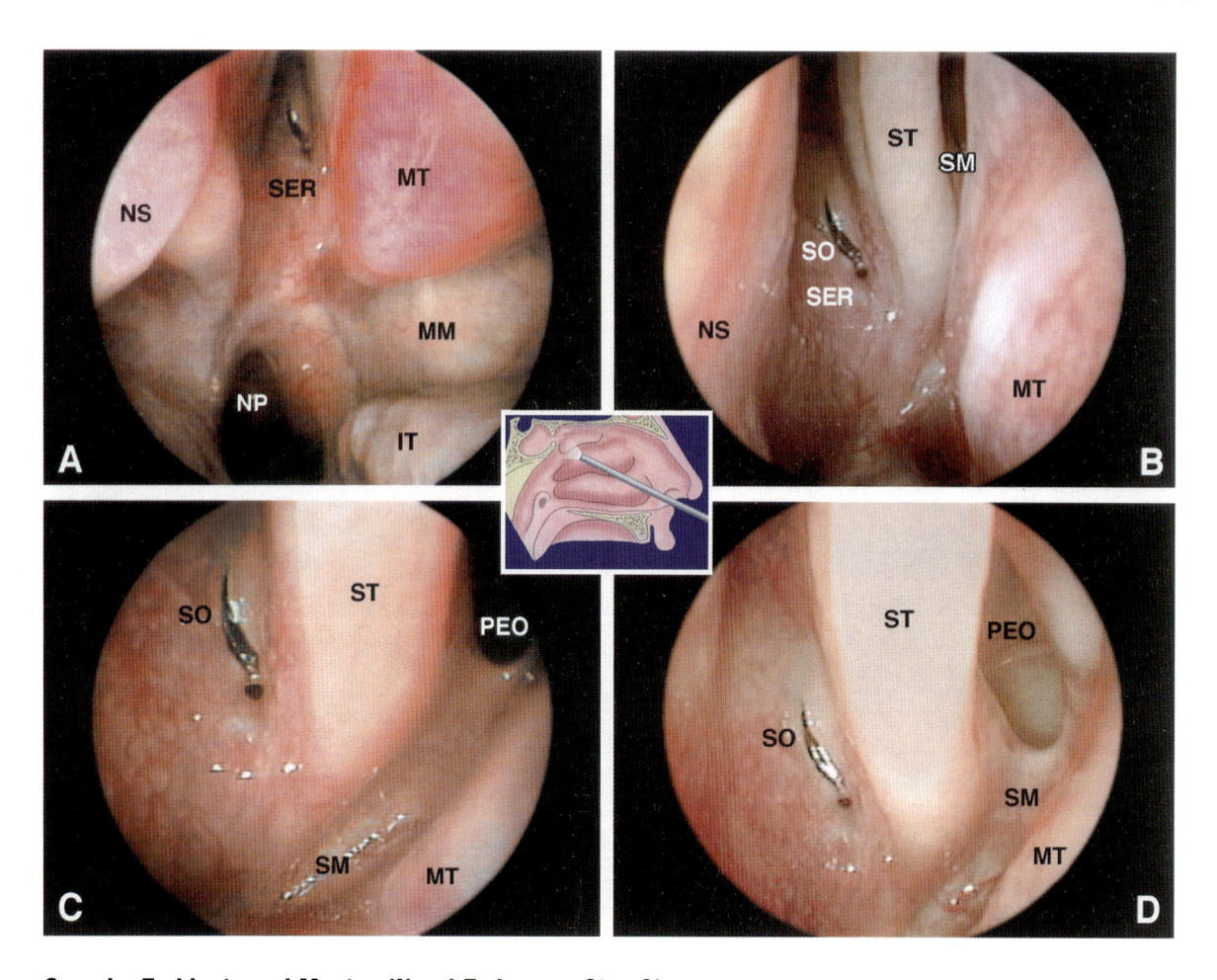

Superior Turbinate and Meatus (Nasal Endoscopy Step 3).

Figure 5-11A.   Sphenoethmoidal recess. The sphenoid sinus ostium is located in the sphenoethmoidal recess in the superior portion of the posterior wall of the nasal cavity. To find the sphenoethmoidal recess during the third step of nasal endoscopy a 0-degree telescope is passed into the nasal cavity (the left side in this case) and advanced toward the nasopharynx between the middle turbinate (MT) and nasal septum (NS). The roof of the choana and the posterior attachment of middle turbinate (MT) are identified. As the scope is advanced superiorly, the sphenoethmoidal recess (SER) is visualized in most cases.

Figure 5-11B.   Sphenoid sinus ostium and superior turbinate. The superior turbinate (ST) is identified between the left middle turbinate (MT) and the nasal septum (NS). The superior meatus (SM) lies between the superior and middle turbinate. The sphenoid sinus ostium (SO) is readily visualized in this left sphenoethmoidal recess (SER) just medial to the attachment of the superior turbinate (ST).

Figure 5-11C.   Sphenoid sinus ostium and superior meatus. As the telescope is advanced, the sphenoid sinus ostium (SO) is clearly visualized. The superior meatus is seen between the superior turbinate (ST) and the middle turbinate (MT).

Figure 5-11D.   Superior meatus and posterior ethmoid sinus ostium. As the 0-degree telescope is directed laterally, a clear picture of the posterior ethmoid sinus ostium (PEO) is recognized in the superior portion of the left superior meatus (SM). The posterior ethmoid cells drain into the superior meatus, while the anterior ethmoid cells open into the hiatus semilunaris of the middle meatus.

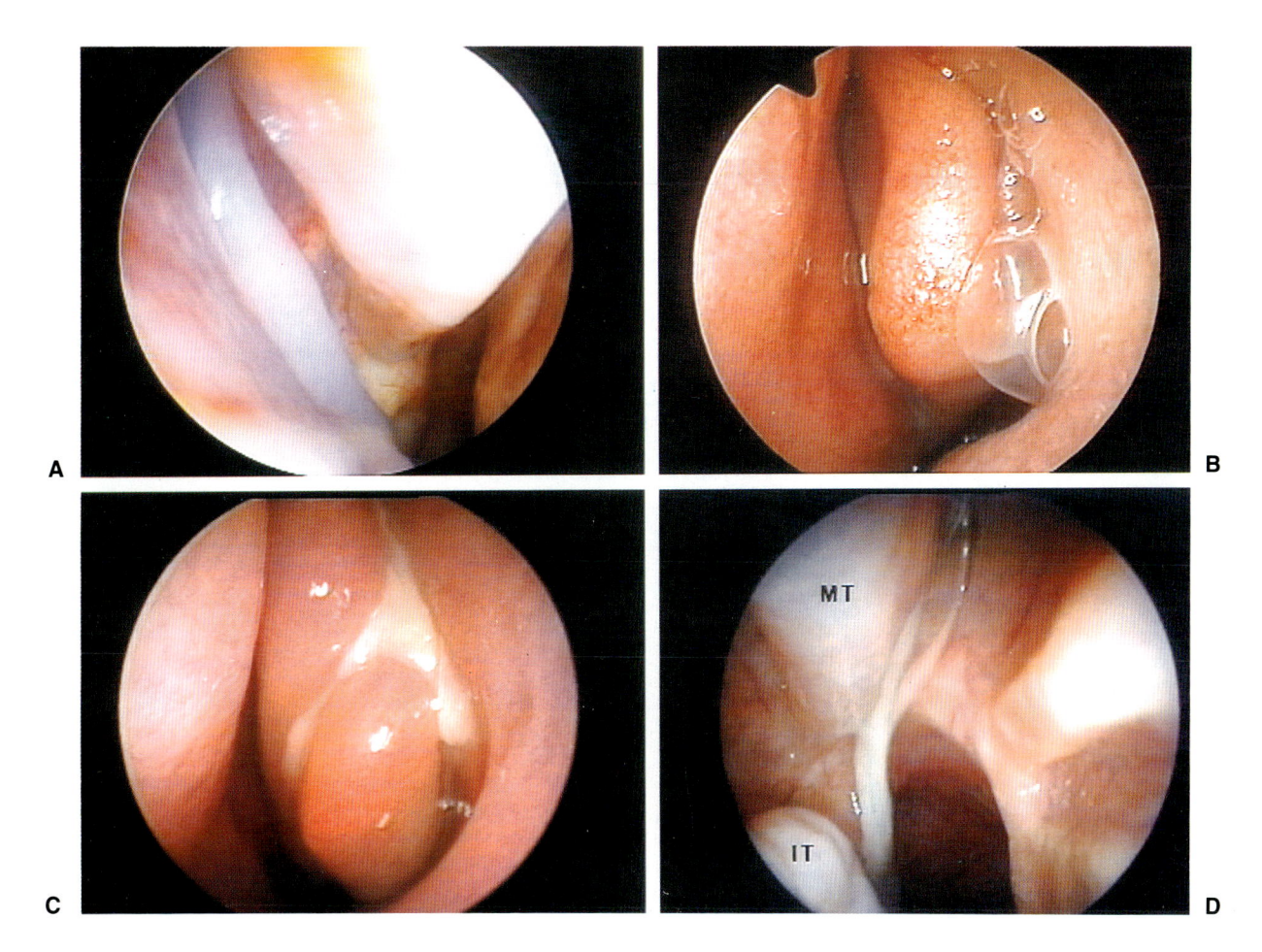

Endoscopy of the Nose (Video Nasal Endoscopy, Videorhinoscopy) 53

DISORDERS OF THE NASAL CAVITY

Sinusitis

Figure 5-12A.   Pus in the middle meatus. A stream of pus can be seen in the right middle meatus originating from the area of hiatus semilunaris draining out toward the nasopharynx. Presence of pus in the middle meatus suggests frontal, maxillary, or anterior ethmoid sinusitis.

Figure 5-12B.   Pus in the middle meatus. The 0-degree telescopy reveals mucopus in the left middle meatus. In this case the sinus x-rays showed left maxillary sinusitis with an air-fluid level.

Figure 5-12C.   Pus in the middle meatus. This patient complained of severe frontal headaches associated with purulent nasal discharge. Nasal endoscopy reveals pus coming out of the superior portion of the left middle meatus around a large middle meatal polyp. Coronal CT scan showed opacification of the left frontal, ethmoidal, and maxillary sinuses.

Figure 5-12D.   Pus from the superior meatus. In the case of acute or chronic sinusitis, the pattern of purulent drainage around the eustachian tube may help to identify the infected sinus. When secretions drain down from the superior meatus and then pass posterior to the torus tubarius as shown in this left nasal cavity, they usually arise from the posterior ethmoid or sphenoid sinuses, indicating infection of these sinuses.

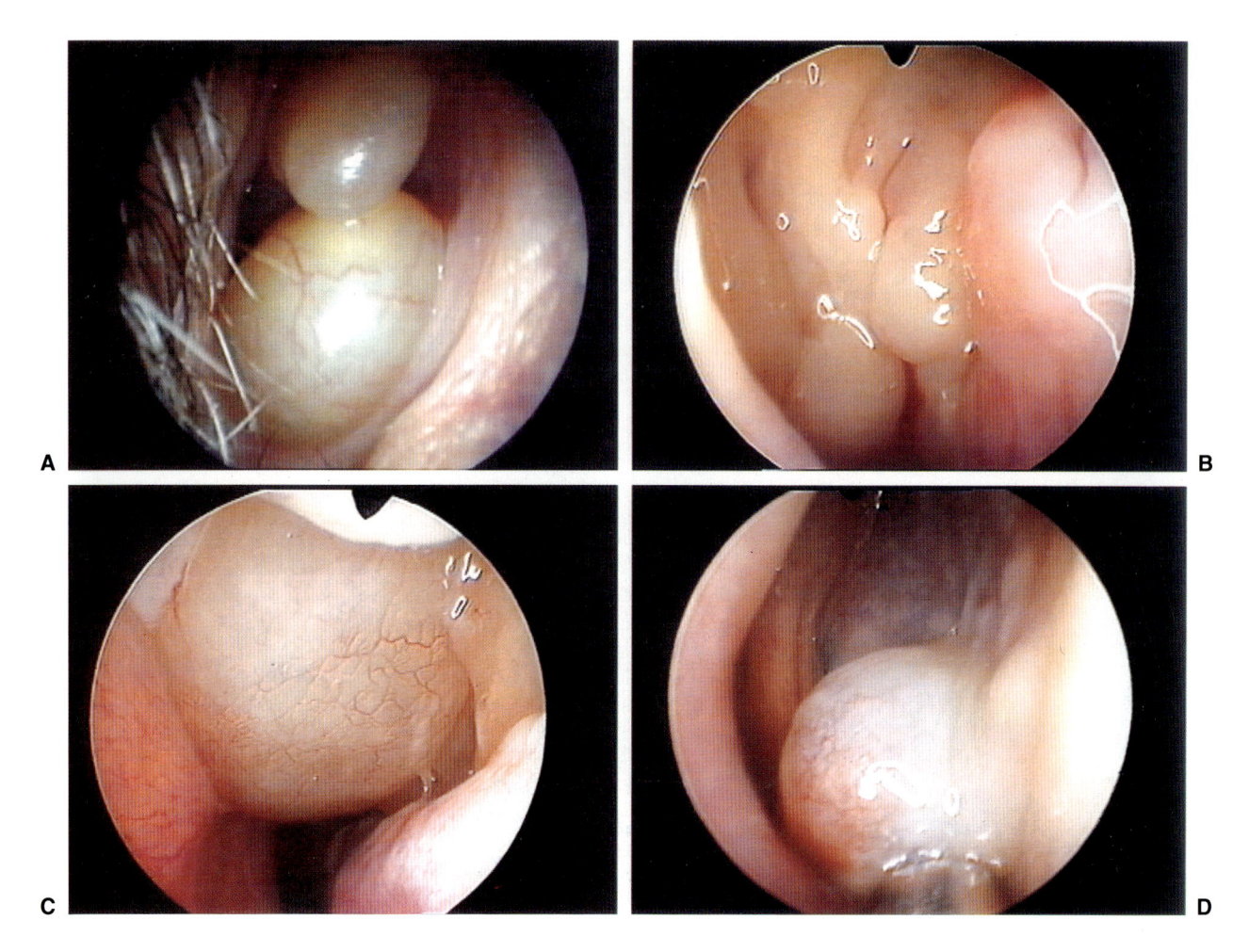

Nasal Polyp

Figure 5-13A. Diffuse nasal polyposis. This patient complained of difficult nasal breathing. Nasal endoscopy reveals obstruction of the right nasal cavity by multiple polyps of varying sizes. Systemic and topical steroids shrunk the polyps to a certain extent. For a lasting relief, the patient required surgical excision of these polyps.

Figure 5-13B. Diffuse nasal polyposis. The 0-degree telescopic view of this patient, who complained of anosmia and difficult nasal breathing, reveals extensive bilateral nasal polyposis. The CT scan revealed opacification of all paranasal sinuses. The patient had only temporaly relief from steroid therapy. His symptoms improved markedly after nasal polypectomy and endoscopic ethmoidectomy. These polyps have a tendency to recur. In patients with recurrent polyps, consider allergic rhinitis, cystic fibrosis, or the aspirin triad (Sampter's triad) as possible etiologies.

Figure 5-13C. Nasal polyp. This large polyp obstructed the superior half of the left nasal cavity. The coronal CT scan showed opacification of the left ethmoid and maxillary sinuses. Polyps were found to originate from the ethmoid sinuses. Polypectomy, anterior ethmoidectomy, and middle meatal antrostomy were carried out with a suction microdébrider. No bleeding was encountered with the use of the microdébrider.

Figure 5-13D. Nasal polyp. The 0-degree telescopic view shows a nasal polyp originating from the posterior superior portion of the nasal septum on the right side. It was in contact with the superior turbinate and a portion of the middle turbinate, obstructing the drainage of the right sphenoid sinus ostium. This polyp was removed with a suction microdébrider.

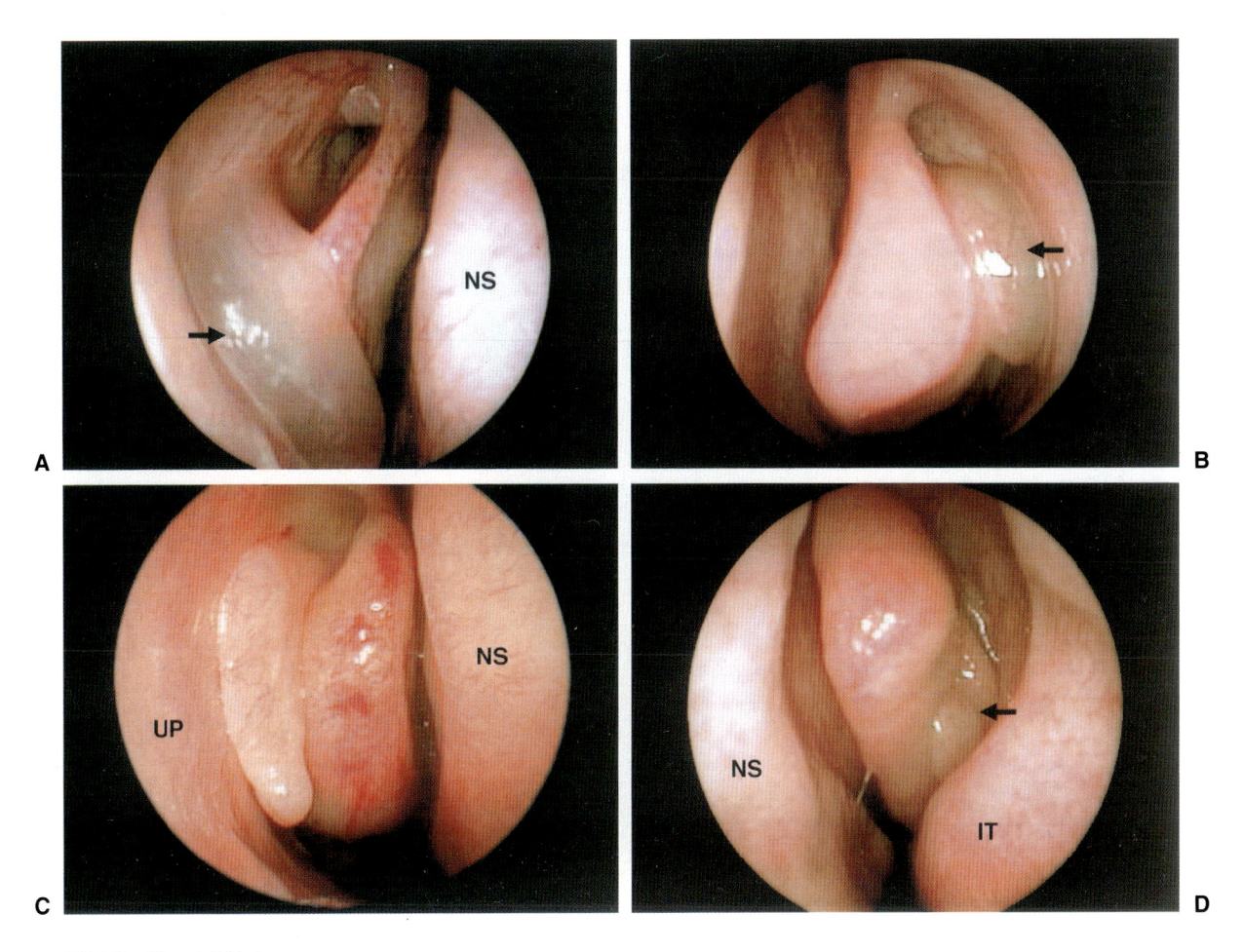

Endoscopy of the Nose (Video Nasal Endoscopy, Videorhinoscopy)

Middle Meatal Polyp

Figure 5-14A. Middle meatal polyp. This patient who previously had a nasal polypectomy and right partial middle turbinectomy developed recurrent right maxillary sinusitis. The 0-degree telescopic examination reveals a medium-sized polyp (*arrow*) with a broad base arising from the right uncinate process. It was endoscopically excised, and a middle meatal antrostomy was performed. No further sinusitis ensued.

Figure 5-14B. Middle meatal polyp. This patient complained of frontal headaches associated with recurrent sinusitis. The 30-degree telescopic examination clearly shows a single polyp (*arrow*) in the left middle meatus arising from the lateral aspect of the midportion of the left middle turbinate. The patient responded well to endoscopic excision with a middle meatal antrostomy and an anterior ethmoidectomy.

Figure 5-14C. Nasal polyp. The 0-degree telescopic view of the right nasal cavity shows a medium-sized middle meatal polyp arising from the ethmoidal bulla. This patient complained of right frontal headaches and recurrent right maxillary sinusitis. An endoscopic excision of this polyp with anterior ethmoidectomy and middle meatal antrostomy markedly improved his symptoms.

Figure 5-14D. Middle meatal polyp. This 0-degree telescopic examination reveals two small polypoid masses (*arrow*) arising from the lateral aspect of the left middle turbinate, obstructing the midportion of the left middle meatus. The coronal CT scan showed complete opacification of the maxillary and ethmoidal sinuses on both sides. This patient responded well to surgical excision of the middle meatal polyps and endoscopic ethmoidectomy and middle meatal antrostomy. Nasal endoscopy plays an important role in the diagnosis of small middle meatal polyps that can produce significant sinus diseases. These polyps can be easily missed by routine anterior rhinoscopy.

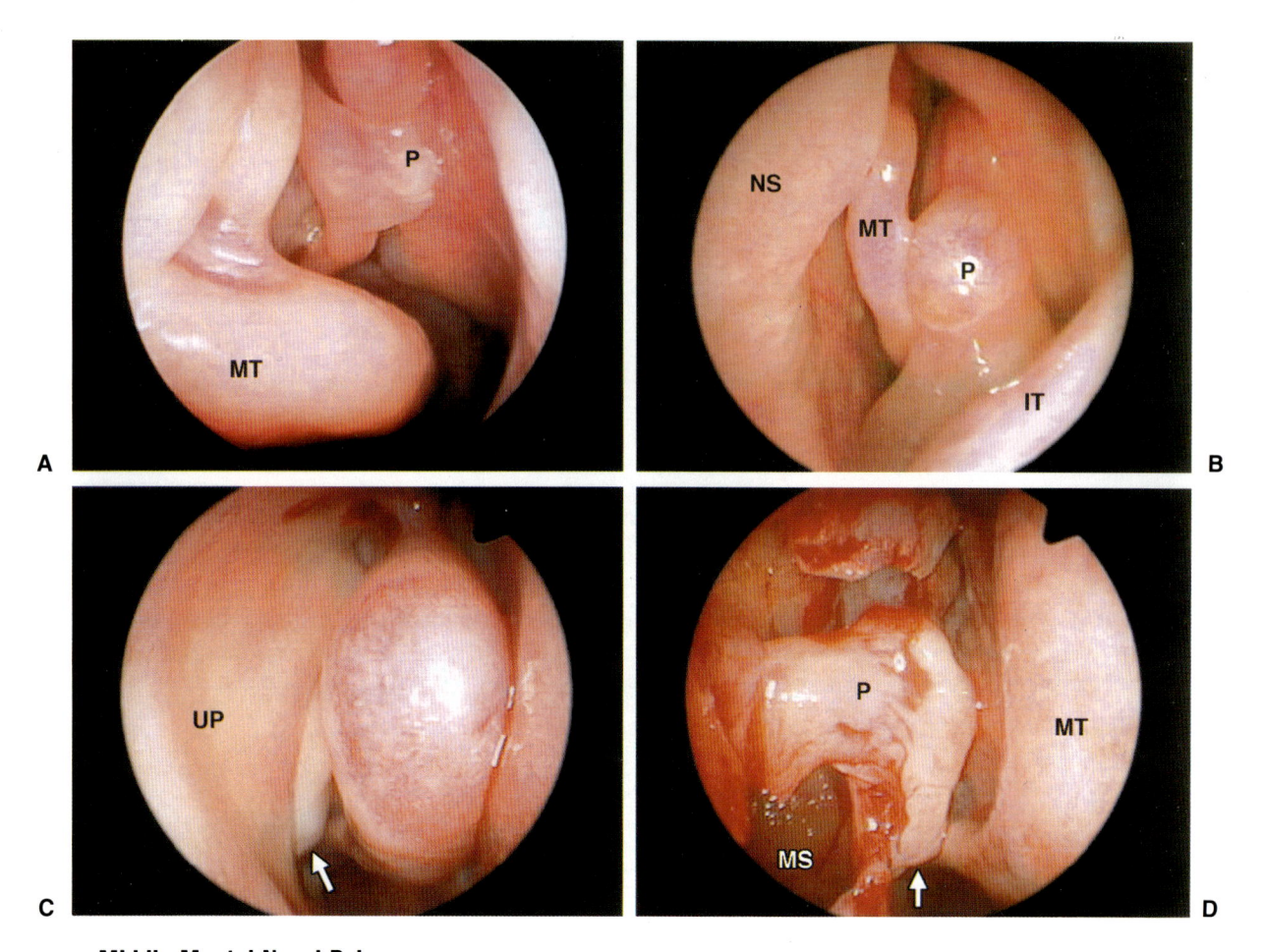

Middle Meatal Nasal Polyp

Figure 5-15A. Middle meatal polyp. The 30-degree nasal telescopic view of the left nasal cavity shows a small polyp (P) in this patient's left middle meatus arising from the hiatus semilunaris. Note the "L-shaped" left middle turbinate (MT).

Figure 5-15B. Middle meatal polyp. This patient complained of recurrent sinusitis and frontal headaches. The 30-degree telescopic examination reveals a medium-sized polyp (P) arising from the anterior surface of the left ethmoid bulla. The patient responded well to endoscopic excision of the polyp and anterior ethmoidectomy.

Figure 5-15C. Antro-middle meatal polyp. The 0-degree telescopic examination of this patient who had recurrent headaches and sinusitis shows a small polypoid lesion (*arrow*) between the posterior margin of the right uncinate process (UP) and the middle turbinate. This lesion obstructed the hiatus semilunaris inferior.

Figure 5-15D. Antro-middle meatal polyp. When the uncinate process of the same patient was endoscopically removed, an antral polyp (P) was found to originate from the roof of the right maxillary sinus (MS) and extend into the middle meatus (*arrow*) via the area of the natural ostium. The antral polyp was excised through the middle meatal antrostomy together with the middle meatal portion of the polyp.

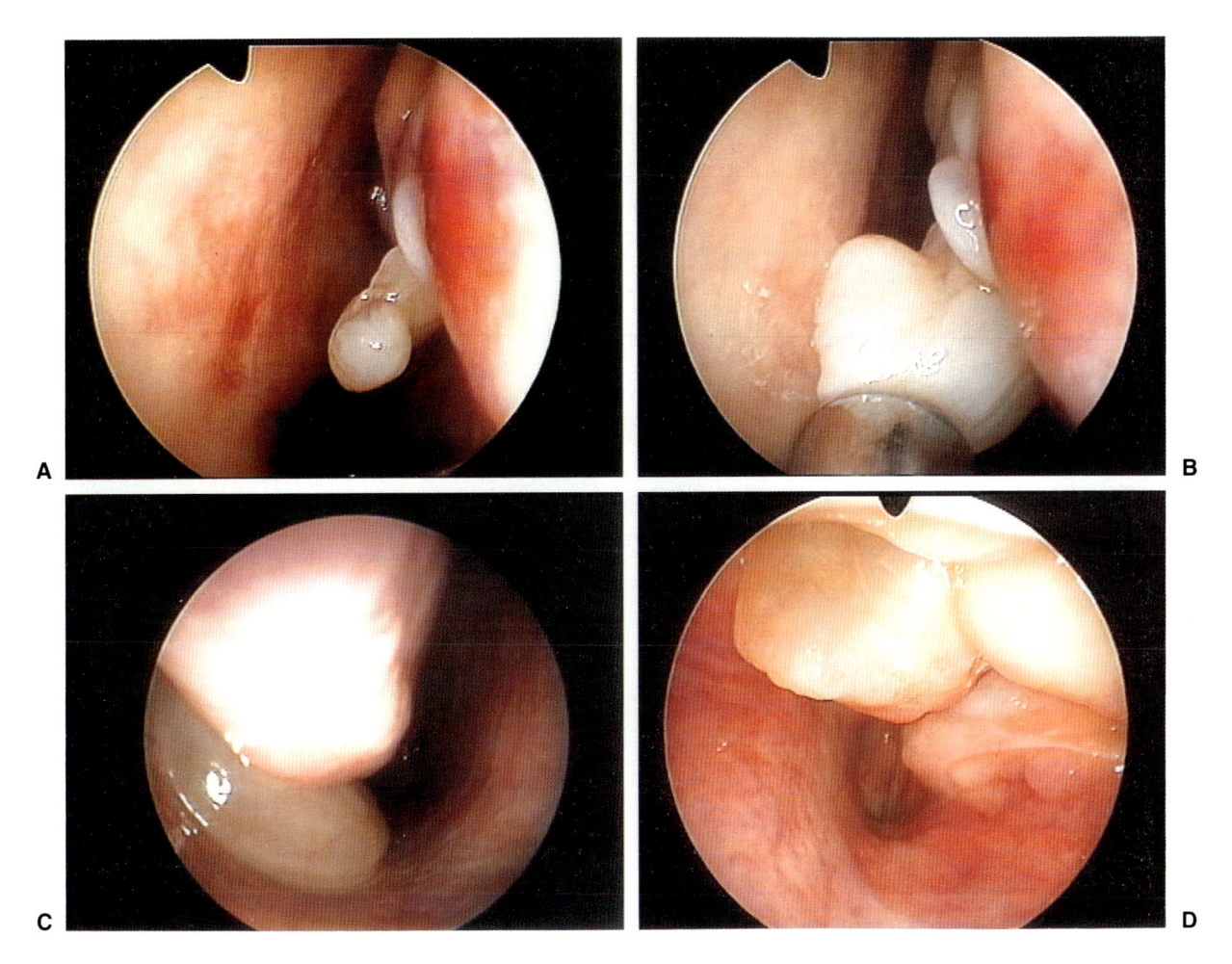

Endoscopy of the Nose (Video Nasal Endoscopy, Videorhinoscopy)

Superior and Inferior Meatal Polyps

Figure 5-16A. Superior meatal polyp. The 0-degree telescopic view demonstrates small polyps arising from the superior portion of the left nasal cavity. These polyps became visible when the suction tip approached the superior nasal cavity.

Figure 5-16B. Superior meatal polyp. Application of the suction tip to the lower portion of the polyp shown in Figure 5-16A unexpectedly exposed several "hidden" polyps from the superior meatus and the sphenoethmoidal recess. Nasal "suction examination" is a useful technique to detect hidden polyps in the nasal cavity. These polyps can be effectively removed by a suction microdébrider or a small upward cutting forceps.

Figure 5-16C. Inferior meatal polyp. The 0-degree telescopic view displays an inferior meatal polyp that originated from the right maxillary sinus via a previously created inferior meatal window.

Figure 5-16D. Inferior meatal polyp. The telescopic view of this patient with diffuse nasal polyposis demonstrates polyps involving the left inferior turbinate and meatus.

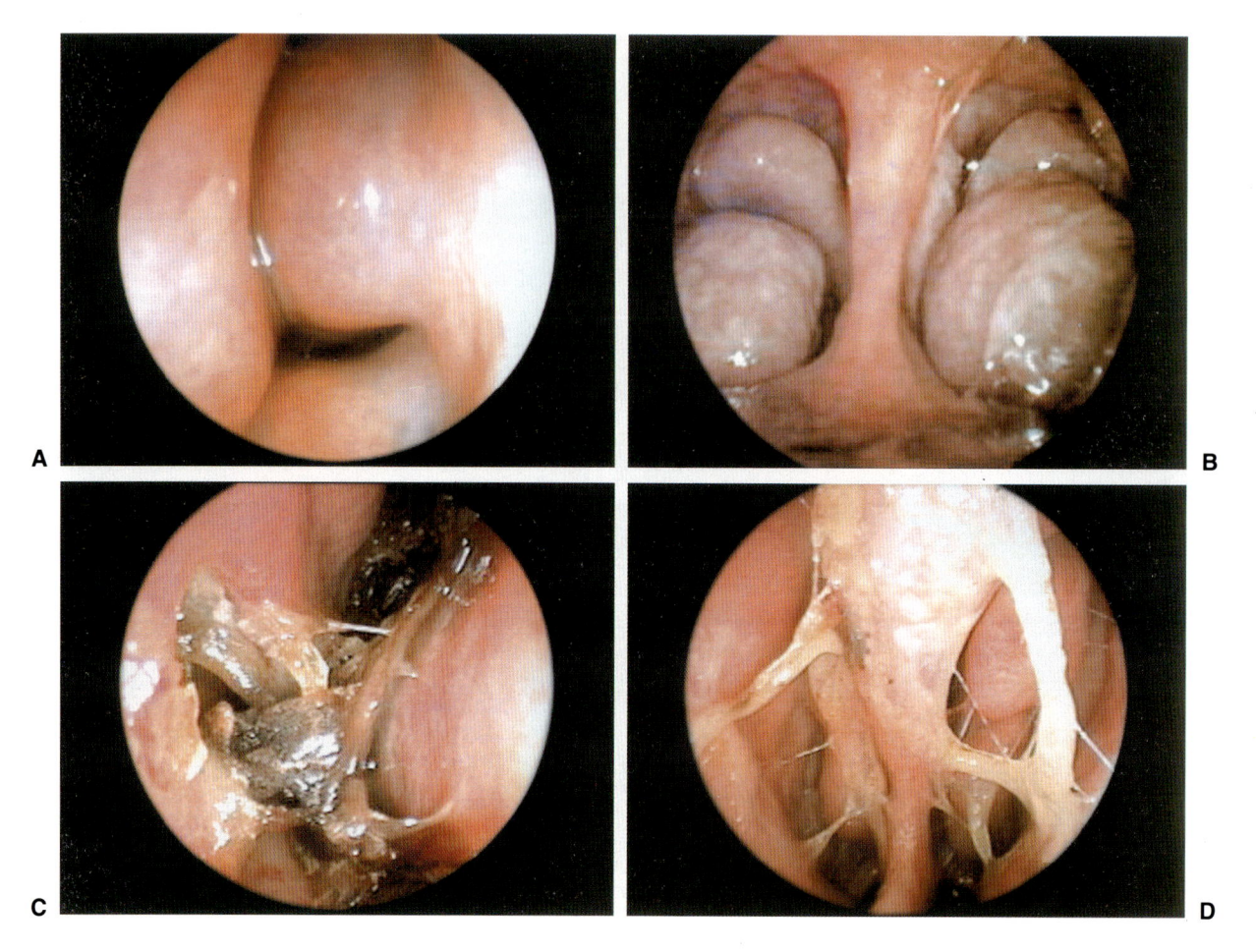

Rhinitis

Figure 5-17A. Allergic rhinitis. This 0-degree telescopic view shows the left inferior turbinate of a patient with allergic rhinitis who suffered from difficult nasal breathing. The inferior turbinate was markedly engorged, pale, and edematous. Clear watery discharge was seen between the turbinate and the nasal septum.

Figure 5-17B. Allergic rhinitis. This patient complained of constant nasal obstruction during allergy season. Transoral 120-degree telescopic examination reveals markedly hypertrophied pale posterior ends of the middle and inferior turbinates on both sides, almost totally obstructing the posterior nasal cavities.

Figure 5-17C. Rhinitis sicca. This patient, who had endoscopic sinus surgery, complained of dryness and difficult nasal breathing. Telescopic examination (0-degree) shows almost complete obstruction of the right nasal cavity with dried crusts. Endoscopic removal of the crusts, topical nasal hydration with nasal spray, and irrigation markedly improved this condition.

Figure 5-17D. Rhinitis sicca. The 0-degree telescopic view shows an example of rhinitis sicca resulting from cocaine use. Note subtotal perforation of the nasal septum with dried crusts.

Endoscopy of the Nose (Video Nasal Endoscopy, Videorhinoscopy)

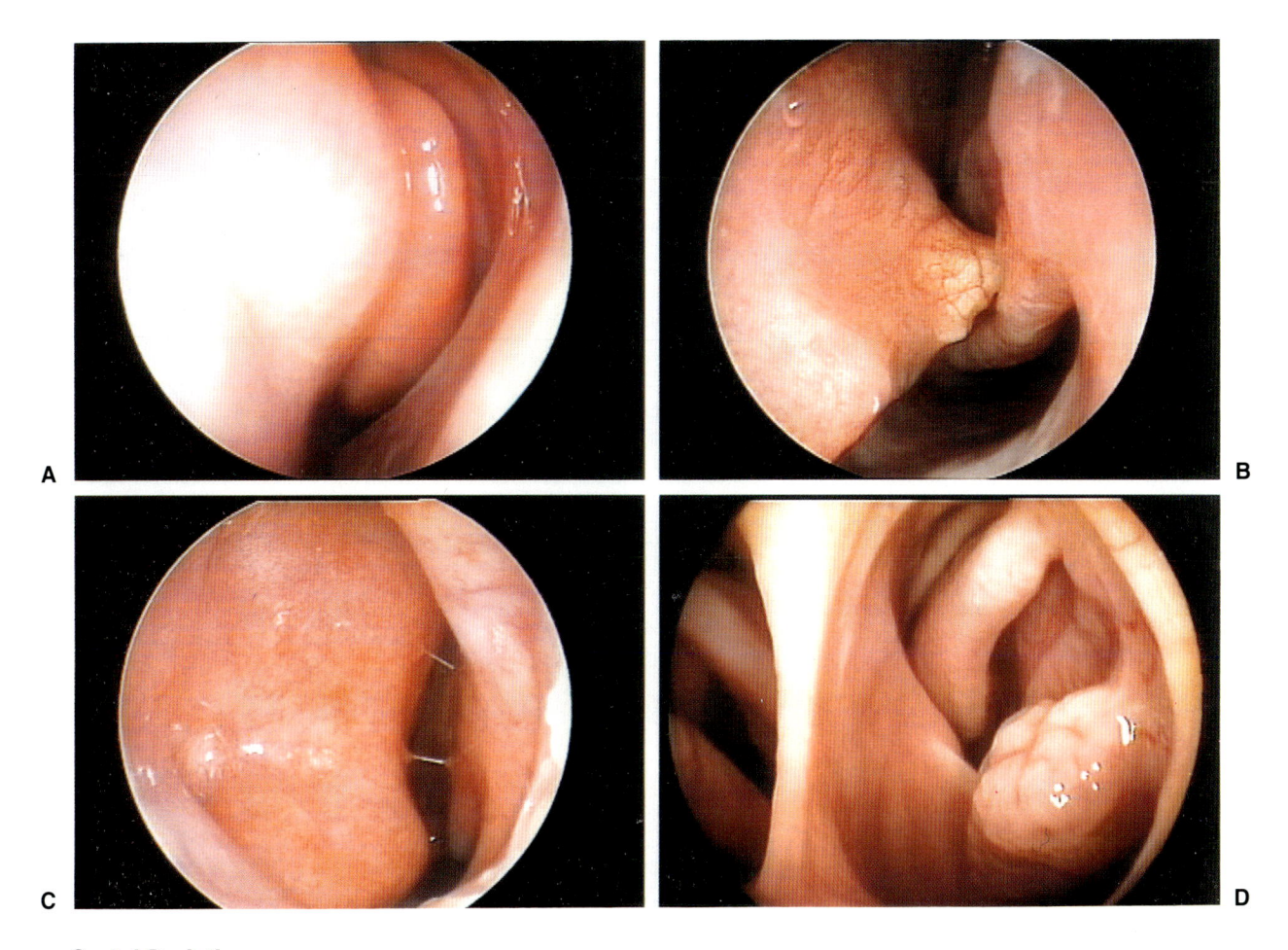

Septal Deviation

Figure 5-18A. Deviated nasal septum. This 0-degree telescopic view shows marked septal deviation toward the left, displacing the left middle turbinate laterally.

Figure 5-18B. Nasal septal spur. This 0-degree telescopic view shows a sharp septal spur projecting into the left inferior turbinate. This patient complained of left-sided facial pain and nasal obstruction. These symptoms disappeared following septoplasty with excision of the spur.

Figure 5-18C. Deviated nasal septum. This 0-degree telescopic view shows an almost total obstruction of the left nasal cavity by a markedly deviated septum.

Figure 5-18D. Posterior septal spur. This patient complained of difficult nasal breathing during allergy season or an upper respiratory infection. Transnasal telescopy (not shown) revealed deviation of the anterior nasal septum toward the left, obscuring the posterior nasal cavity. This 90-degree transoral retrograde telescopic nasopharyngoscopy shows a posterior septal spur on the left side in direct contact with the left inferior turbinate with mulberry hypertrophy.

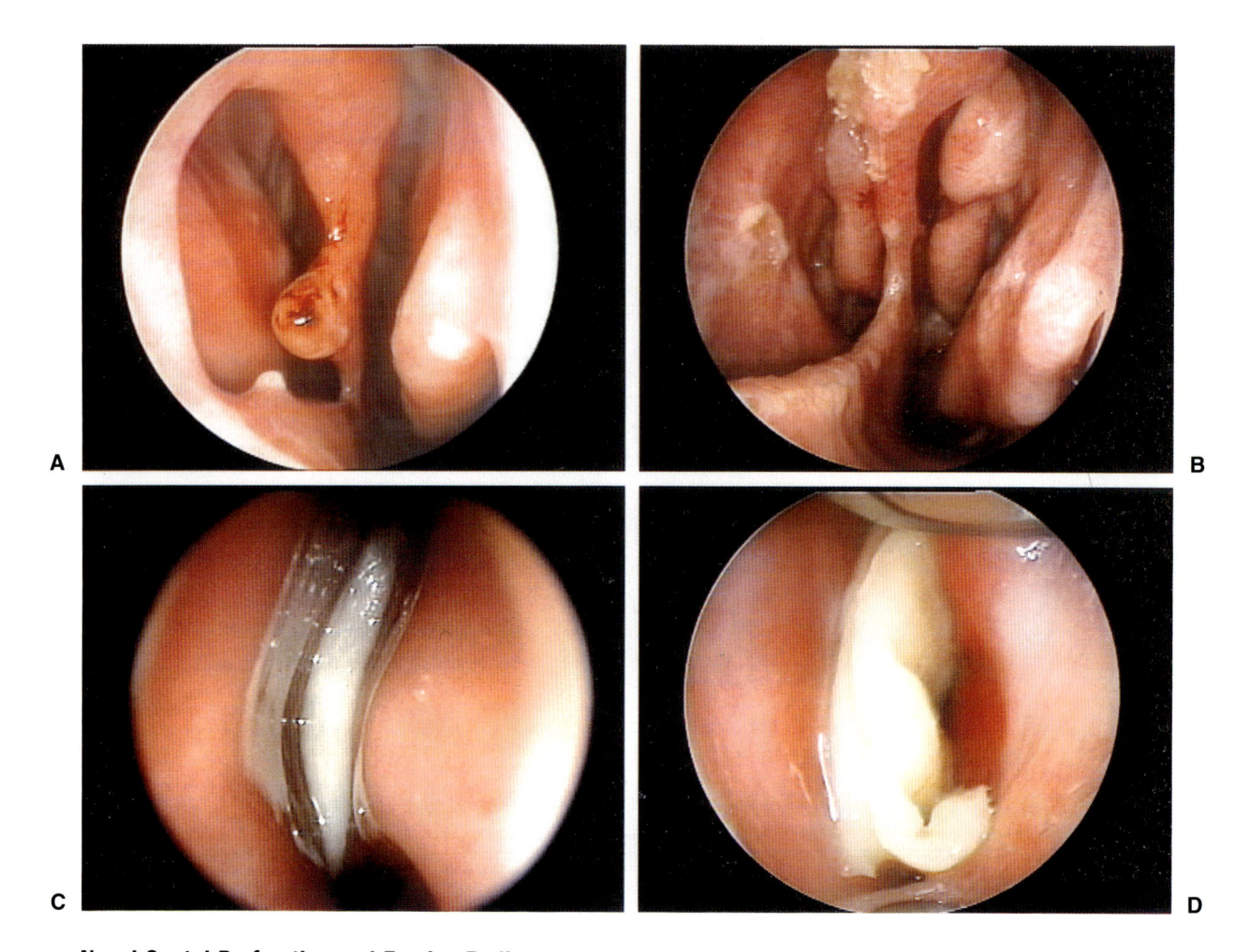

Nasal Septal Perforation and Foreign Bodies

Figure 5-19A. Nasal septal perforation. This 0-degree telescopic view shows a subtotal perforation of the nasal septum with a granuloma on the posterior edge of the perforation.

Figure 5-19B. Septal perforation. This 0-degree left nasal telescopy demonstrates a nearly total perforation of the nasal septum of this patient who complained of "difficult nasal breathing."

Figure 5-19C. Foreign body. This 4-year-old boy had a one-month history of left-sided malodorous rhinorrhea and intermittent anterior epistaxis. Anterior rhinoscopy revealed marked bilateral inferior turbinate hypertrophy. Sinus x-ray showed a left maxillary sinus air-fluid level. Nasal endoscopy (0-degree 4-mm) after the nose was sprayed with topical decongestant and anesthetics reveals a foreign body (sponge) in the midportion of the left nasal cavity. The foreign body was removed and the patient became asymptomatic. A nasal foreign body should always be considered when unilateral foul smelling rhinorrhea persists. In order to make a correct diagnosis of a foreign body, decongesting the turbinates is essential.

Figure 5-19D. Foreign body. This patient, who had removal of nasal packing one week after the endoscopic nasal surgery, complained of a left-sided foul smelling discharge and difficult nasal breathing. Nasal endoscopy after shrinkage of the inflamed inferior turbinate reveals an obvious foreign body obstructing the left nasal cavity. It was a portion of the nasal packing (Telfa sheet) placed in the middle meatus to prevent postoperative synechiae. The patient became symptom free following removal of this foreign body.

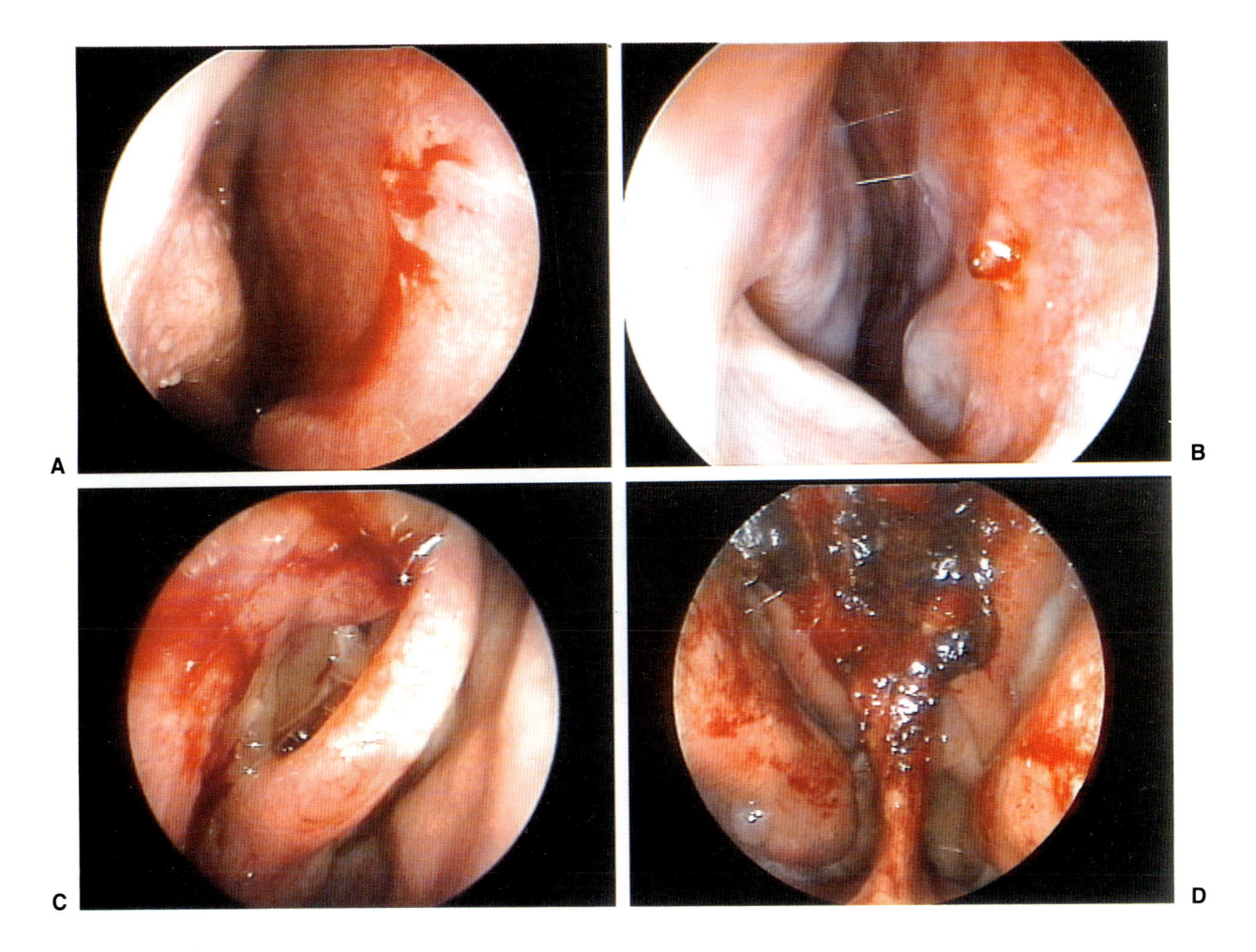

Endoscopy of the Nose (Video Nasal Endoscopy, Videorhinoscopy)

Epistaxis

Figure 5-20A. Anterior epistaxis. The most frequent site of epistaxis is from the anterior nasal septum (Kiesselbach's plexus). This 0-degree nasal telescopic examination reveals active bleeding from Kiesselbach's plexus on the right nasal septum. It was controlled by silver nitrate cautery and packing.

Figure 5-20B. Anterior epistaxis. This patient had recurrent epistaxis from the right side of the nose. Nasal endoscopy shows a fresh blood clot in the area of the right Kiesselbach's plexus. Active bleeding started when this was touched with an instrument and was controlled with electrocautery.

Figure 5-20C. Anterior ethmoidal epistaxis. This patient who had endoscopic anterior ethmoidectomy experienced repeated postoperative epistaxis from the right side. This endoscopic view shows active bleeding from the superior medial portion of the right middle meatus just medial to the superior attachment of the remaining middle turbinate. This was controlled by electrocautery followed by selective anterior packing.

Figure 5-20D. Osler–Weber–Rendu disease. This patient had recurrent epistaxis for many years from both sides of the nasal cavities and underwent multiple surgical procedures including repeated electrocautery to the nasal septum, septodermoplasty, and anterior ethmoidal and internal maxillary artery ligations. The 0-degree telescopy shows near-total absence of the nasal septum with recent blood clots in the superior portion of the posterior edge of the septal perforation. This patient also bled from the middle turbinate. She was treated with both CO_2 and Yag laser with only a temporary control. Repeated anterior and posterior packings were necessary.

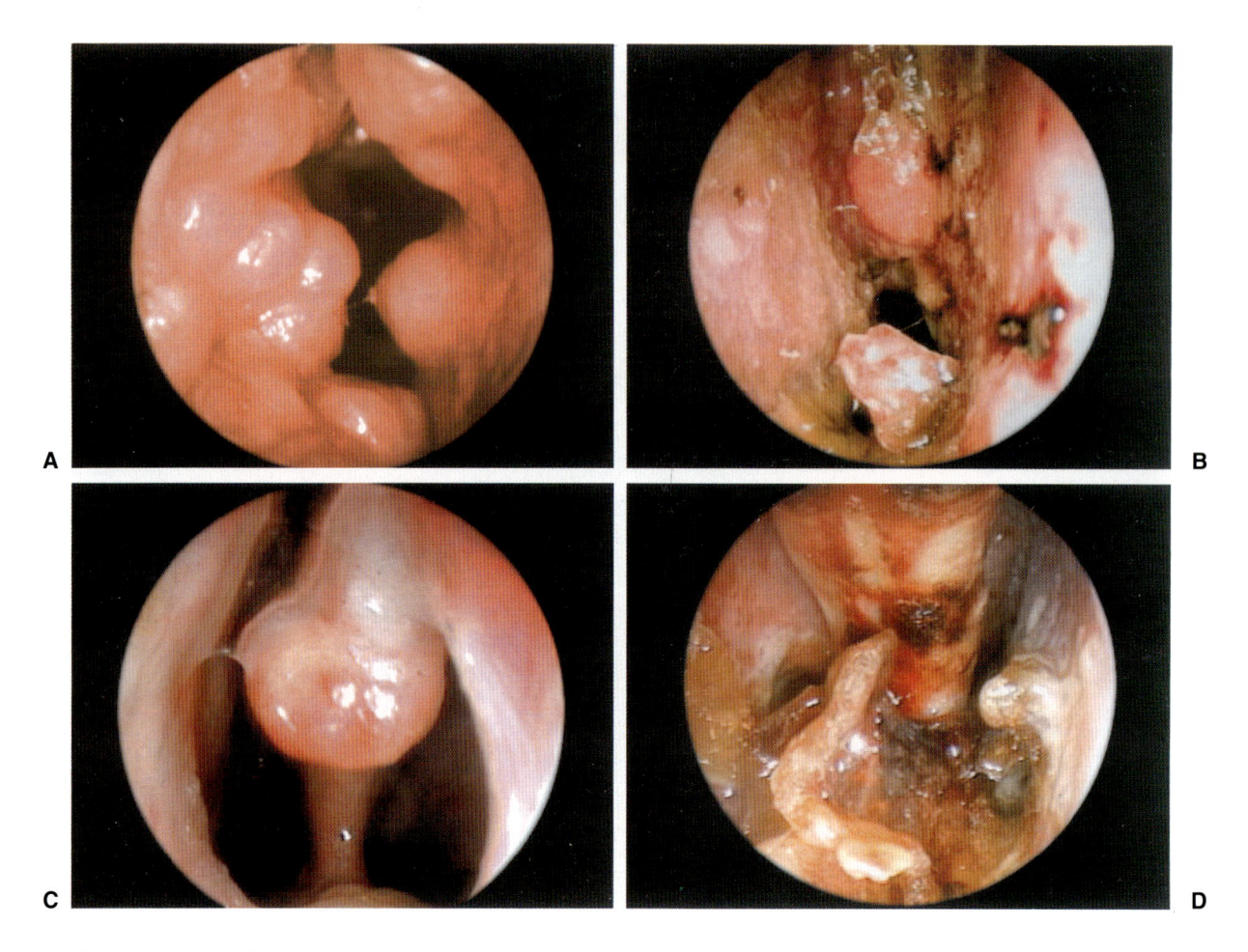

Granulomatous Disease

Figure 5-21A. Nasal sarcoidosis. Sarcoidosis is a granulomatous disease involving the upper and lower respiratory tracts, including the nasal cavity. Here the 0-degree telescopic examination of the right nasal cavity reveals nodular masses arising from the right inferior turbinate and the nasal septum. Biopsy confirmed the diagnosis of sarcoidosis. This patient also had pulmonary sarcoidosis.

Figure 5-21B. Nasal sarcoidosis. This patient complained of bilateral nasal obstruction associated with crusting and recurrent sinusitis. Nasal endoscopy of the right nasal cavity shows multiple granulomatous lesions arising from the nasal septum, the floor of the nose, and the middle turbinate. There was an excessive amount of dried crusts. Repeated removal of crusts, steroid nasal spray, and antibiotic treatments provided symptomatic relief.

Figure 5-21C. Granuloma of the nasal septum. The 0-degree nasal telescopy displays a large granuloma on the superior portion of a septal perforation. This was an inflammatory granuloma and responded well to electrocautery excision and antibiotics.

Figure 5-21D. Cocaine rhinitis. This patient, who gave a history of cocaine use for many years, complained of difficult nasal breathing and recurrent sinus infections. The 0-degree nasal endoscopy reveals almost total absence of the nasal septum and almost total obstruction of the posterior nasal cavity on both sides with crusts and purulent material. Symptomatic relief was obtained by repeated mechanical cleaning, antibiotics, nasal irrigation, and topical steroid nasal sprays.

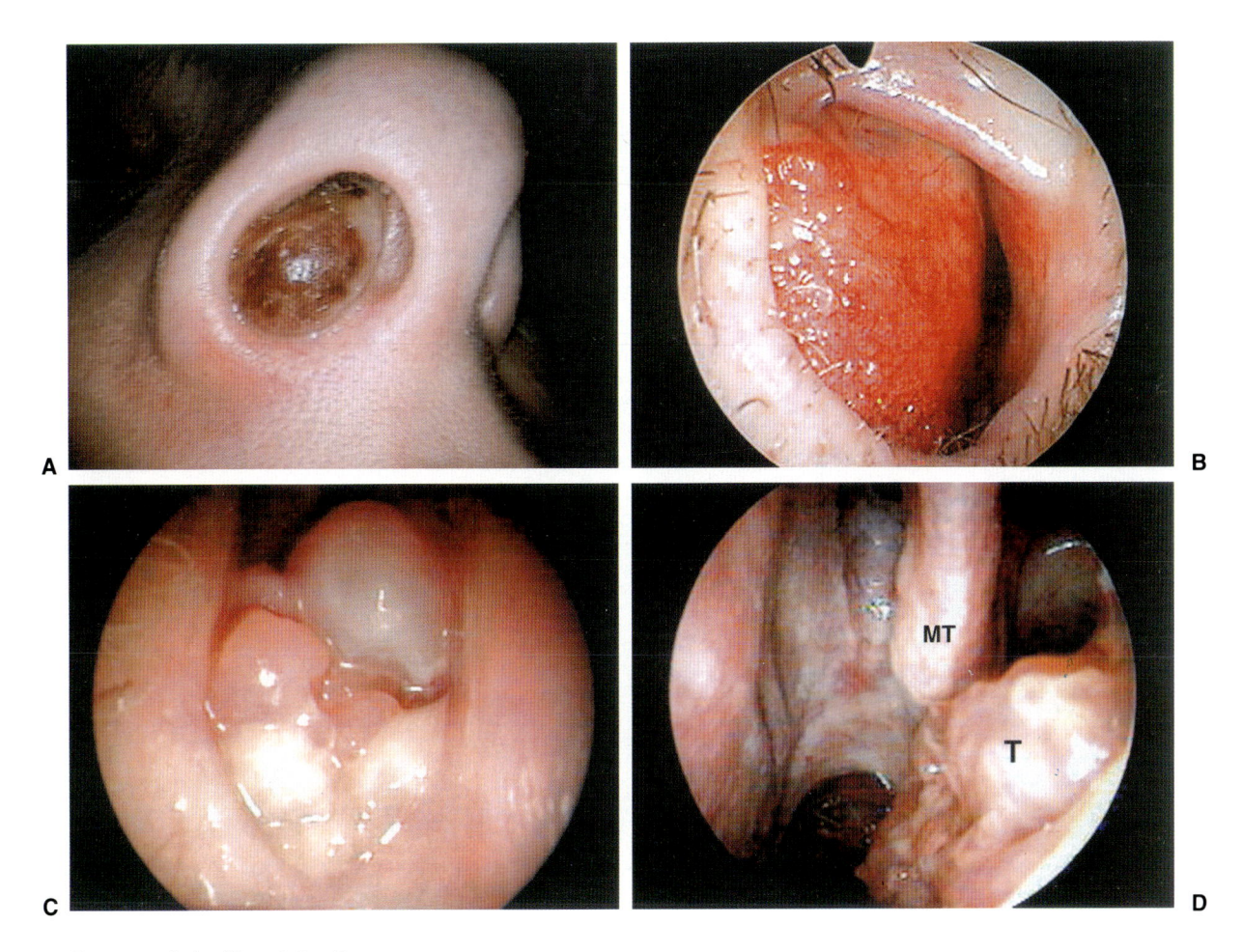

Endoscopy of the Nose (Video Nasal Endoscopy, Videorhinoscopy)

Tumors of the Nasal Cavity

Figure 5-22A. Hemangioma of the nasal septum. This vascular tumor arising from the anterior inferior portion of the right nasal septum was cured with electrocautery excision.

Figure 5-22B. Papilloma of the nasal septum. This papilloma involving the deviated portion of the anterior nasal septum on the left side was excised together with a cartilaginous portion of the nasal septum.

Figure 5-22C. Inverting papilloma of the nasal cavity. This patient complained of nasal obstruction on the right side. Nasal endoscopy reveals multiple polyps of different sizes completely obstructing the right nasal cavity. Biopsy showed inverting papilloma. Treatment consisted of endoscopic excision of the intranasal tumors and lateral rhinotomy with excision of the medial wall of the right maxillary sinus.

Figure 5-22D. Inverting papilloma of the nasal cavity. This patient developed a recurrent lateral wall inverting papilloma after an endoscopic excision of the inverting papilloma. The 30-degree telescopy reveals recurrent tumor (T) involving the lateral wall of the nasal cavity between the middle turbinate (MT) and the inferior turbinate. This patient was successfully treated with a lateral rhinotomy and excision of the lateral wall of the left nasal cavity.

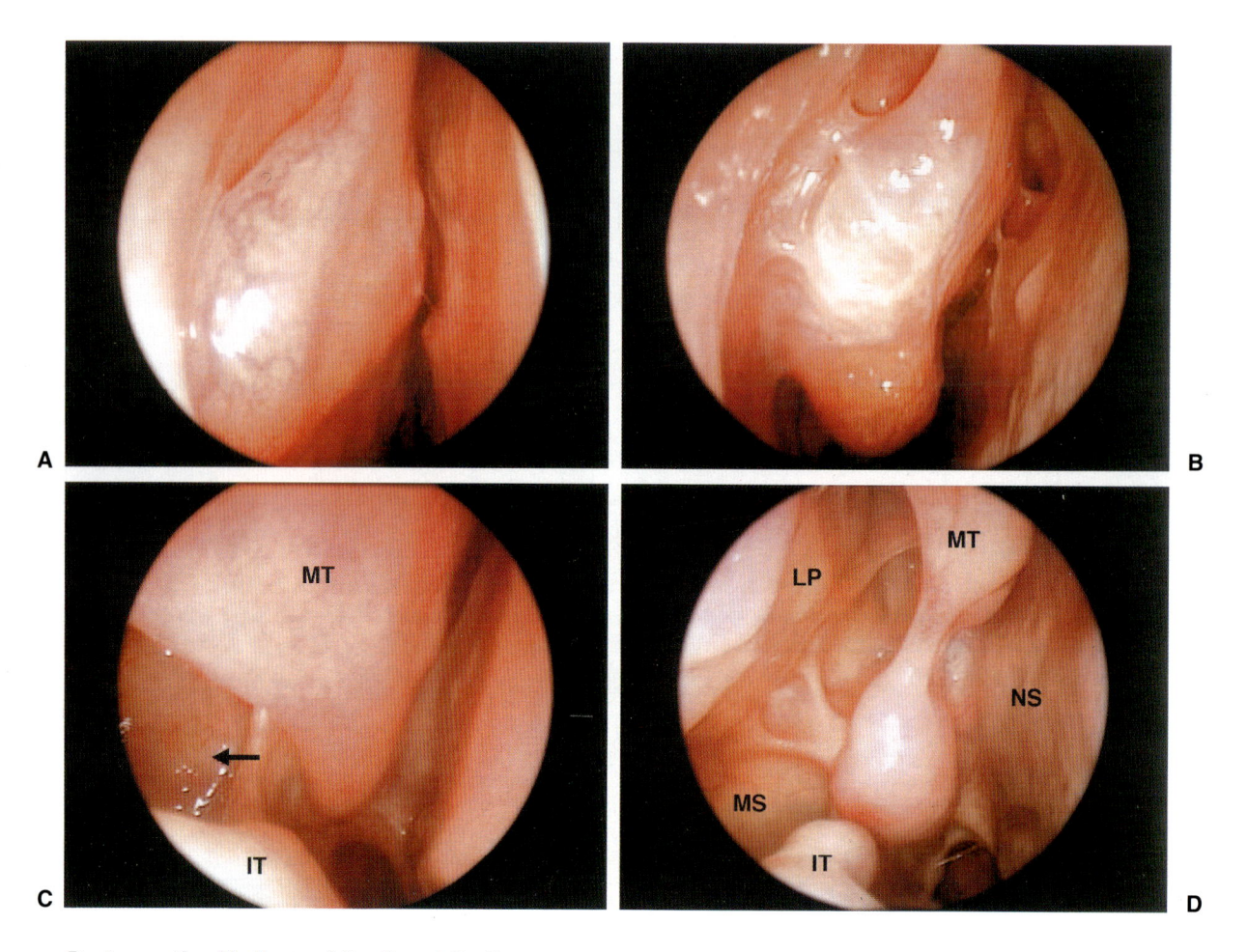

Postoperative Findings of the Nasal Cavity

Figure 5-23A. Postoperative synechiae. Most intranasal synechiae develop following surgery. In this case the inferior lateral portion of the right middle turbinate adhered to the lateral wall of the nose. However, this patient was asymptomatic because the synechia involved only the anterior portion of the middle turbinate and no treatment was required.

Figure 5-23B. Postoperative synechiae. More extensive synechiae between the lateral aspect of the right middle turbinate and the lateral wall of the nose is seen here following endoscopic sinus surgery. The middle meatal window created at the initial surgery was completely closed. This patient developed recurrent sinusitis with headaches. Revision surgery included endoscopic separation of the synechiae, middle meatal antrostomy, and insertion of a Silastic sheet between the middle turbinate and the lateral nasal wall. The anterior end of the Silastic sheet was sutured to the nasal septum and removed 6 weeks later.

Figure 5-23C. Middle meatal antrostomy. A patient's well-healed middle meatal antrostomy opening is seen (*arrow*) between the inferior and middle turbinate on the right side.

Figure 5-23D. Postoperative ethmoidectomy cavity. This picture displays a well-healed postoperative ethmoidectomy cavity. The lamina papyracea (LP) is seen laterally, remnants of the middle turbinate (MT) are viewed in the middle, the nasal septum (NS) is located medially, and the maxillary sinus (MS) is seen inferolaterally. Note the upper border of the inferior turbinate (IT) is also seen.

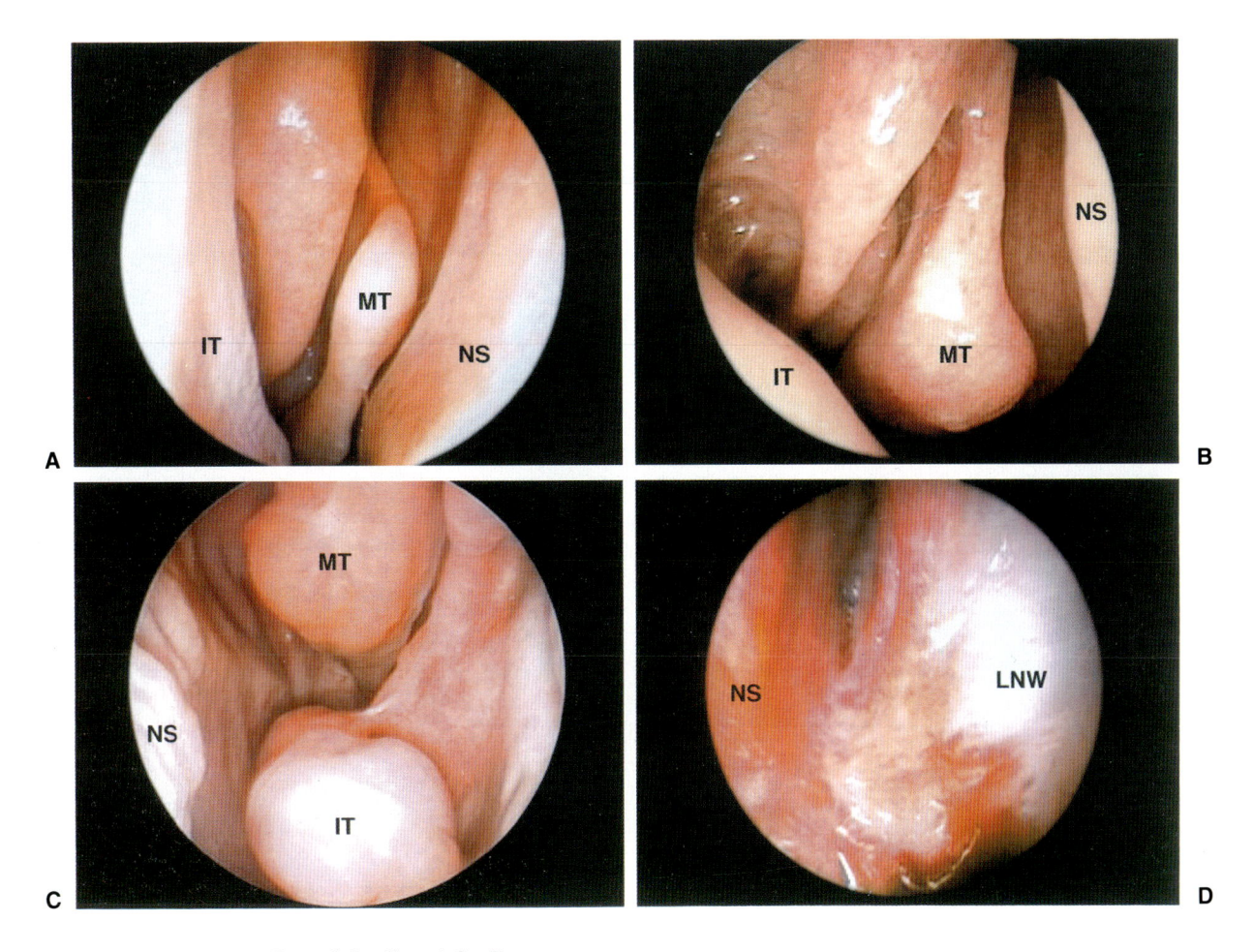

Endoscopy of the Nose (Video Nasal Endoscopy, Videorhinoscopy)

Congenital Anomalies of the Nasal Cavity

Figure 5-24A. Medially bent large uncinate process. A large, prominent, medially bent right uncinate process is seen between the inferior turbinate (IT) and the medially displaced small middle turbinate (MT). The nasal septum (NS) is seen medial to the right middle turbinate.

Figure 5-24B. Medially bent uncinate process. This medially bent right uncinate process may be interpreted as a "double" or "clefted" middle turbinate. The patient was asymptomatic and required no treatment.

Figure 5-24C. Deformed inferior turbinate. This abnormal left inferior turbinate (IT) arose from a broad bony projection of the lateral nasal wall, leaving only a slit-like middle meatus. The anterior portion of this left middle turbinate was abnormally enlarged. This patient was asymptomatic.

Figure 5-24D. Choanal atresia. The 0-degree telescopic examination of the left nasal cavity shows a complete closure of the left posterior choana.

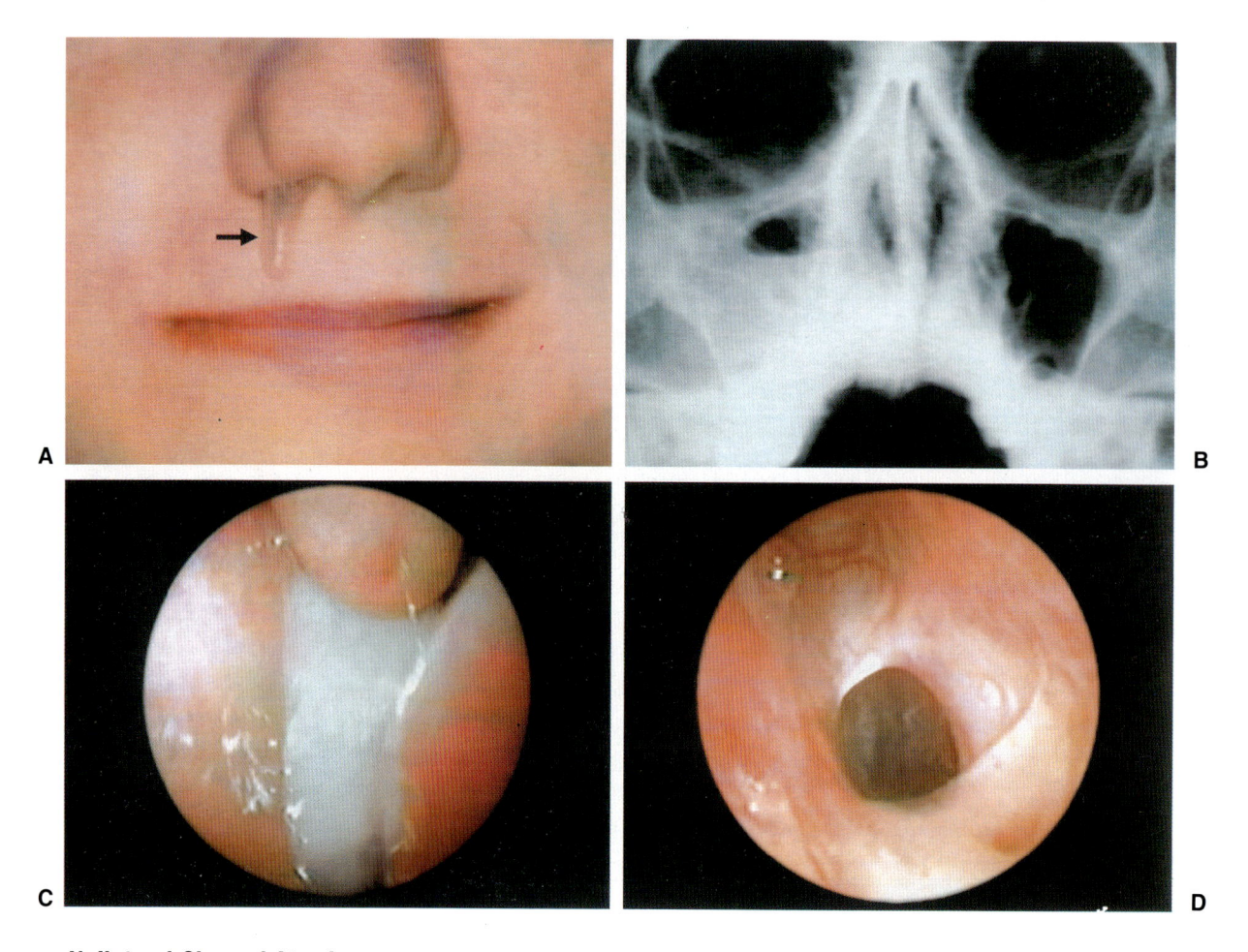

Unilateral Choanal Atresia

Figure 5-25A. Unilateral Choanal atresia. This 17-year-old female complained of recurrent right-sided purulent uncontrollable rhinorrhea (*arrow*) and difficult nasal breathing associated with persistent right-sided maxillary sinusitis and serous otitis media. She was unable to blow out nasal secretions or to draw them back into the nasopharynx.

Figure 5-25B. Unilateral choanal atresia with sinusitis. The Waters' view of this patient's sinuses shows right maxillary sinusitis with an air-fluid level.

Figure 5-25C. Choanal atresia. Anterior rhinoscopy reveals purulent discharge filling the right posterior nasal cavity. A right nasal antrostomy was carried out. While irrigating the right nasal cavity it was noted that the solution did not drain down to the pharynx. A flexible catheter could not be passed to the nasopharynx. Closer microscopic examination reveals complete bony atresia of the right choana. The atresia plate was removed. A plastic stent was placed in the reconstructed choana and was removed 6 weeks postoperatively.

Figure 5-25D. Postoperative choanal atresia. Twenty years later the patient continued to be free of nasal symptoms. The 0-degree telescopy reveals a patent right posterior choana. Unilateral choanal atresia (two-thirds are unilateral, one-third is bilateral) should be suspected in the presence of uncontrollable unilateral nasal discharge, persistent unilateral sinusitis, and serous otitis media resistant to medical treatment. The diagnosis can be confirmed with nasal endoscopy, CT, or contrast x-ray study.

Chapter 6

Endoscopy of the Paranasal Sinuses (Videosinoscopy)

Sinoscopy is the examination of the interior of paranasal sinuses and their ostia with a rigid telescope through external or intranasal approaches. When sinoscopic findings are documented with a video camera, the procedure is called *videosinoscopy*.

Videosinoscopy is a valuable method of examining and documenting anatomy and pathology of the paranasal sinuses. Some of the important structures seen on sinoscopy include (a) natural and accessory ostia as well as surgical ostia created to improve drainage, (b) sinus mucosa, and (c) intrasinus neurovascular structures (infraorbital nerve in maxillary sinus; optic nerve and carotid artery in sphenoid sinus). A variety of pathologic conditions as well as mucociliary movement within the sinuses are also well seen on videosinoscopy.

The maxillary sinuses can be visualized through external (canine fossa) or intranasal approaches (inferior or middle meatal antrostomy), and the frontal sinus can be seen through external (Lynch approach) and intranasal (trans-middle meatal) approaches. The ethmoid and sphenoid sinuses can be seen endoscopically via intranasal approaches only after these sinuses are opened surgically.

The sinoscopy of the sphenoid sinus can also be performed by passing a long trocar and a 4-mm telescope through its anterior wall, but it should be done only by an experienced endoscopic sinus surgeon. There is a significant risk of injury to the optic nerve and carotid artery, which lie in the lateral wall of the sphenoid sinus. Do not touch the lateral wall of this sinus!

Equipment required for sinoscopy includes: (1) 4-mm 0-, 30-, 70-, and 120-degree nasal telescopes, (2) light source, (3) bone drill with 4 to 5-mm bit, (4) trocars (Karl Storz 8.5-cm × O.D. 5-mm for 4-mm telescope for maxillary sinus and 11-cm × O.D. 5-mm for sphenoid sinus), and (5) topical and injectable local anesthetics and decongestant. Videosinoscopy also requires (1) a video camera, (2) a video recorder, (3) a video monitor, and (4) a video printer.

Sinoscopy is most valuable for evaluation of the maxillary sinus, where it is relatively easy to obtain views through both external and intranasal approaches. Intranasal sinoscopy is also particularly useful for postoperative evaluations of the interior of sinuses.

In this chapter, not only sinoscopic views of the paranasal sinuses, but also intranasal telescopic views of the anatomy and pathology of natural and accessory ostia of the sinuses, will be shown.

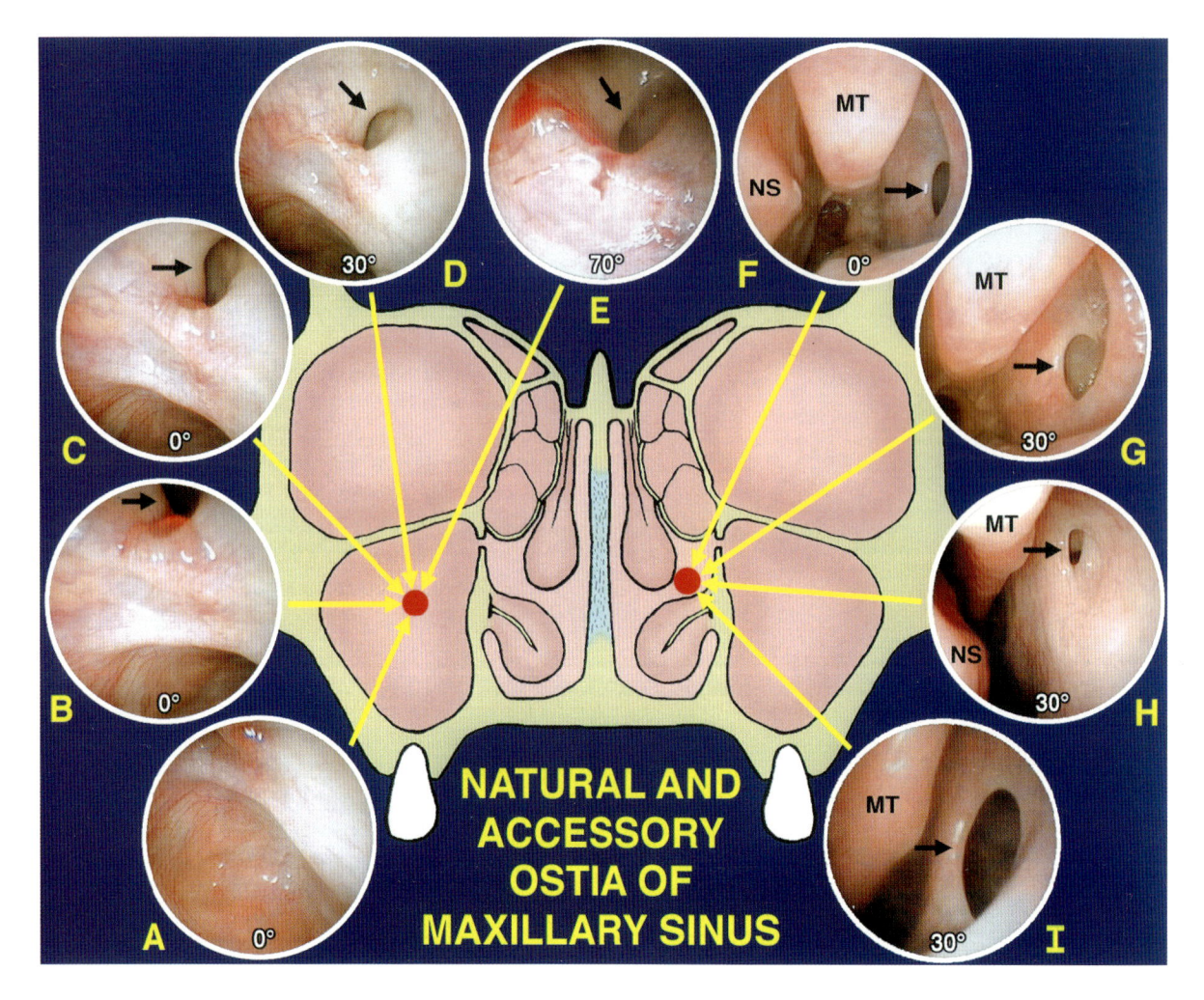

OVERVIEW OF PARANASAL SINUS ANATOMY

Natural and Accessory Ostia of the Maxillary Sinus

Figure 6-1A. Maxillary sinoscopy. This 0-degree sinoscopic view of the right maxillary sinus via the canine fossa demonstrates the posterior superior medial aspect of this normal antrum.

Figure 6-1B. Maxillary sinoscopic view of the right natural ostium. As the 0-degree telescope is advanced superiorly, the natural ostium comes into view (*arrow*). Note the flow of clear mucus to the natural ostium by ciliary action.

Figure 6-1C. Maxillary sinoscopic view of the right natural ostium. Further upward advancement of the 0-degree telescope clearly reveals the natural ostium (*arrow*).

Figure 6-1D. Maxillary sinoscopic view of the natural ostium. The 30-degree sinoscopic view of the same sinus via the canine fossa fully displays the natural ostium (*arrow*).

Figure 6-1E. Maxillary sinoscopic view of the right natural ostium. The natural ostium is seen in the same maxillary sinus viewed with the 70-degree telescope via the canine fossa.

Figure 6-1F. Nasal telescopic view of accessory ostium of the left maxillary sinus. The 0-degree nasal telescopy demonstrates a normal accessory ostium of the left maxillary sinus (*arrow*). This view also displays the inferior aspect of the middle turbinate (MT) and meatus, the superior aspect of the inferior turbinate, and a septal spur on the nasal septum (NS).

Figure 6-1G. Accessory ostium. The 30-degree nasal telescope gives a closer view of the same left accessory ostium as shown in Figure 6-1F (*arrow*) in the inferior aspect of the left middle meatus.

Figure 6-1H. Accessory ostium. Another 30-degree telescopic view demonstrates the accessory ostium of the left maxillary sinus (*arrow*) from below.

Figure 6-1I. Accessory ostium. The 30-degree nasal telescopy gives a full view of this large left accessory ostium (*arrow*).

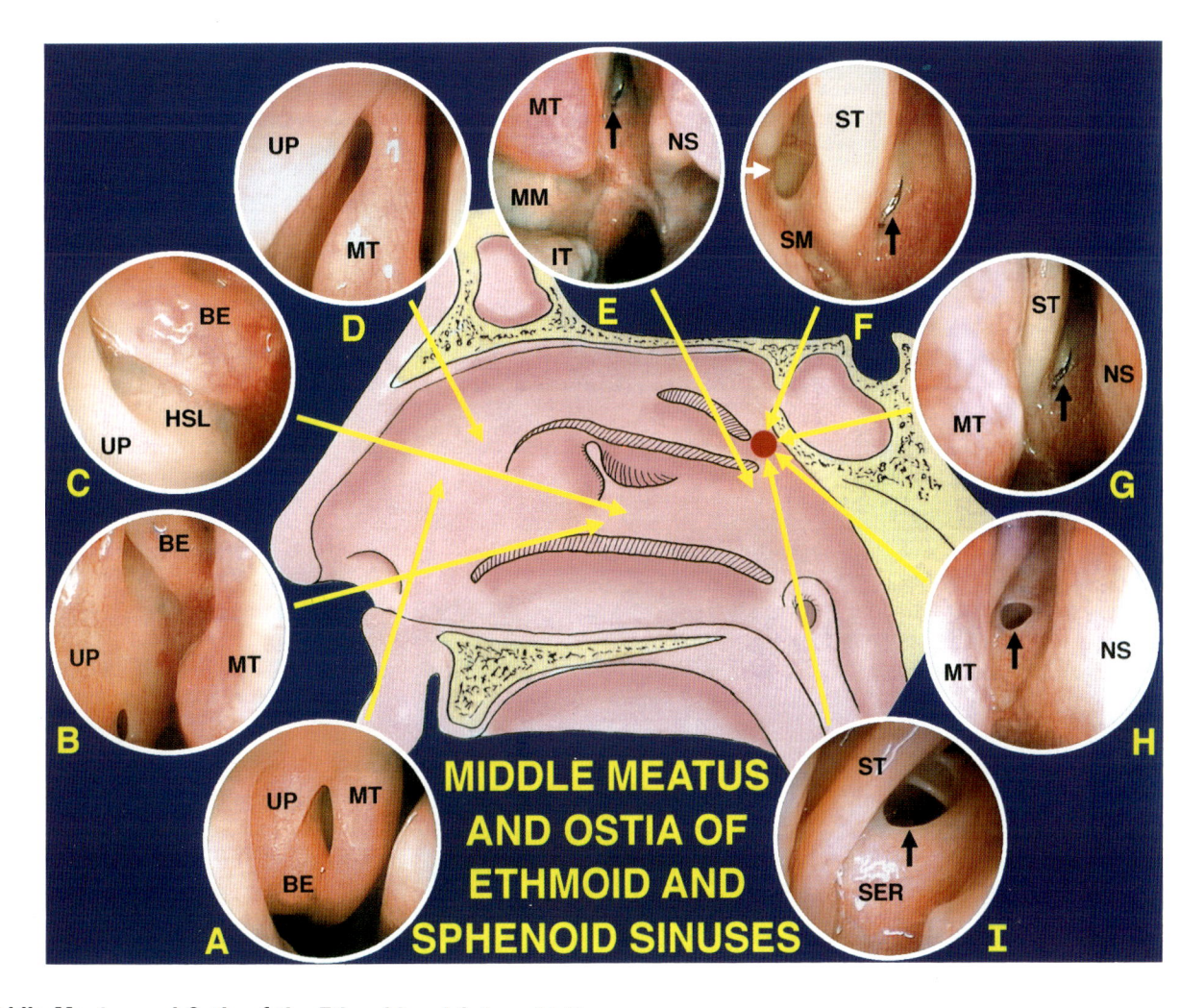

Middle Meatus and Ostia of the Ethmoid and Sphenoid Sinuses

Figure 6-2A. Middle meatus. The 0-degree nasal telescope views the right middle turbinate (MT) and meatus. Clearly seen in the middle meatus are the uncinate process (UP) and the ethmoid bulla, also called the bulla ethmoidalis (BE).

Figure 6-2B. Middle meatus. The 0-degree nasal telescope is advanced into the right middle meatus yielding a closer view of the middle turbinate (MT), uncinate process (UP), and ethmoid bulla (BE). Also seen on this view are an accessory ostium of the right maxillary sinus (*bottom left of view*) and the bottom of the hiatus semilunaris inferior (*upper left of view*).

Figure 6-2C. Middle meatus. Further advancement of the 0-degree nasal telescope demonstrates the right hiatus semilunaris inferior (HSL) lying between the uncinate process (UP) and the ethmoid bulla (BE).

Figure 6-2D. Middle turbinate. The uncinate process (UP) meets the anterior base of the right middle turbinate (MT) on this 0-degree nasal telescopic view.

Figure 6-2E. Sphenoethmoidal recess. The sphenoethmoidal recess lies behind the superior turbinate. The sphenoid sinus ostium (*arrow*) lies in this recess medial to the superior turbinate. In this panoramic 0-degree telescopic view of the posterior right nasal cavity, one clearly sees the inferior turbinate (IT), middle meatus (MM), middle turbinate (MT), nasal septum (NS), and nasopharynx (*dark area bottom of view*). One also begins to see the right superior turbinate (*light area just medial to the top of the middle turbinate at the top of the view*), the sphenoethmoidal recess (*dark area at the top of the view*), and the slit-like sphenoid sinus ostium (*arrow*).

Figure 6-2F. Superior meatus, superior turbinate, and sphenoid sinus ostium. The 0-degree nasal telescope now views the right posterior superior nasal cavity demonstrating the superior meatus (SM) into which the posterior ethmoid sinus ostium opens (*white arrow*), the superior turbinate (ST), and the sphenoethmoidal recess into which the slit-like sphenoid sinus ostium opens (*black arrow*).

Figure 6-2G. Sphenoid sinus ostium. Another 0-degree nasal telescopic view of the right posterior superior nasal cavity shows the middle turbinate (MT), superior turbinate (ST), sphenoid sinus ostium (*arrow*), and nasal septum (NS).

Figure 6-2H. Sphenoid sinus ostium. The round right sphenoid sinus ostium (*arrow*) is displayed in a different patient, on posterior superior 0-degree nasal telescopy.

Figure 6-2I. Sphenoid sinus ostium. The 0-degree nasal telescope reveals the right superior turbinate (ST), the open sphenoid sinus ostium (*arrow*), and the sphenoethmoidal recess (SER).

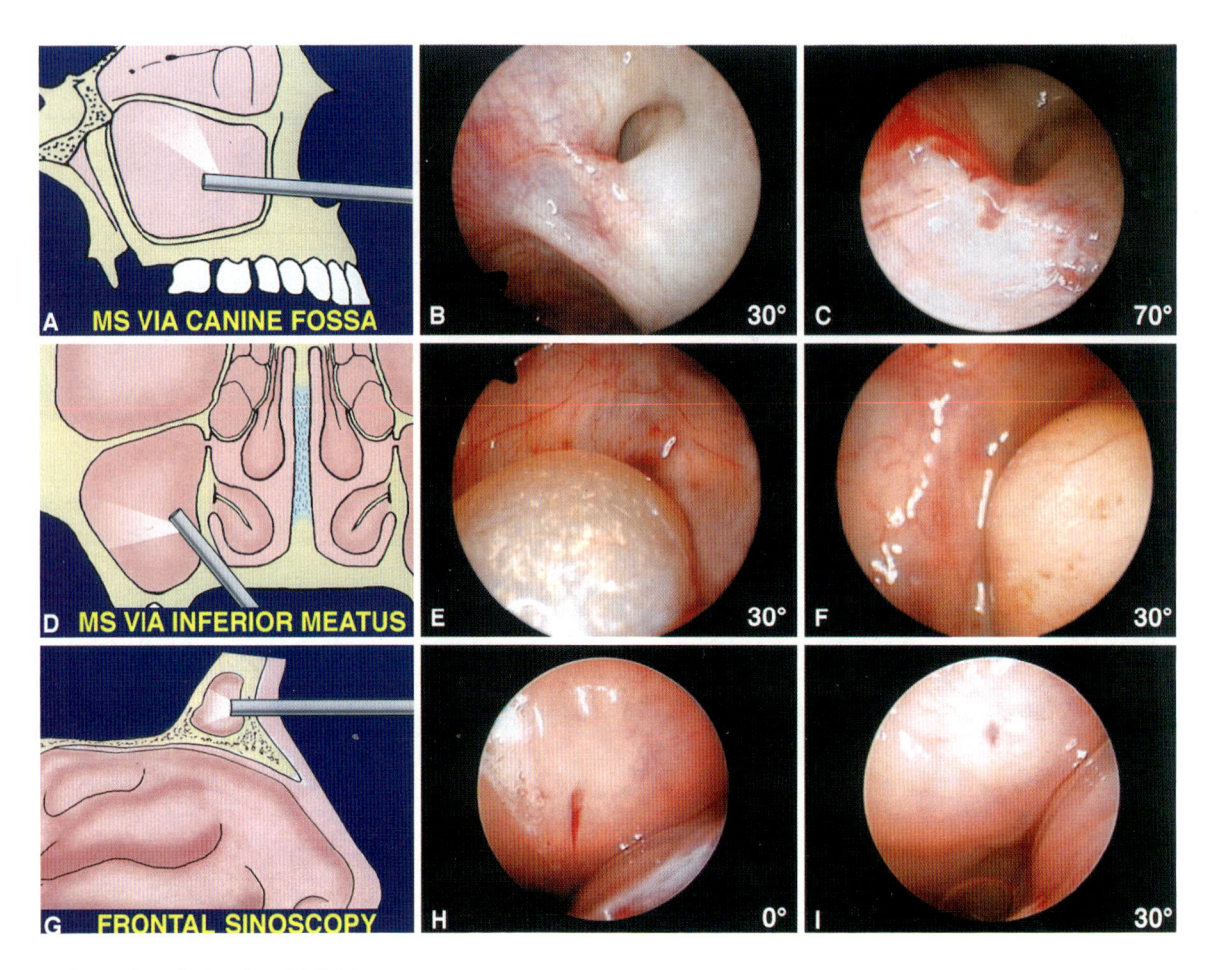

TECHNIQUES OF SINOSCOPY

Figure 6-3. *Top row:* Maxillary sinoscopy via the canine fossa. After the canine fossa is locally anesthetized a maxillary sinus trocar with its sheath is inserted into the maxillary sinus via the canine fossa. A careful to-and-fro rotating movement is applied to the trocar. The trocar is removed upon entry into the sinus, while its sheath is left in the sinus. The 4-mm 0-, 30-, and/or 70-degree telescopes are passed into the maxillary sinus through the sheath to view the mucosa, ostia, and pathologic conditions. The natural ostium of the maxillary sinus is best seen with the 30-degree (Figure 6-3B) or 70-degree (Figure 6-3C) telescopes. *Middle row:* Maxillary sinoscopy via the inferior meatus. After the nasal mucosa is decongested and anesthetized both topically and by injection, a maxillary sinus trocar is inserted through the inferior meatus at least 2 cm deep to the anterior face of the inferior turbinate (to avoid the nasolacrimal duct). The maxillary sinus is then examined with the 4-mm telescope. A large inferior maxillary sinus cyst is well demonstrated on 30-degree maxillary sinoscopy via the inferior meatus (Figures 6-3E and 6-3F). *Bottom row:* Frontal sinoscopy. A small anterior frontal sinusotomy allows telescopic access to the frontal sinus. The 0-, 30-, and 70-degree 4-mm telescopes are introduced into the frontal sinus via the small drill hole created in the anterior wall of the frontal sinus. A preoperative sinus CT scan is necessary to define the frontal sinus bony anatomy prior to creating a sinusotomy drill hole. Edematous mucosa of the sinus and the frontal sinus ostium are shown with the 0-degree (Figure 6-3H) and 30-degree (Figure 6-3I) telescopes.

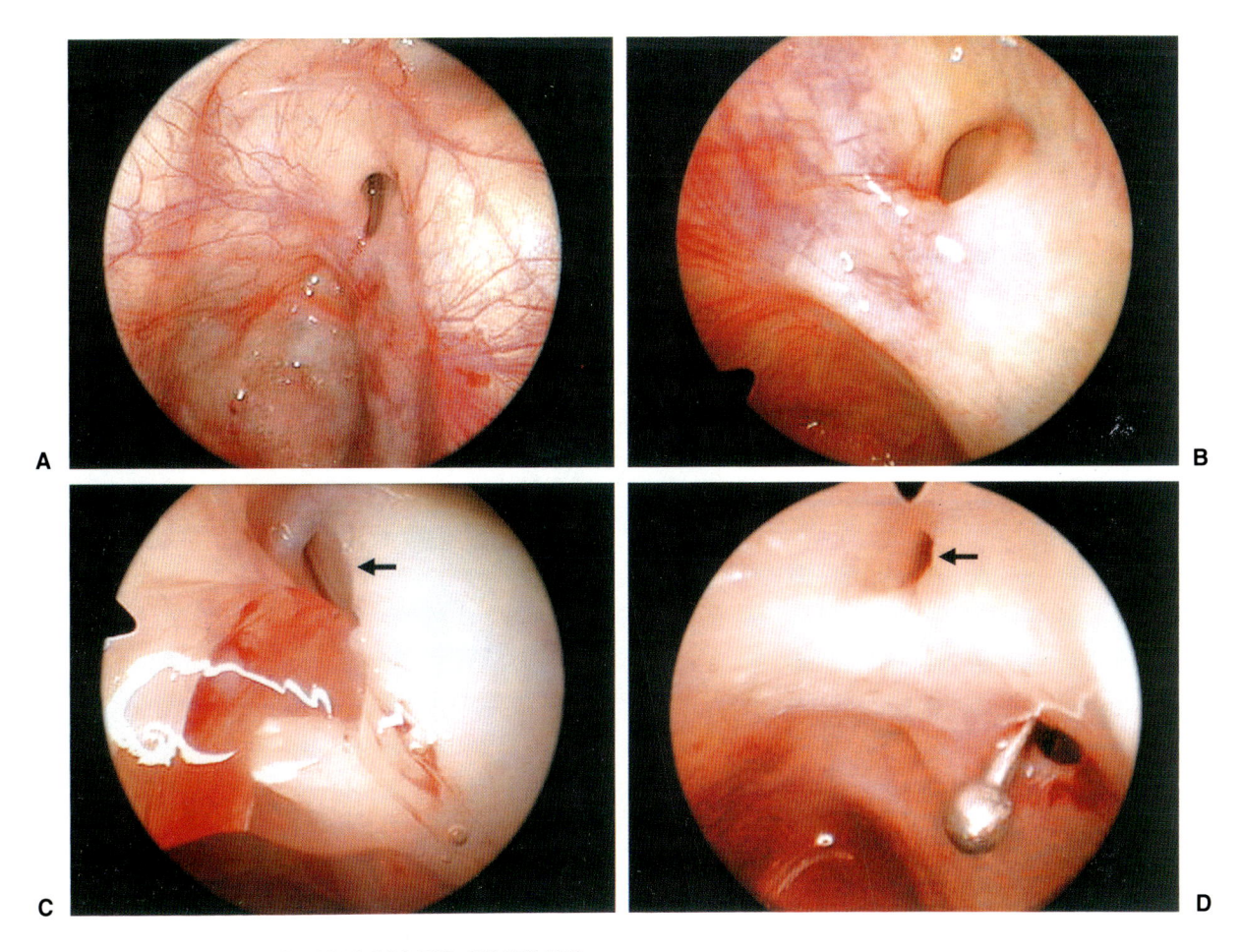

Endoscopy of the Paranasal Sinuses (Videosinoscopy)

PARANASAL SINUS ENDOSCOPIC ANATOMY

Natural Maxillary Sinus Ostia on Maxillary Sinoscopy Via the Canine Fossa

Figure 6-4A. Maxillary sinus ostium. The natural ostium is usually found in the medial posterosuperior corner of the maxillary sinus. This 0-degree sinoscopy via the canine fossa clearly shows the natural ostium of the right maxillary sinus in the medial posterosuperior portion of the sinus.

Figure 6-4B. Maxillary sinus ostium. This is a close-up view of the right maxillary sinus natural ostium seen on the 30-degree canine fossa telescopic sinoscopy. Note that the mucosal fold is often seen just below the natural ostium.

Figure 6-4C. Maxillary sinus ostium. Blood-tinged mucus flows by ciliary action to the natural ostium of this normal right maxillary sinus viewed with a 0-degree telescope through the canine fossa.

Figure 6-4D. Maxillary sinus ostia. This 30-degree telescopic sinoscopy via the canine fossa displays the right maxillary sinus natural ostium (*arrow*) and an accessory ostium (*ball-tipped probe passed transnasally*). Accessory ostia should be connected to the natural ostium during endoscopic sinus surgery in order to prevent the recirculation of sinus secretions (directed out the natural ostium by ciliary transport and flowing back in the accessory ostium).

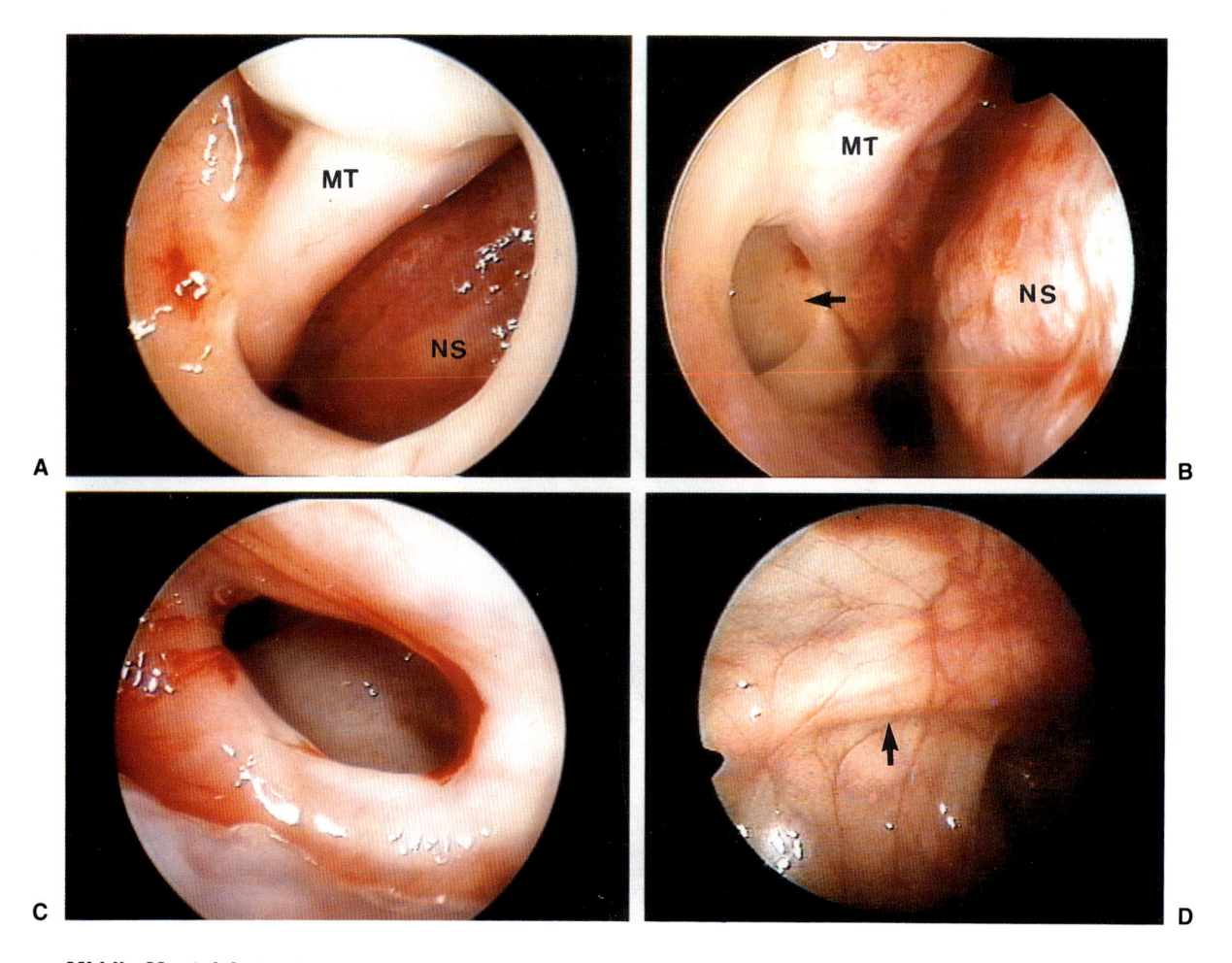

Middle Meatal Antrostomy

Figure 6-5A. Maxillary sinoscopic view of middle meatal antrostomy. The right middle turbinate (MT) and nasal septum (NS) are clearly seen through a wide middle meatal antrostomy viewed on 0-degree maxillary sinoscopy via the canine fossa.

Figure 6-5B. Transnasal telescopic view of middle meatal antrostomy. The 0-degree nasal telescopic exam demonstrates a right middle meatal antrostomy (*arrow*).

Figure 6-5C. Maxillary sinoscopic view of middle meatal antrostomy. The blood-tinged mucus flows by ciliary action to the middle meatal antrostomy (where the natural ostium was) seen on 30-degree canine fossa maxillary sinoscopy.

Figure 6-5D. Middle meatal sinoscopic view of infraorbital nerve. The 30-degree maxillary sinoscopic view through a middle meatal antrostomy demonstrates the left infraorbital nerve (*arrow*) in the roof of the left maxillary sinus.

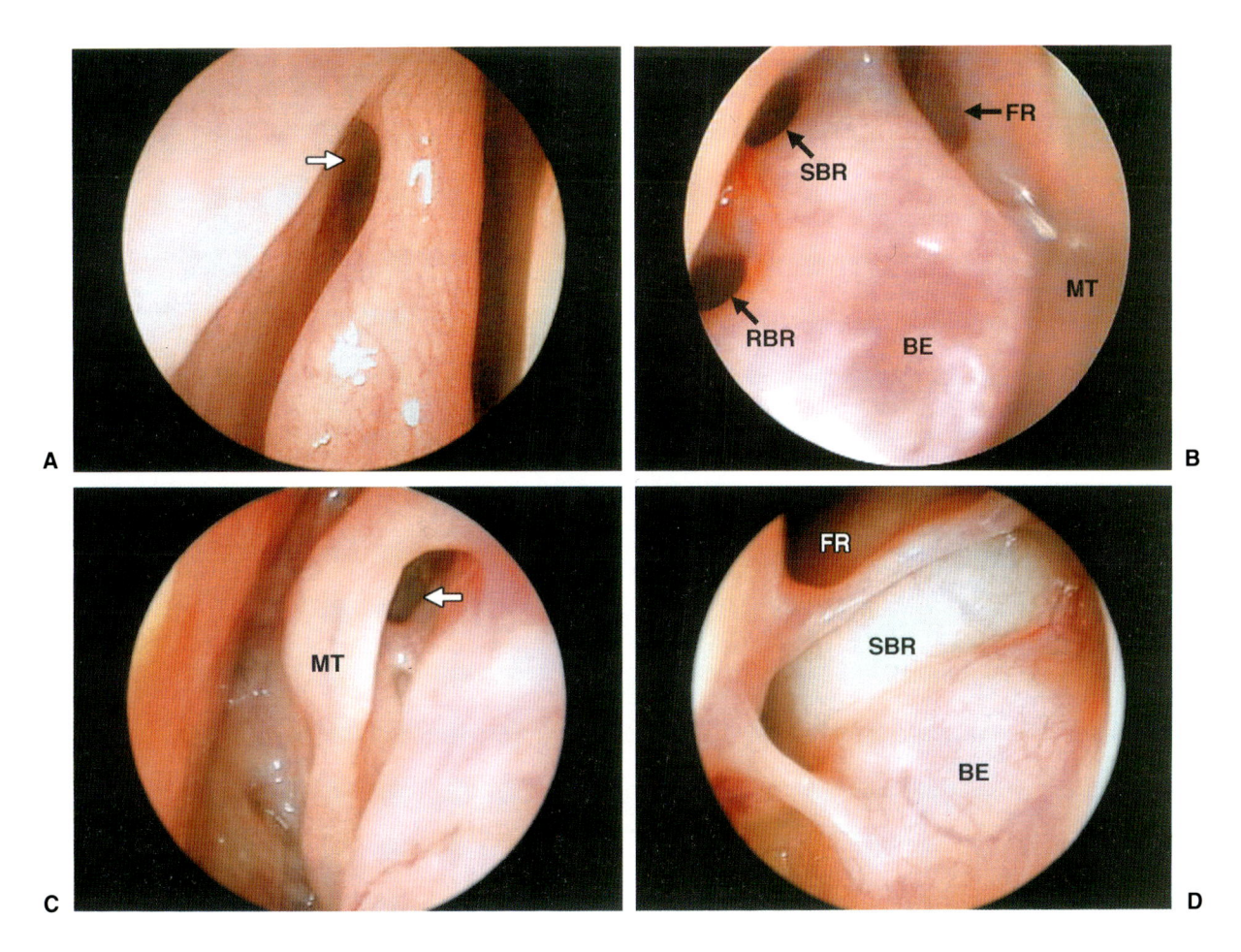

Frontal Sinus Recess

Figure 6-6A. Frontal recess. The 0-degree nasal telescope demonstrates the right frontal recess (*arrow*) at the top of the right middle meatus.

Figure 6-6B. Frontal recess, suprabullar recess, and retrobullar recess. This 30-degree nasal telescopic view of the superior part of the right middle meatus prominently displays the ethmoid bulla (BE). The cleft between the superior aspect of the middle turbinate and the ethmoid bulla, called the *hiatus semilunaris superior,* leads to the frontal recess (FR). The space that forms behind and above the ethmoidal bulla, termed the *retrobullar recess* and the *suprabullar recess,* respectively (also called *sinus lateralis*), is of variable size and shape from person to person. In this patient the retrobullar recess (RBR) and suprabullar recess (SBR) are separate with narrow openings into the middle meatus.

Figure 6-6C. Frontal recess. The postoperative nasal telescopic exam of the left middle meatus reveals a patent frontal recess (*arrow*).

Figure 6-6D. Frontal recess and suprabullar recess. The 30-degree nasal telescopic view of the superior aspect of the left middle meatus demonstrates a widely patent frontal recess (FR) and an open suprabullar recess (SBR) above the ethmoid bulla (BE).

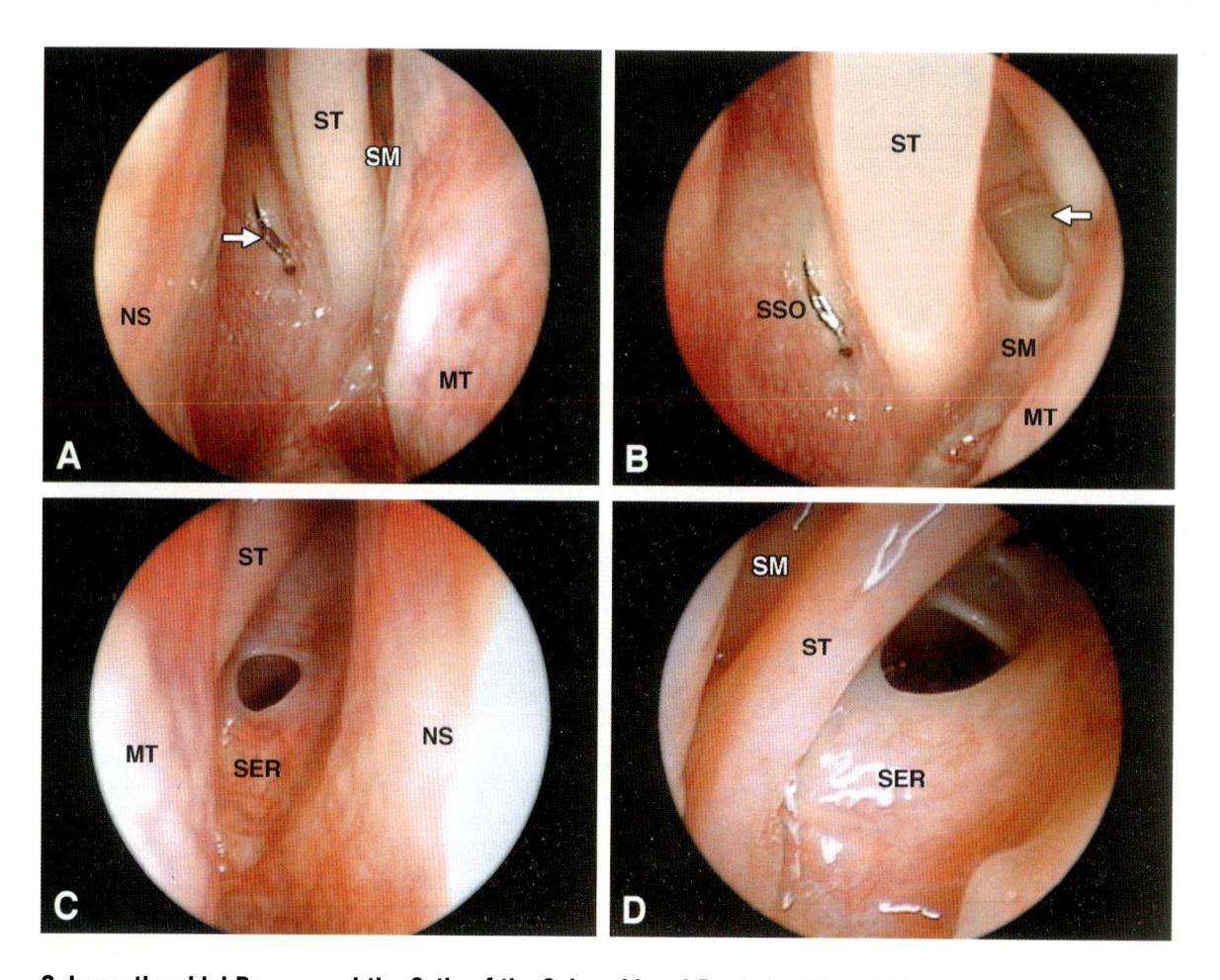

Sphenoethmoidal Recess and the Ostia of the Sphenoid and Posterior Ethmoid Sinuses

Figure 6-7A.   Sphenoethmoidal recess and sphenoid sinus ostium. The posterior left nasal cavity seen through a 0-degree nasal telescope contains the sphenoethmoidal recess medial to the superior turbinate (ST). Within the sphenoethmoidal recess along the posterior superior nasal cavity lies the slit-like sphenoid sinus ostium (*arrow*). The superior meatus (SM) is the space between the superior turbinate (ST) and the middle turbinate (MT).

Figure 6-7B.   Sphenoid and posterior ethmoid sinus ostia. Advancement of the nasal telescope to the left superior meatus (SM) reveals a large open posterior ethmoid sinus ostium (*arrow*). The sphenoid sinus ostium (SSO) is also clearly seen.

Figure 6-7C.   Sphenoid sinus ostium. Another posterior superior 0-degree nasal telescopic exam displays the right middle turbinate (MT), posterior nasal septum (NS), superior turbinate (ST), sphenoethmoidal recess (SER), and oval sphenoid sinus ostium.

Figure 6-7D.   Sphenoid sinus ostium. This close-up 0-degree nasal telescopic view of the posterior superior right nasal cavity displays the superior meatus (SM), superior turbinate (ST), sphenoethmoidal recess (SER), and a widely patent sphenoid sinus ostium.

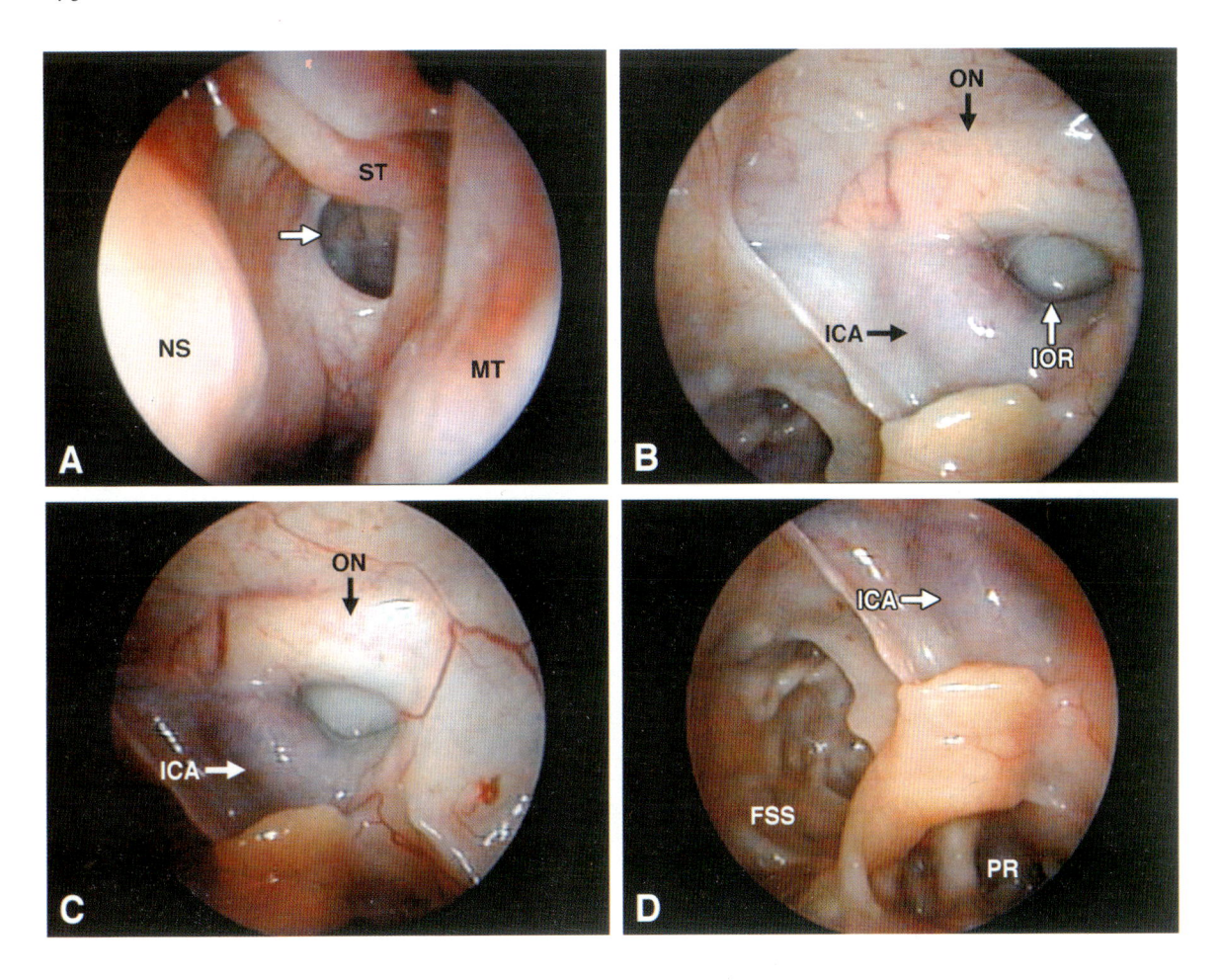

Endoscopic View of the Sphenoid Sinus Cavity

Figure 6-8A. Sphenoidotomy opening. The 0-degree nasal telescopic exam reveals a widely patent left sphenoidotomy opening (*arrow*) in the sphenoethmoidal recess inferomedial to the left superior turbinate (ST).

Figure 6-8B. Optic nerve and internal carotid artery. This 0-degree nasal telescopic superolateral view of the left sphenoid sinus cavity through the sphenoidotomy dramatically reveals the left internal carotid artery (ICA), which was visibly pulsatile and thus dehiscent, and the left optic nerve (ON). The infraoptic recess (IOR) seen between the optic nerve and internal carotid artery is formed by pneumatization of the anterior clinoid process of the sphenoid bone.

Figure 6-8C. Optic nerve and internal carotid artery. The 30-degree nasal telescope directed laterally within the left sphenoid sinus clearly demonstrates the optic nerve (ON) and internal carotid artery (ICA).

Figure 6-8D. Internal carotid artery and pterygoid recess. The 30-degree nasal telescope directed inferiorly within the left sphenoid sinus shows the main cavity of the sinus and its floor (FSS) medially, the internal carotid artery (ICA) superolaterally, and the pterygoid recess (PR) inferolaterally. The pterygoid recess represents the pneumatized pterygoid process of the sphenoid bone.

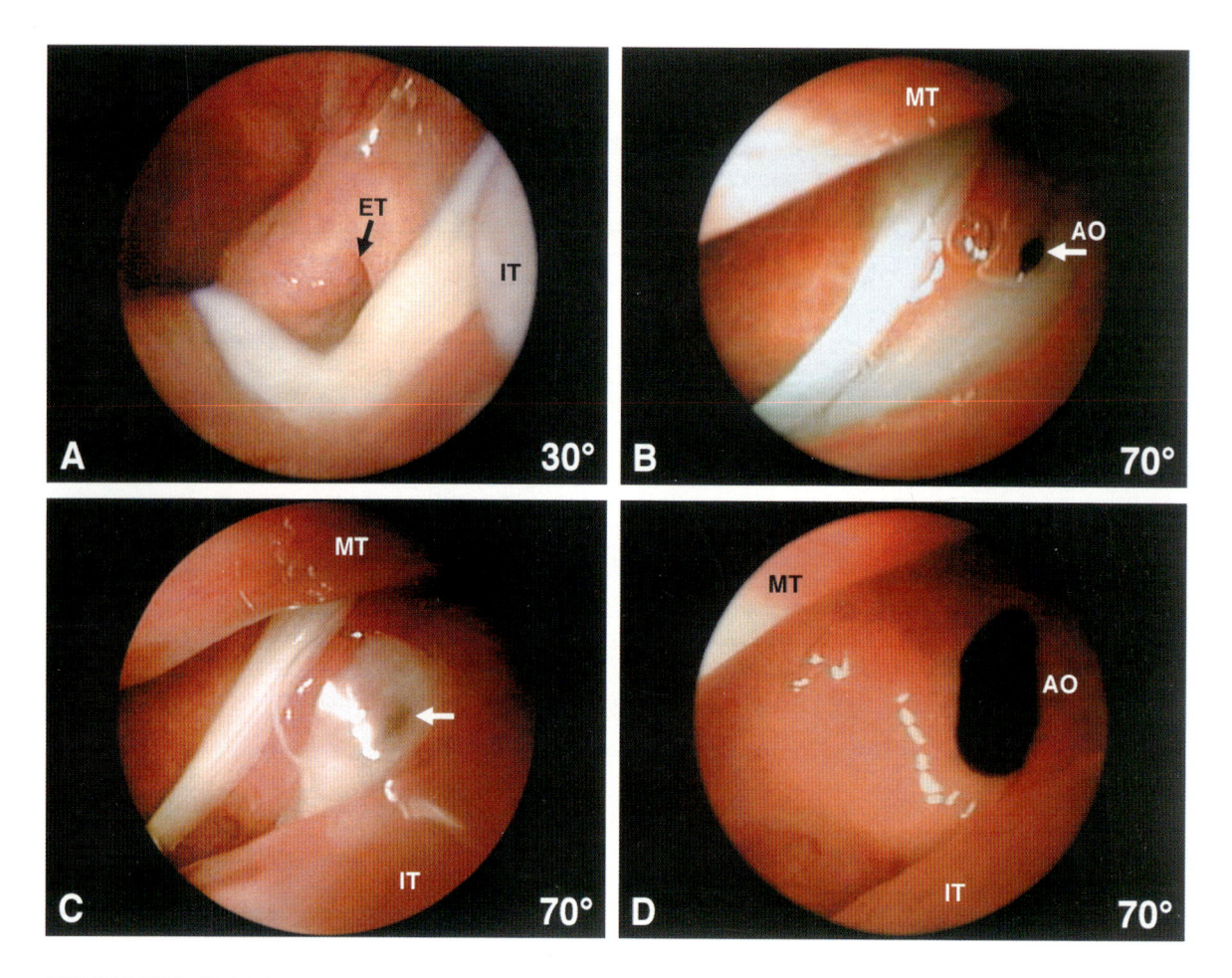

DISORDERS OF THE PARANASAL SINUSES

Acute Maxillary Sinusitis

Figure 6-9A. Acute maxillary sinusitis. This patient complained of a two-week history of left headache, left facial pain, nasal congestion, and postnasal discharge. The 30-degree transnasal telescopic exam of the left posterior nasal cavity displays a stream of purulent discharge flowing from the posterior middle meatus into the nasopharynx just anterior to the eustachian tube orifice.

Figure 6-9B. Acute maxillary sinusitis. The 70-degree nasal telescopy of the left lateral nasal cavity of the same patient reveals two streams of mucopus between the inferior turbinate and middle turbinate (MT) flowing posteriorly. The top stream appeared to flow from the natural ostium of the left maxillary sinus and the bottom stream from an accessory ostium (AO).

Figure 6-9C. Acute maxillary sinusitis. Air escaped from the left maxillary sinus accessory ostium, creating a bubble in the mucopus.

Figure 6-9D. Treated acute maxillary sinusitis. Two weeks later, after treatment with oral antibiotics, oral steroids, and topical steroid spray, the patient's symptoms cleared. Follow-up 70-degree nasal telescopy demonstrates a widely patent accessory ostium (AO) of the left maxillary sinus and complete disappearance of purulent drainage.

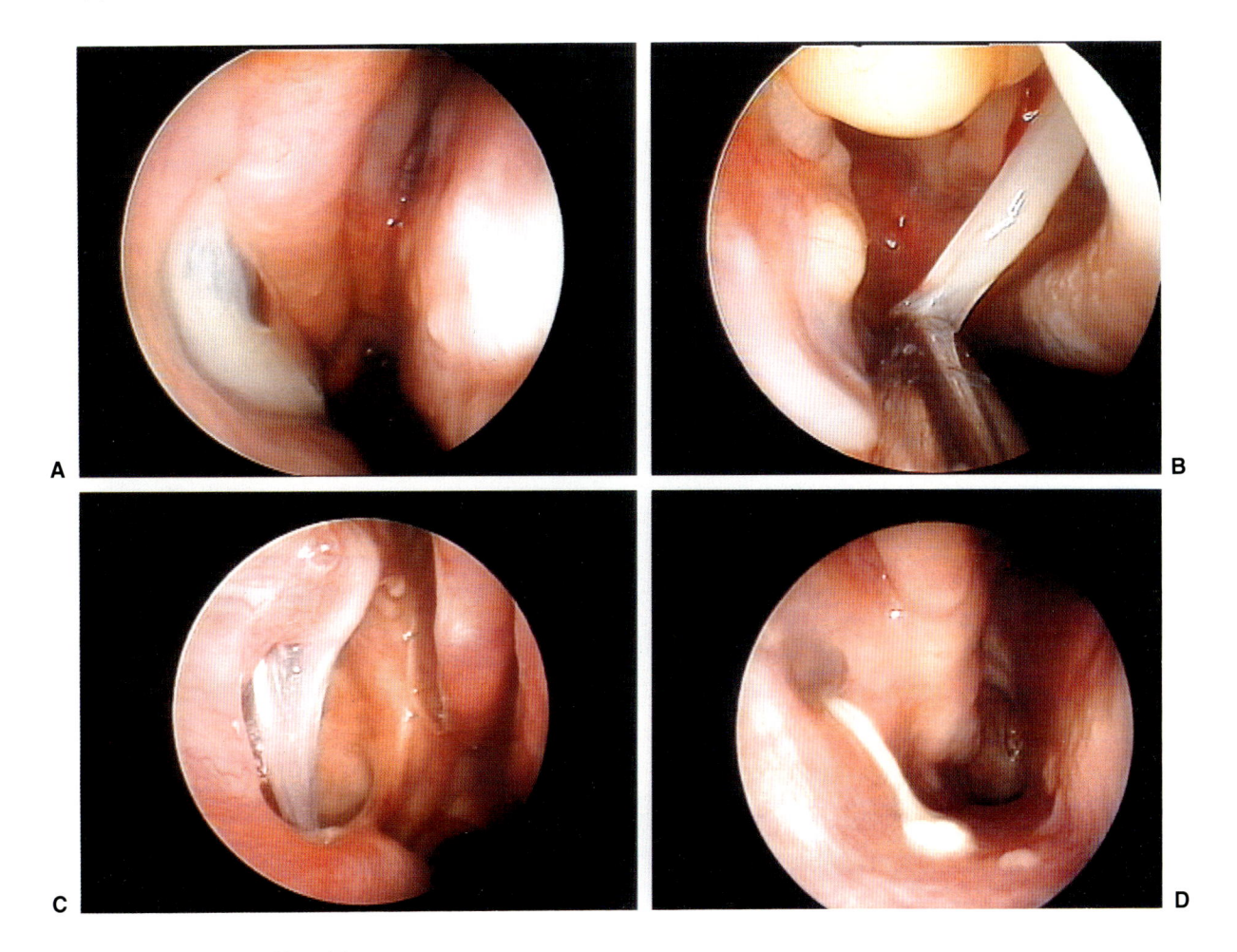

Endoscopy of the Paranasal Sinuses (Videosinoscopy) 77

Chronic Maxillary Sinusitis

Figure 6-10A. Chronic maxillary sinusitis. Despite treatment, this patient had persistent mucopurulent drainage from his right maxillary sinus filling the middle meatus, seen here on 0-degree nasal telescopy.

Figure 6-10B. Chronic maxillary sinusitis. Even after undergoing endoscopic sinus surgery, this patient had persistent left maxillary sinus pus suctioned from the left middle meatal antrostomy while viewed through the 0-degree nasal telescope.

Figure 6-10C. Recirculation of maxillary sinus drainage. Mucopurulent drainage from the natural ostium of the right maxillary sinus flows down and back into the same sinus through a large antrostomy, as seen through the 30-degree nasal telescope. This example demonstrates the importance of connecting an accessory ostium to the natural ostium during a middle meatal antrostomy procedure.

Figure 6-10D. Chronic maxillary sinusitis. Mucopus flows from a stenotic right inferior meatal antrostomy seen on 30-degree nasal telescopy.

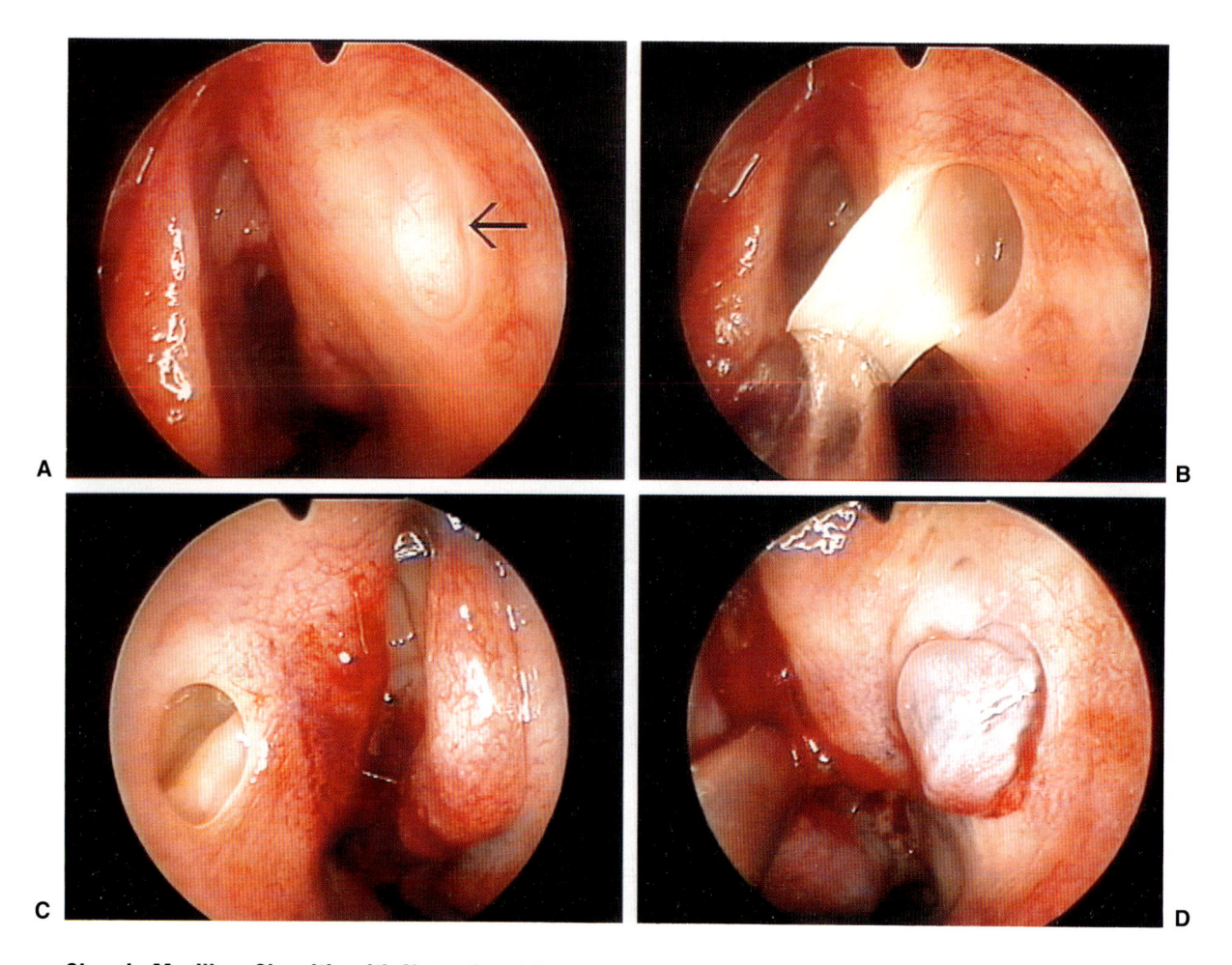

Chronic Maxillary Sinusitis with Natural and Accessory Ostial Disease

Figure 6-11A. Chronic maxillary sinusitis. Polyps obstructed the left maxillary sinus natural ostium in this patient who suffered from chronically obstructed and infected maxillary sinuses. The 0-degree nasal telescopic exam of the left middle meatus reveals a bulging anterior fontanelle. The accessory ostium (*arrow*) was also obstructed by an antral polyp.

Figure 6-11B. Chronic maxillary sinusitis. The suction retracted the obstructing polyp, opening the accessory ostium and revealing left maxillary sinus mucosal edema and mucopus. A large middle meatal antrostomy connecting the natural and accessory ostia should be part of the treatment in this situation.

Figure 6-11C. Chronic maxillary sinusitis. The 0-degree nasal telescopic exam of the right middle meatus in another patient similarly demonstrates polyps overlying the area of the natural ostium and thick maxillary sinus mucosa and mucopus seen through an accessory ostium.

Figure 6-11D. Chronic maxillary sinusitis. The left accessory maxillary ostium in this patient is completely obstructed by an antral polyp that protrudes through this ostium.

Endoscopy of the Paranasal Sinuses (Videosinoscopy) 79

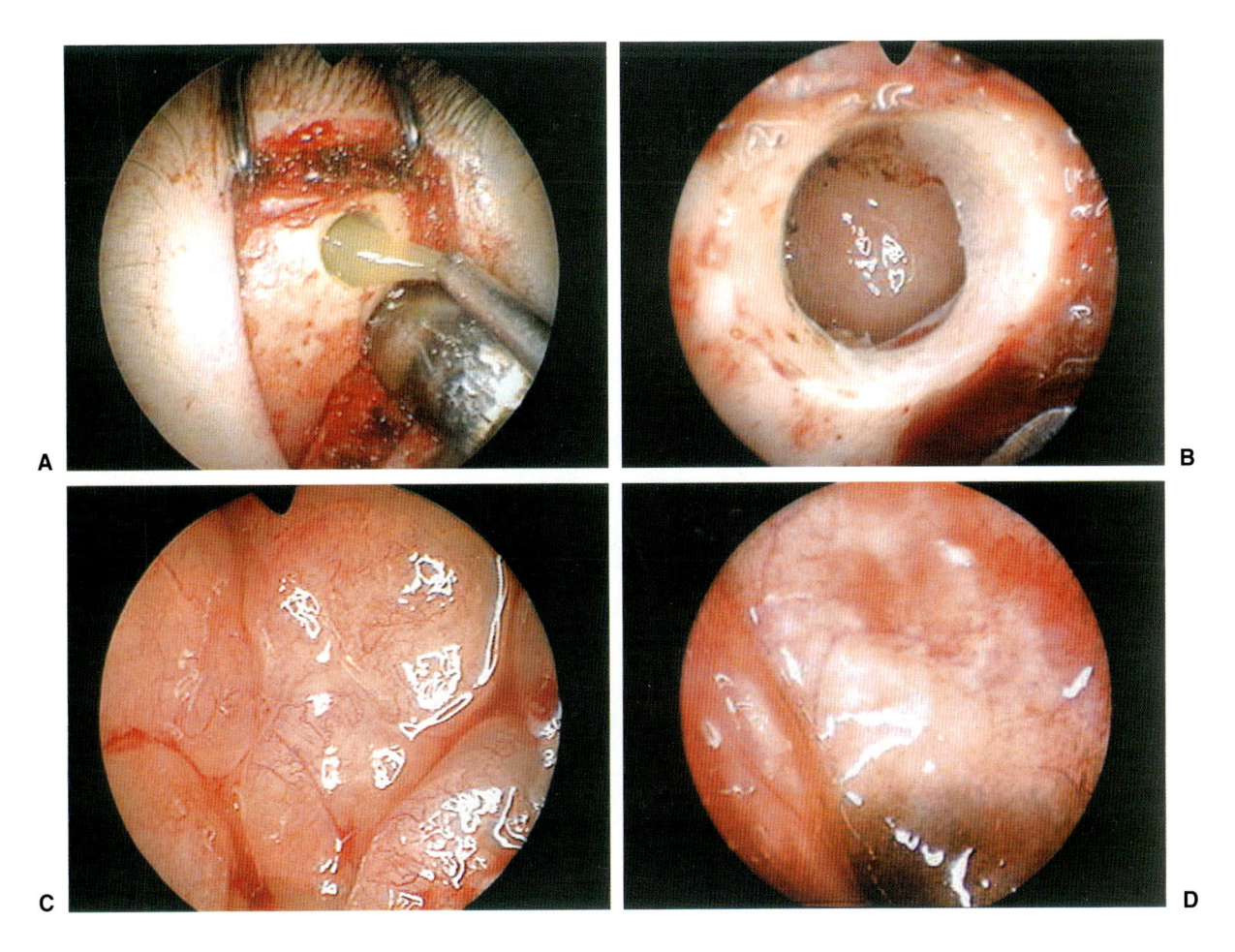

Frontal Sinusitis

Figure 6-12A. Frontal sinusitis. Right frontal sinus pus is suctioned from an anterior frontal sinusotomy opening created for frontal sinoscopy. The right eyebrow is seen at the top of the view, and the bridge of the nose is seen at the right of the view.

Figure 6-12B. Frontal sinusitis. After removal of the frontal sinus mucopus, 0-degree telescopy from just outside the frontal sinus reveals edematous frontal sinus mucosa.

Figure 6-12C. Frontal sinusitis. Zero-degree frontal sinoscopy demonstrates red, injected, markedly edematous sinus mucosa in the same patient. The frontal ostium begins at the bottom of this view.

Figure 6-12D. Frontal sinusitis. A similar view of thick, edematous, injected frontal sinus mucosa of another patient is demonstrated on 0-degree frontal sinoscopy after aspiration of the mucopus. Note the remaining dark mucopus at the frontal sinus ostium.

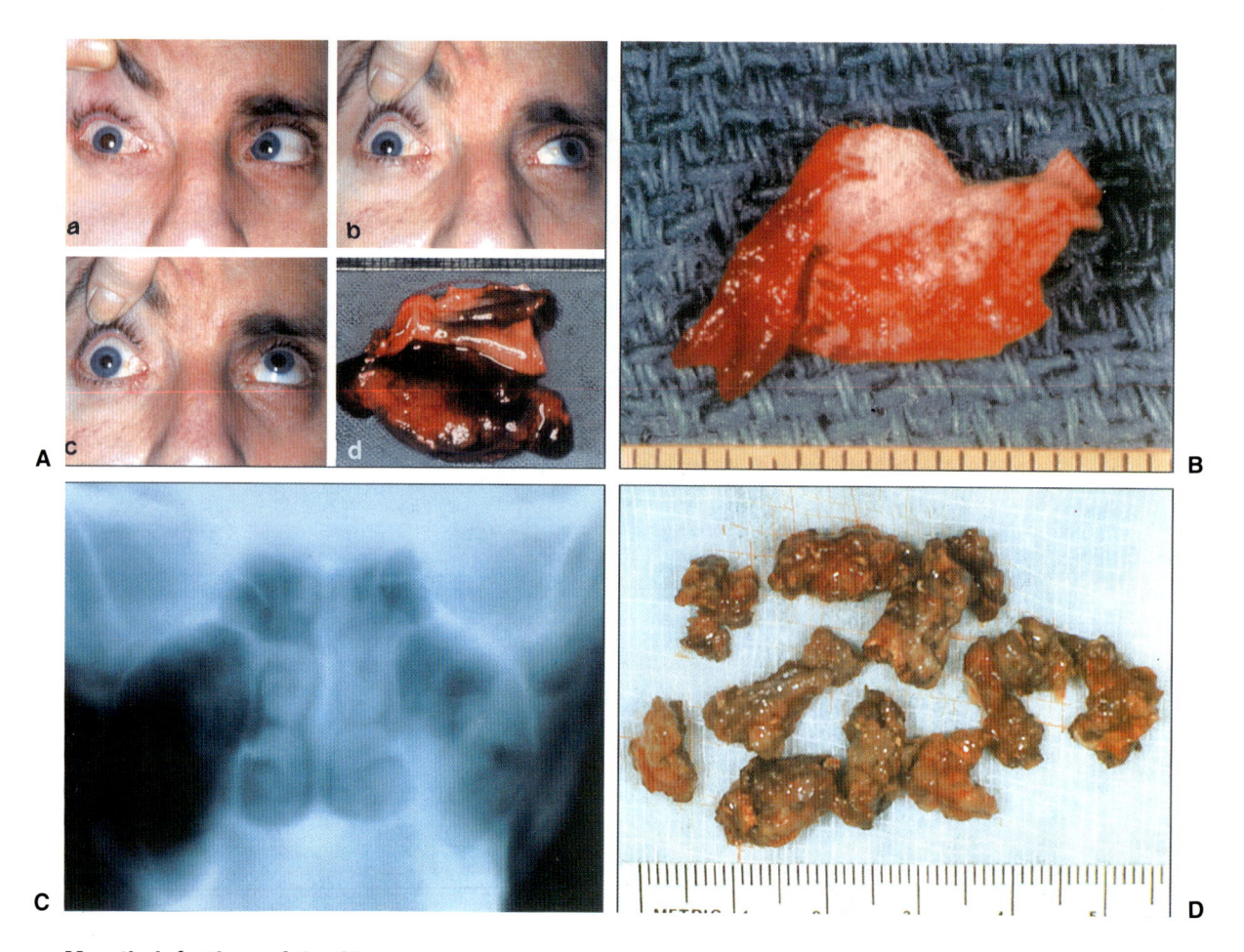

Mycotic Infections of the Sinuses

Figure 6-13A. Mucormycosis. This diabetic patient developed a complete right ophthalmoplegia associated with acute sinusitis (a-c). Mucormycosis invades and obstructs mucosal vasculature, resulting first in pale mucosa and then in the classic necrotic "black turbinate." The black middle turbinate is shown (d) from a different patient who suffered aggressive mucormycosis. (Courtesy of Howard W. Smith, M.D.)

Figure 6-13B. Fungus ball. The mass of pure fungus was removed from the sphenoid sinus of a diabetic patient with mucormycosis.

Figure 6-13C. Maxillary sinus aspergillosis. Polytomography of the sinuses demonstrates irregular soft tissue masses in the left maxillary sinus suggestive of fungal infection.

Figure 6-13D. Maxillary sinus aspergillosis. The brown "peanutbuttery" fungal debris was removed from the patient infected with *Aspergillus* shown in Figure 6-13C.

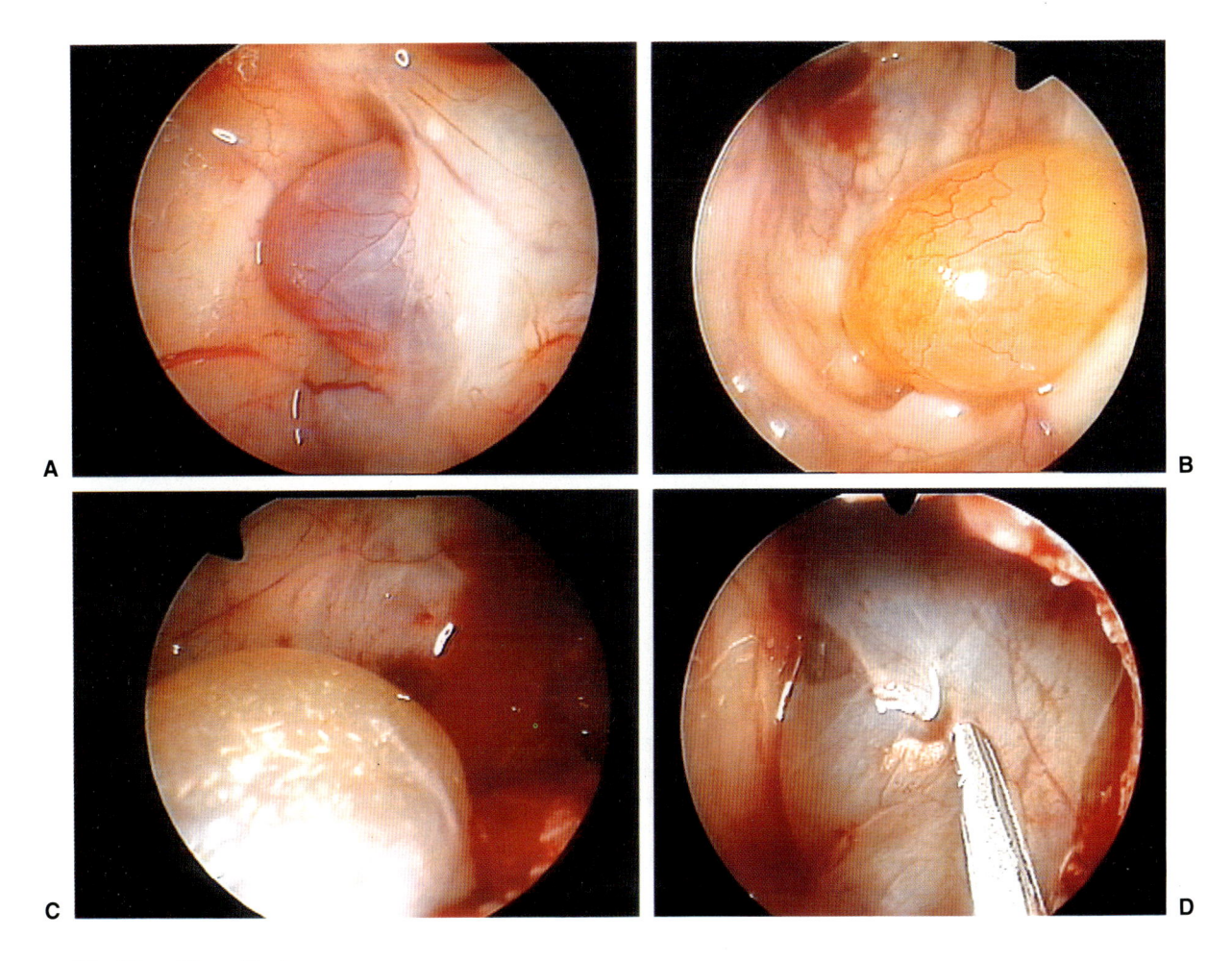

Maxillary Sinus Cysts

Figure 6-14A. Maxillary sinus cyst. Zero-degree right maxillary sinoscopy via the canine fossa displays a medium-sized medial antral cyst. This cyst was excised via a middle meatal antrostomy.

Figure 6-14B. Maxillary sinus cyst. Zero-degree left maxillary sinoscopy via the canine fossa reveals a large lateral wall antral cyst. Its contents was aspirated via the canine fossa sinoscopy, and the cyst was removed via the left middle meatal antrostomy.

Figure 6-14C. Maxillary sinus cyst. The 25-degree inferior meatal telescopy reveals a large inferior cyst of the right maxillary sinus. This symptomatic cyst was removed through an inferior meatal antrostomy.

Figure 6-14D. Maxillary sinus cyst. This huge left maxillary sinus cyst fills the whole sinus, viewed with 0-degree sinoscopy through a Caldwell–Luc approach. This large cyst was excised after it was decompressed by aspiration of its contents.

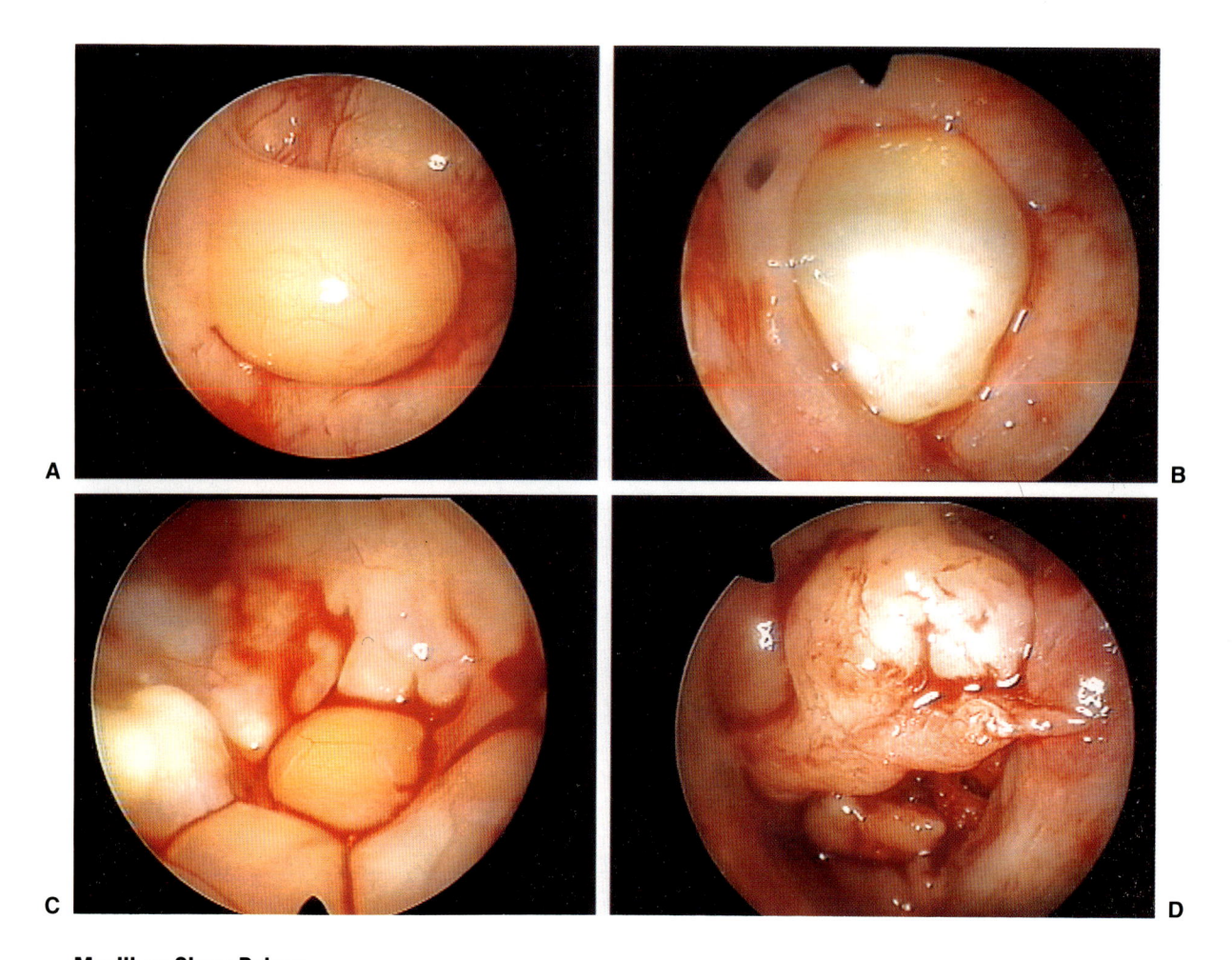

Maxillary Sinus Polyps

Figure 6-15A. Maxillary sinus polyp. The 0-degree maxillary sinoscopy via the canine fossa reveals a large polyp arising from the lateral wall of the right maxillary sinus. This can be excised endoscopically via middle meatal antrostomy.

Figure 6-15B. Maxillary sinus polyp. The medial superior left maxillary sinus polyp is seen on the 0-degree maxillary sinoscopy through the canine fossa. An accessory ostium is visible at the upper medial aspect of the left maxillary sinus. The polyp was removed via middle meatal antrostomy.

Figure 6-15C. Maxillary sinus polyps. There are multiple polyps along the floor and posterior wall of the left maxillary sinus seen via the canine fossa 0-degree maxillary sinoscopy. Middle meatal antrostomy was performed.

Figure 6-15D. Maxillary sinus polyps. Multiple large polyps stemming from the left antral roof are visible on the 0-degree maxillary sinoscopy via a left Caldwell–Luc approach. Its attachment to the antral roof was incised, and the entire mass of polyps was removed.

Endoscopy of the Paranasal Sinuses (Videosinoscopy) 83

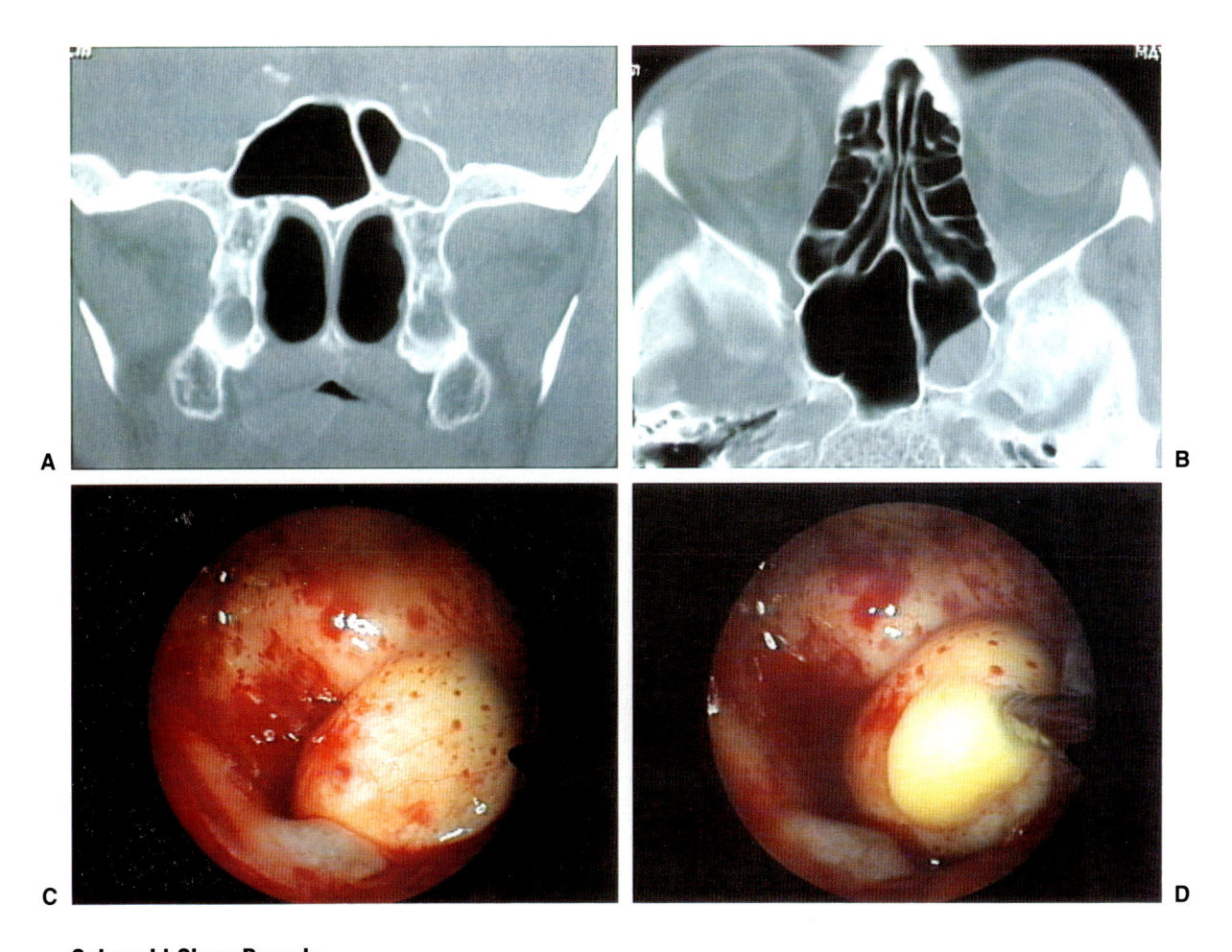

Sphenoid Sinus Pyocele

Figure 6-16A. Sphenoid sinus pyocele. The coronal sinus CT scan demonstrates a soft tissue mass in the lateral part of the left sphenoid sinus. The bony sinus is intact.

Figure 6-16B. Sphenoid sinus pyocele. The axial sinus CT scan displays the soft tissue mass in the posterolateral part of the left sphenoid sinus.

Figure 6-16C. Sphenoid sinus pyocele. The round soft tissue mass lies on the lateral posterior floor of the left sphenoid sinus, seen on transnasal 0-degree telescopy through the left sphenoidotomy.

Figure 6-16D. Sphenoid sinus pyocele. Compression of the soft tissue mass expresses the creamy purulent contents.

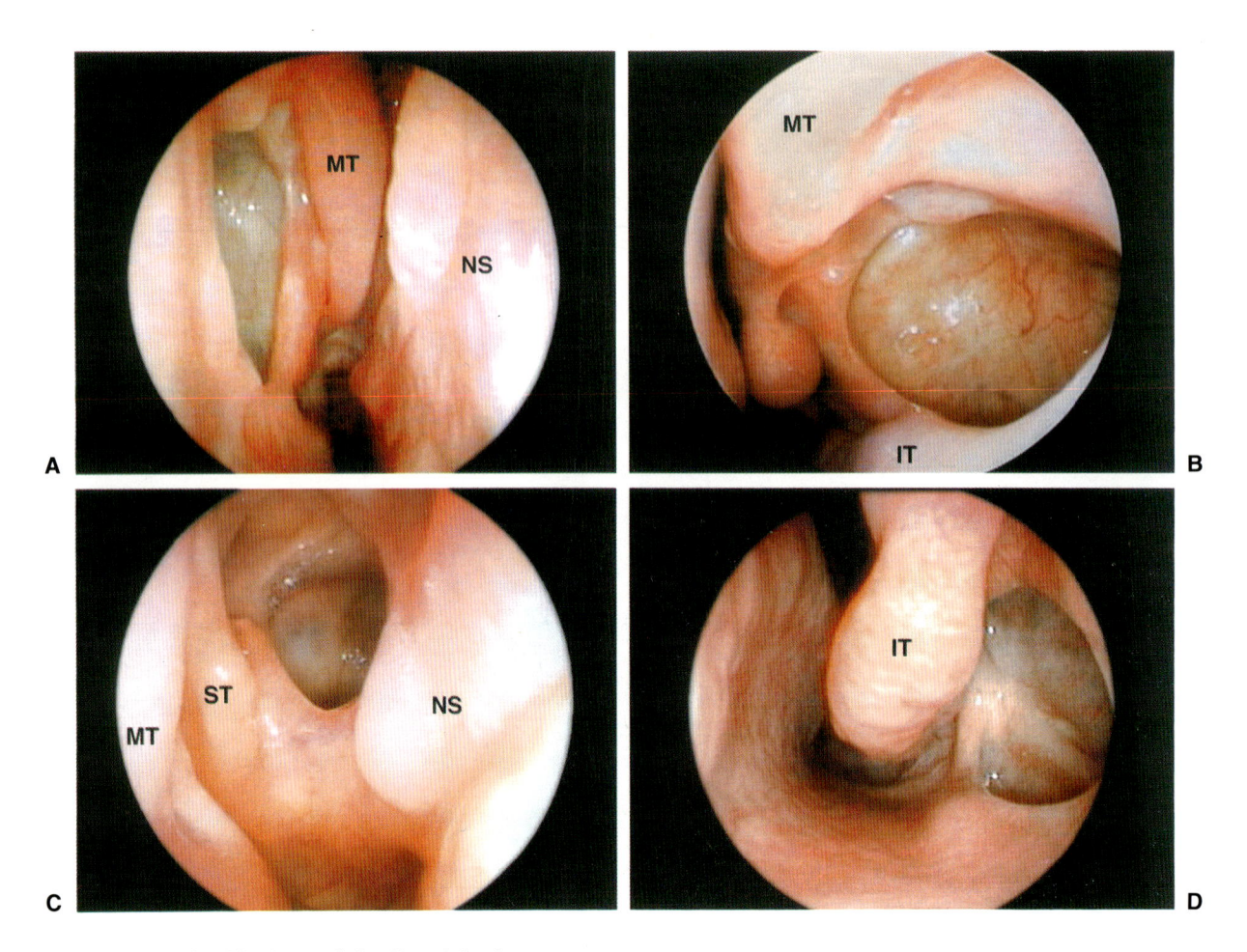

Postoperative Findings of the Nasal Cavity

Figure 6-17A. Middle meatal antrostomy. The 0-degree nasal telescopic exam of the right nasal cavity demonstrates a well-healed wide middle meatal antrostomy with healthy maxillary sinus mucosa.

Figure 6-17B. Middle meatal antrostomy. The 30-degree nasal telescopy of the left middle meatus displays a large left antrostomy with healthy maxillary sinus mucosa. The well-healed partial middle turbinectomy leaves the antrostomy unobstructed.

Figure 6-17C. Sphenoid sinusotomy. The right sphenoid sinus remains open and well-aerated after sphenoid sinusotomy. This 0-degree nasal telescopic exam also shows the superior turbinate (ST), middle turbinate (MT), and nasal septum (NS), all with normal mucosa.

Figure 6-17D. Inferior meatal antrostomy. This wide-open left inferior meatal antrostomy is easily appreciated on 0-degree nasal telescopy.

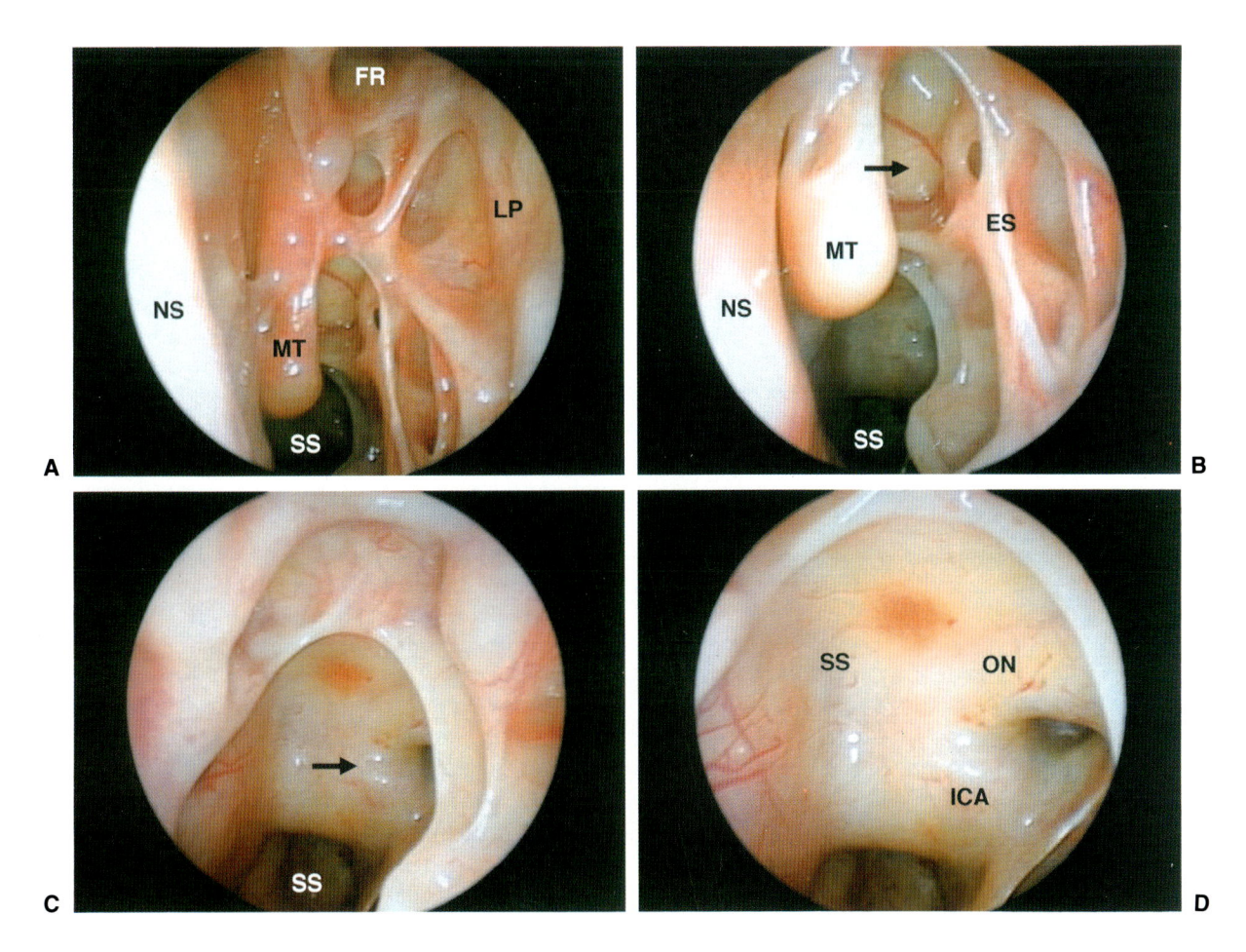

Endoscopy of the Paranasal Sinuses (Videosinoscopy)

Postoperative Sphenoethmoidectomy Findings

Figure 6-18A. Postoperative sphenoethmoidectomy findings. This patient underwent multiple sinus operations for recurrent ethmoid and frontal sinusitis. Follow-up 0-degree nasal telescopic examination of the left posterior nasal cavity displays the middle turbinate remnant (MT) adherent to the nasal septum (NS). The sphenoid sinus (SS) was wide open. The lamina papyracea (LP) was exposed and the frontal recess (FR) was open. The mucosa was well-healed.

Figure 6-18B. Postoperative sphenoethmoidectomy findings. Deeper 0-degree nasal telescopic examination demonstrates scar bands within the open ethmoid sinus cavity (ES). The posterior ethmoidal artery or its branch is seen in the roof of the posterior ethmoidal sinus cavity (*arrow*). Note that the anterior sphenoid wall is absent.

Figure 6-18C. Post operative sphenoethmoidectomy findings. Still deeper 0-degree telescopy displays the large sphenoidotomy opening. The sphenoid sinus cavity (SS) appears healthy. The optic nerve (*above the arrow*) and the internal carotid artery (*below the arrow*) are visible.

Figure 6-18D. Optic nerve and internal carotid artery in postoperative sphenoid sinus cavity. The 0-degree telescope is directed into the left sphenoid sinus (SS), more clearly showing the optic nerve (ON) and internal carotid artery (ICA) in the posterolateral sphenoid sinus. When cleaning the postoperative deep sinus cavity with a suction tip or a pointed instrument, always remember that the vital structures within the sphenoid sinus may be exposed by previous procedures. In this case the anterior wall of the sphenoid sinus was almost totally absent, exposing the optic nerve and the internal carotid artery. Note a small area of mucosal erythema near the optic nerve which was touched by a suction tip. Postoperative cleaning of the posterior ethmoid and sphenoid sinus cavity should always be carried out under telescopic (or microscopic) observation.

Chapter 7
Endoscopy of the Nasopharynx (Videonasopharyngoscopy)

Nasopharyngoscopy is the examination of the nasopharynx using a rigid telescope or a flexible fiberscope via a transnasal or transoral approach. When the nasopharyngoscopic findings are documented with a video camera, the procedure is called *videonasopharyngoscopy*. It can also be accomplished transorally with a mirror using a microscope to which a video camera is attached.

This procedure allows in-depth examination and documentation of the anatomy and pathology of nasopharyngeal structures such as the posterior choanae, eustachian tube orifices, tori tubarii, Rosenmüller's fossae, velopharyngeal isthmus, and posterior wall of the nasopharynx.

The equipment used for nasopharyngoscopy includes (1) 0-, 30-, 70-, 90-, and 120-degree rigid telescopes (4 mm in adults, 2.7 mm in children), (2) a flexible fiberoptic nasal endoscope such as Olympus ENF P3 (3.6 mm), (3) a surgical microscope (250 to 300-mm lens), (4) a light source, and (5) a nasal topical anesthetic and decongestant. Videonasopharyngoscopy also requires (1) a video camera, (2) a video recorder, (3) a video monitor, and (4) a video printer.

This procedure is usually accomplished by a rigid telescope or a flexible fiberscope passed transnasally and a rigid retrograde telescope transorally. Videonasopharyngoscopy affords a very clear view of the nasopharynx which allows for accurate diagnosis of pathologic conditions and full appreciation of anatomic relationships and physiological functions of nasopharyngeal structures. It is an excellent mechanism for teaching patients and students about the nasopharynx and for detailed medical documentation.

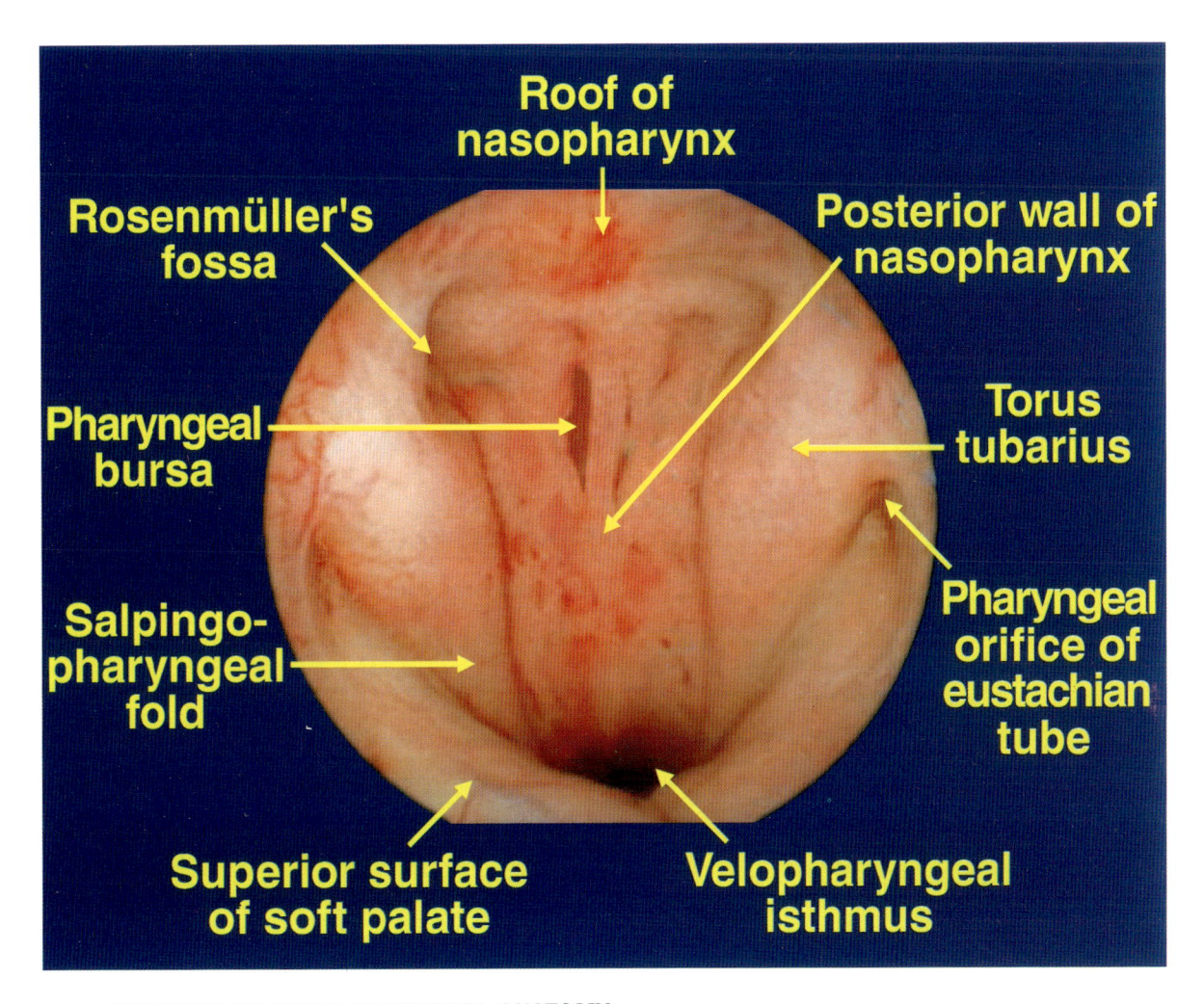

Endoscopy of the Nasopharynx (Videonasopharyngoscopy)

OVERVIEW OF NASOPHARYNGEAL ANATOMY

Figure 7-1. Transnasal telescopic view of the nasopharynx. A panoramic view of the nasopharynx including its roof, its lateral and posterior walls, and its velopharyngeal isthmus is shown (4-mm 30-degree telescope).

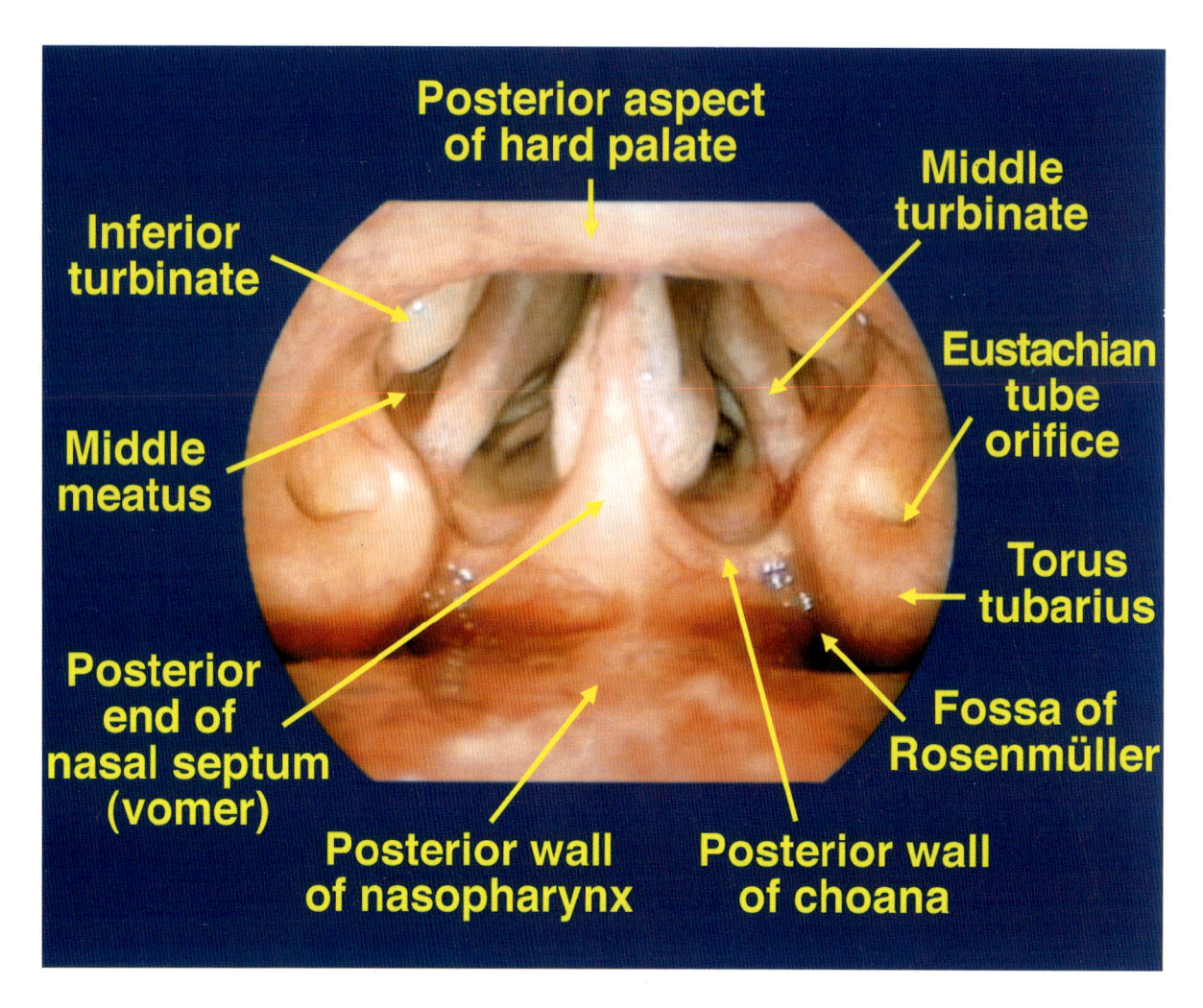

Figure 7-2. Transoral telescopic view of the nasopharynx. The posterior nasal cavities, posterior end of the nasal septum, eustachian tube orifices, tori tubarii, Rosenmüller's fossae, and the posterior wall of the nasopharynx are shown (120-degree telescope).

Endoscopy of the Nasopharynx (Videonasopharyngoscopy) 89

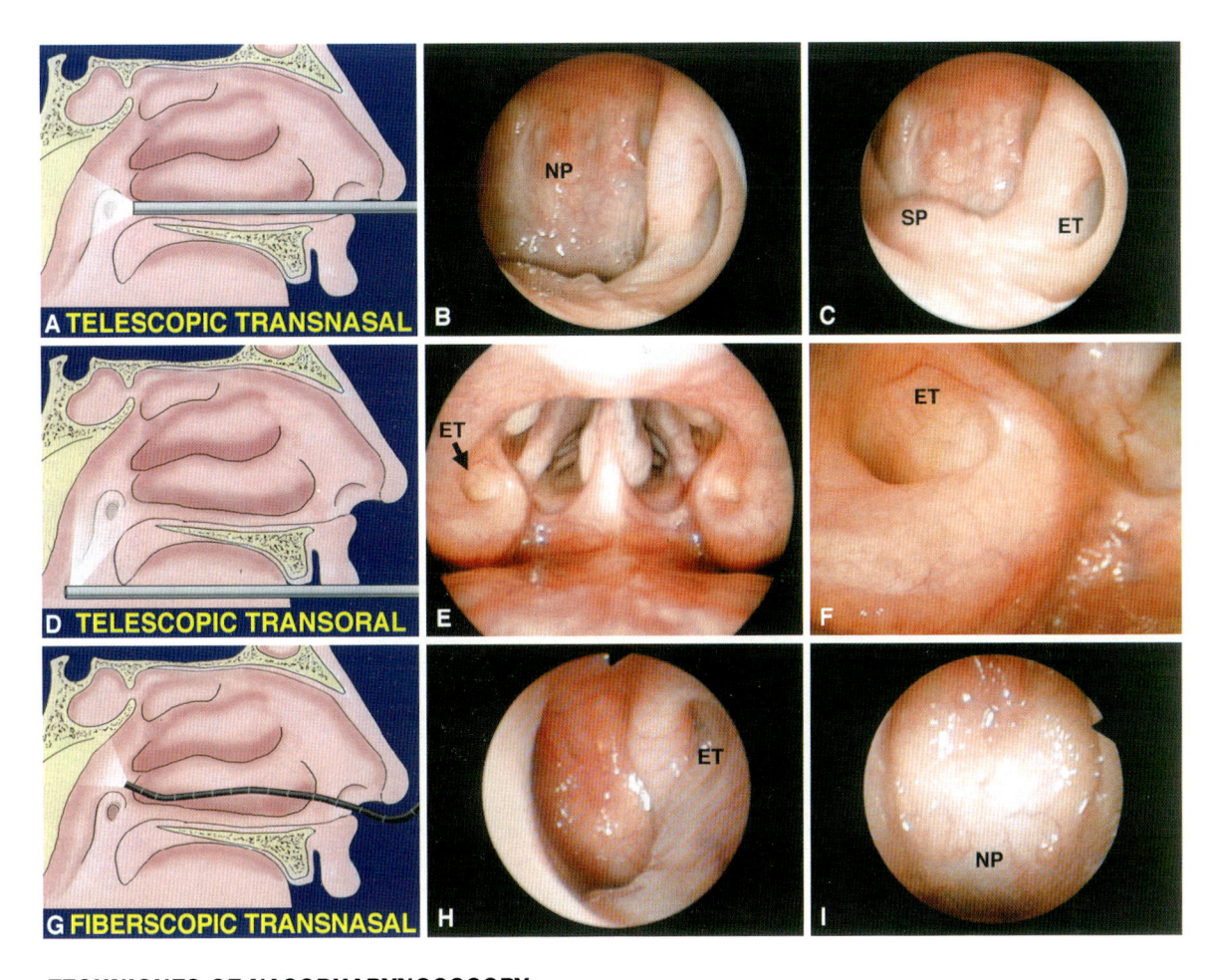

TECHNIQUES OF NASOPHARYNGOSCOPY

Figure 7-3. *Top row:* Transnasal telescopic nasopharyngoscopy. After the nasal turbinates are decongested and topically anesthetized, a 0-, 30-, or 70-degree telescope (4 mm for adults, 2.7 mm for children) is passed into the nasal cavity between the inferior turbinate and the nasal septum toward the nasopharynx. The anatomical structures and pathological conditions of the nasopharynx are then examined. The eustachian tube orifice and the nasopharynx are examined during phonation and swallowing. Figure 7-3B shows the eustachian tube orifice on phonation "M," while Figure 7-3C shows the same eustachian tube orifice on phonation "K." *Middle row:* Transoral telescopic nasopharyngoscopy. The posterior oropharynx is first sprayed with a topical anesthetic. Then a 90- or 120-degree telescope is passed into the oral cavity and carefully placed behind the soft palate. The anatomical structures and pathological conditions of the nasopharynx are then examined. It may become necessary to use the soft palate retractor. In such an event, the posterior aspect of the soft palate must be anesthetized both through the nasal cavity from above and through the oral cavity from below. While the specially designed nasopharyngoscope can be used, a standard 90- or 120-degree Karl Storz telescope can also be used with the distal lens turned upward. Figure 7-3E shows the panoramic view of the nasopharynx as seen from below. Posterior structures of the nasal cavity, eustachian tube orifices, tori tubarii, Rosenmüller's fossae, and the posterior wall of the nasopharynx are well visualized. Figure 7-3F shows a closer view of the eustachian tube orifice on the right side. *Bottom row:* Transnasal fiberscopic nasopharyngoscopy. In case telescopic examinations cannot be performed due to either anatomical reasons or a hyperactive gag reflex, the nasopharynx can be examined using a flexible fiberscope. The fiberscopic examination, however, produces images that are less clear and more distorted than the images obtained by telescopic examination due to the wide-angled lens of the fiberscope.

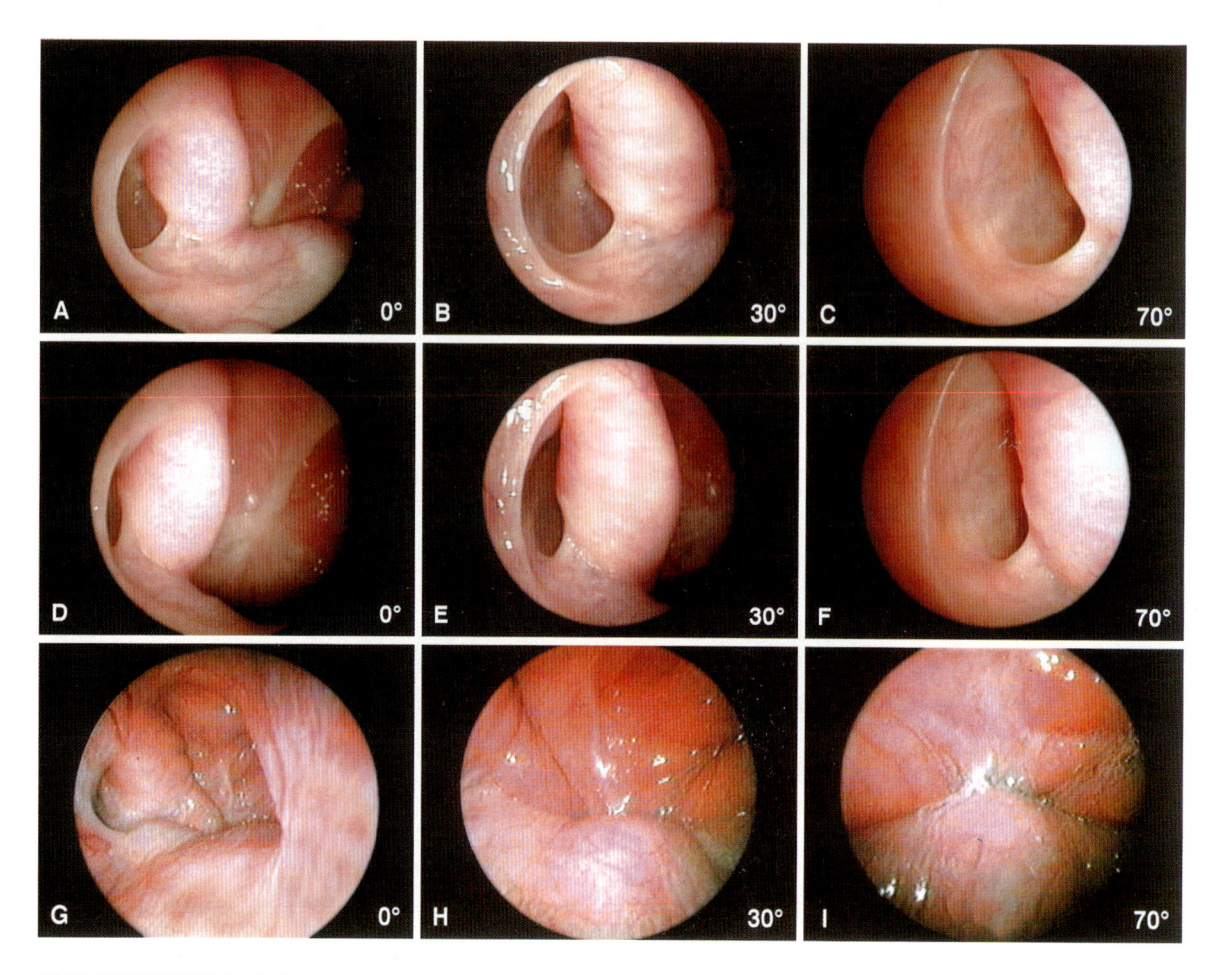

NASOPHARYNGEAL ENDOSCOPIC ANATOMY

Eustachian Tubes and Velopharyngeal Port

Figure 7-4. *Top row:* Transnasal views of the eustachian tube orifice obtained by 0-, 30-, and 70-degree telescopes. The right eustachian tube orifice opens during phonation "K," viewed with a 0-degree telescope (Figure 7-4A), a 30-degree telescope (Figure 7-4B), and a 70-degree telescope (Figure 7-4C). Although in the lateral view of the eustachian tube orifice there is a difference from patient to patient, the best view of the lumen of the eustachian tube orifice is obtained by the 30-degree telescope in the majority of cases. *Middle row:* Transnasal views of the eustachian tube orifice obtained by 0-, 30-, and 70-degree telescopes. Views of the same right eustachian tube orifice as shown in the top row now during phonation "M" by a 0-degree telescope (Figure 7-4D), a 30-degree telescope (Figure 7-4E), and a 70-degree telescope (Figure 7-4F) are shown. *Bottom row:* Transnasal views of the velopharyngeal port during swallowing. Transnasal views of the velopharyngeal port (isthmus) during swallowing by a 0-degree telescope (Figure 7-4G), a 30-degree telescope (Figure 7-4H), and a 70-degree telescope (Figure 7-4I) are shown. The best view of the opening and closure of the velopharyngeal opening is obtained by a 70-degree telescope.

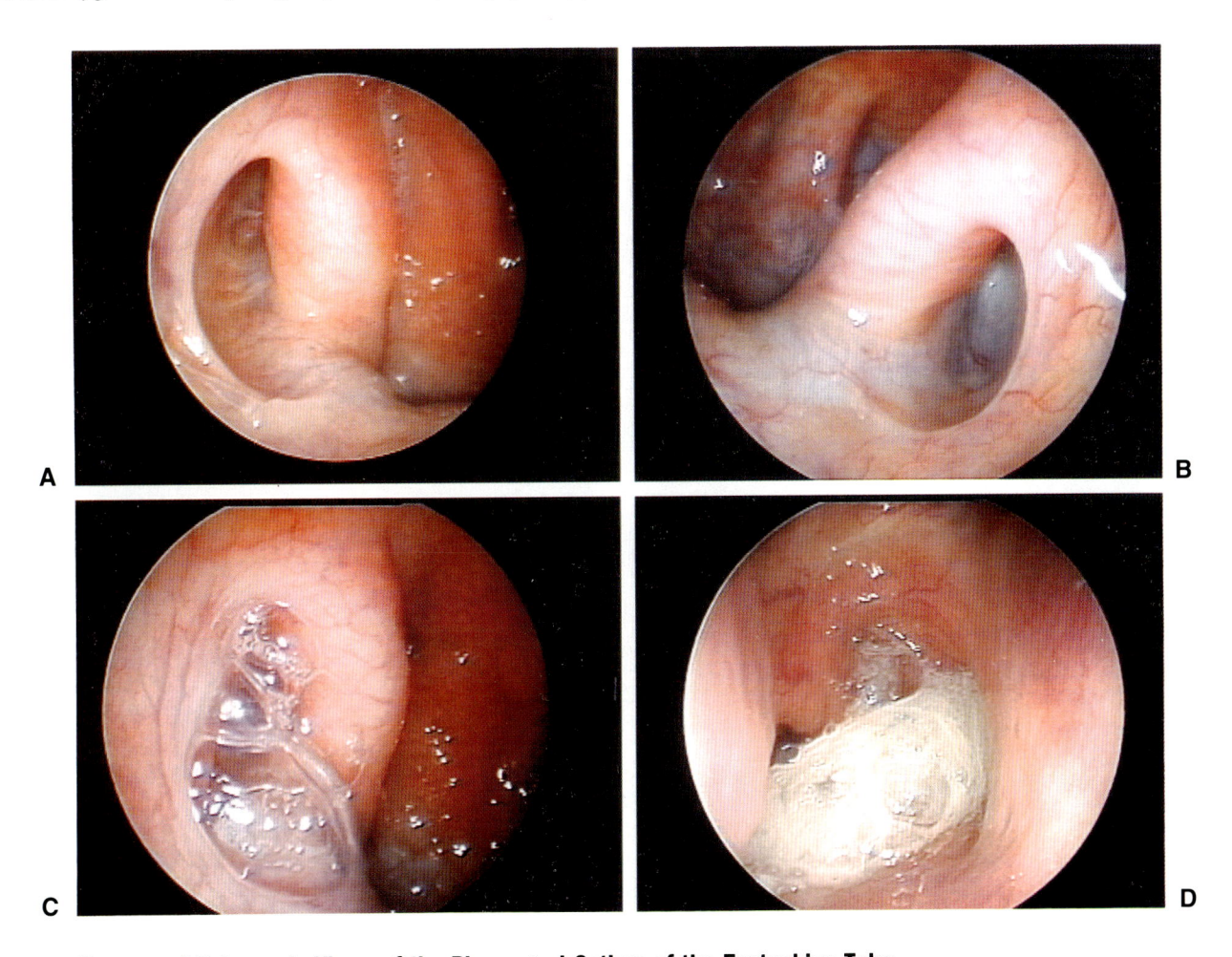

Endoscopy of the Nasopharynx (Videonasopharyngoscopy)

Transnasal Telescopic Views of the Pharyngeal Ostium of the Eustachian Tube

Figure 7-5A. Right eustachian tube orifice. The 30-degree telescopic view of the nasopharynx demonstrates the right eustachian tube orifice and lumen. Note the horizontal scar band visible within the eustachian tube lumen.

Figure 7-5B. Left eustachian tube orifice. This 30-degree telescopic view displays the normal left eustachian tube orifice and lumen.

Figure 7-5C. Right eustachian tube orifice. Air escaping from the right middle ear space through the right eustachian tube creates bubbles in the clear mucus overlying the right eustachian tube orifice.

Figure 7-5D. Left eustachian tube orifice. Mucopus from a left acute sinusitis obstructs the left eustachian tube orifice, resulting in eustachian tube dysfunction.

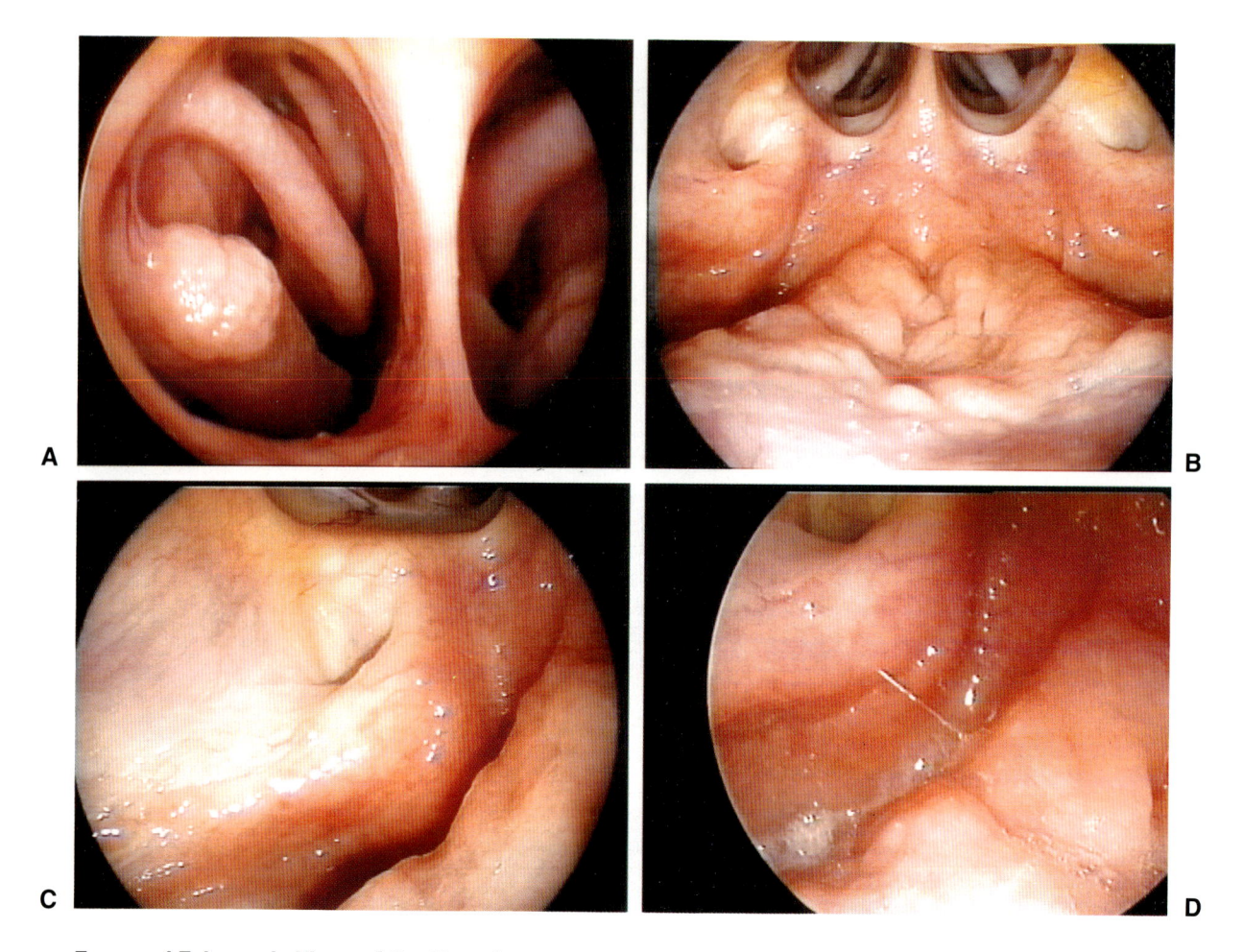

Transoral Telescopic Views of the Nasopharynx

Figure 7-6A. Turbinates. The transoral 110-degree Nagashima SFN telescope delivers an upright mirror image of the right choana displaying the superior, middle, and inferior turbinates and meatus. Note the mulberry hypertrophy of the posterior end of the inferior turbinate.

Figure 7-6B. Eustachian tube, torus tubarius, and Rosenmüller's fossa. This is a broad inverted view of the normal nasopharynx by the transoral 120-degree Karl Storz telescope. It demonstrates the roof of the nasopharynx in the middle of the view, bilateral Rosenmüller fossae, tori tubarii, and eustachian tube orifices. The superior aspect of the choanae are seen at the top of the view.

Figure 7-6C. Eustachian tube, torus tubarius, and Rosenmüller's fossa. A close-up transoral 90-degree Karl Storz telescopic view shows the right eustachian tube orifice, the torus tubarius, and Rosenmüller's fossa, which appears as a deep crevice.

Figure 7-6D. Rosenmüller's fossa. A closer view with the transoral 90-degree telescope demonstrates the floor of the right Rosenmüller's fossa with the right eustachian tube orifice seen in the upper left aspect of this view.

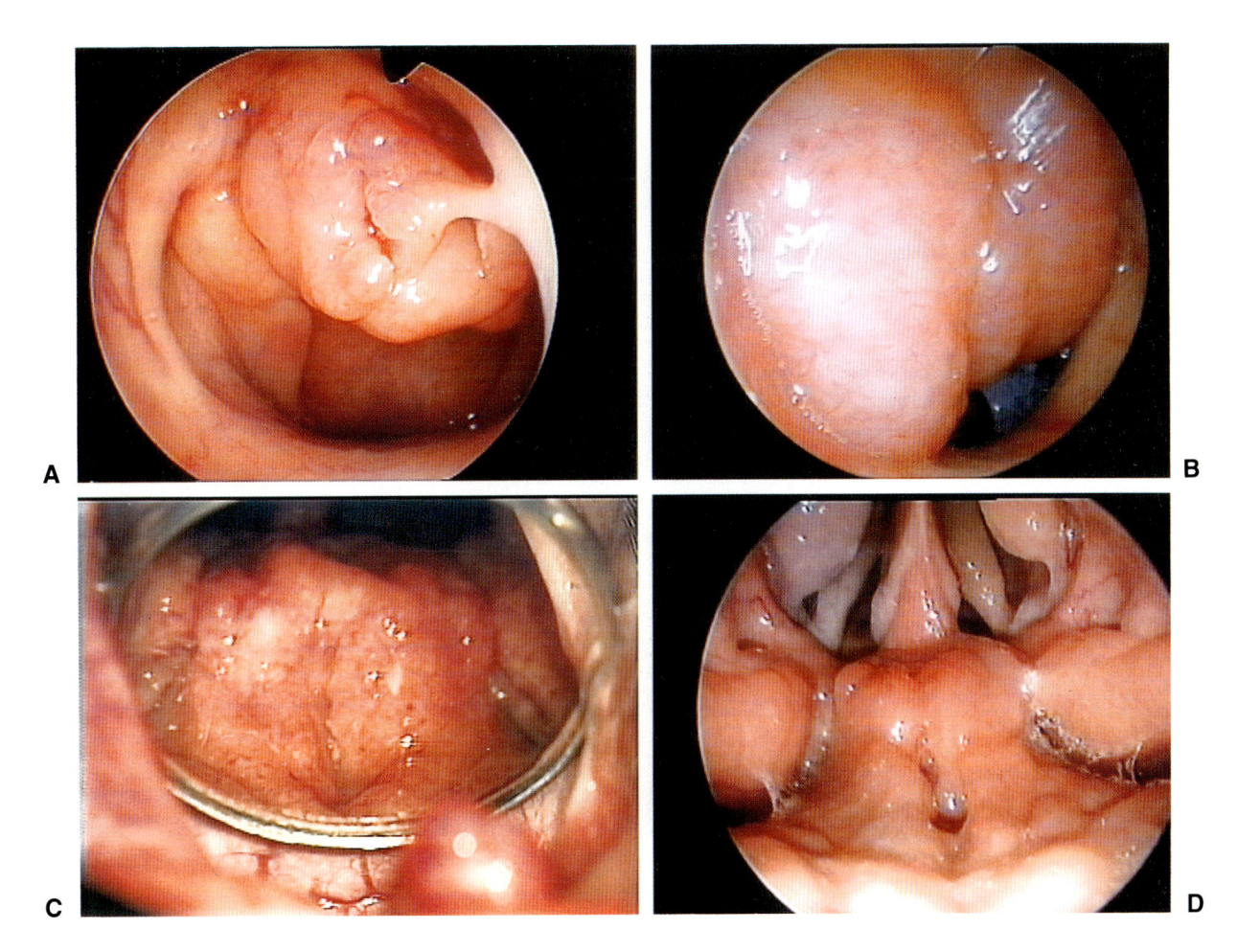

Endoscopy of the Nasopharynx (Videonasopharyngoscopy)

Examination of the Adenoids

Figure 7-7A. Transnasal telescopic examination of adenoids. This patient complained of obstructed nasal breathing after undergoing adenoidectomy. This transnasal 0-degree telescopic examination demonstrates residual adenoid tissue arising from the right superior nasopharynx with a scar band to the posterior nasal septum.

Figure 7-7B. Transnasal telescopic examination of adenoids. This huge adenoid nearly completely obstructs the left nasal passage as it projects into the left choana, seen through the transnasal 0-degree telescope.

Figure 7-7C. Transoral microscopic mirror examination of adenoids. This large adenoid pad partially obstructs the choanae as seen in this common mirror view of the adenoids. The uvula is seen at the bottom of the view. The right choana and the vomer are seen at the top of the mirror view, and the pharyngeal bursa is visible at the bottom of the mirror view.

Figure 7-7D. Transoral telescopic examination of adenoids. The transoral 90-degree telescopic view widely displays the nasopharynx with the moderate-sized adenoid in the center of the view. The middle and superior turbinates are clearly seen through the unobstructed choanae. The eustachian tube orifices, tori tubarii, and Rosenmüller's fossae are visible laterally.

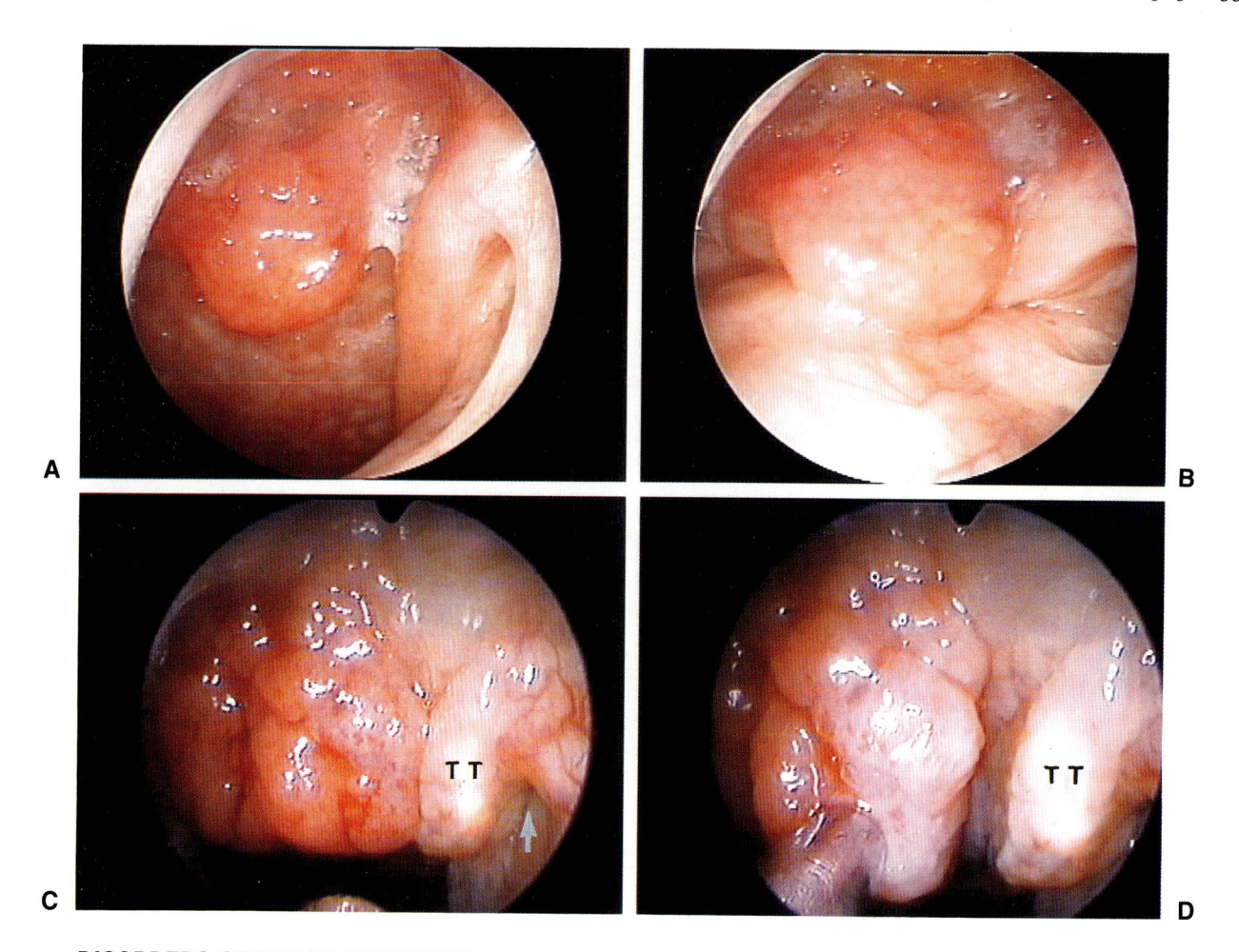

DISORDERS OF THE NASOPHARYNX

Hypertrophied Adenoids

Figure 7-8A. Adenoid before swallowing. The transnasal 0-degree telescopic examination just before swallowing reveals a medium-sized adenoid mass extending inferiorly to the level of the soft palate. A similar view is obtained on phonation "M." Note that the soft palate descends, opening the velopharyngeal port. The left torus tubarius and eustachian tube orifice are seen laterally, and the soft palate is visible at the bottom right edge of this view.

Figure 7-8B. Adenoid on swallowing. On swallowing, the adenoid shown in Figure 7-8A now rests on the elevated posterior soft palate. A similar view is obtained on phonation "K." Note also the opening of the left eustachian tube.

Figure 7-8C. Torus tubarius in adenoiditis. The torus tubarius (TT) can be difficult to distinguish from inflamed hypertophic adenoid, as is the case with this left torus tubarius on transnasal 0-degree telescopic examination. The arrow points to the eustachian tube orifice.

Figure 7-8D. Torus tubarius in adenoiditis. Retraction of the hypertrophic adenoid medially distinguishes the torus tubarious (TT) from the adenoid. This technique is useful during adenoidectomy to avoid injury to the torus tubarius.

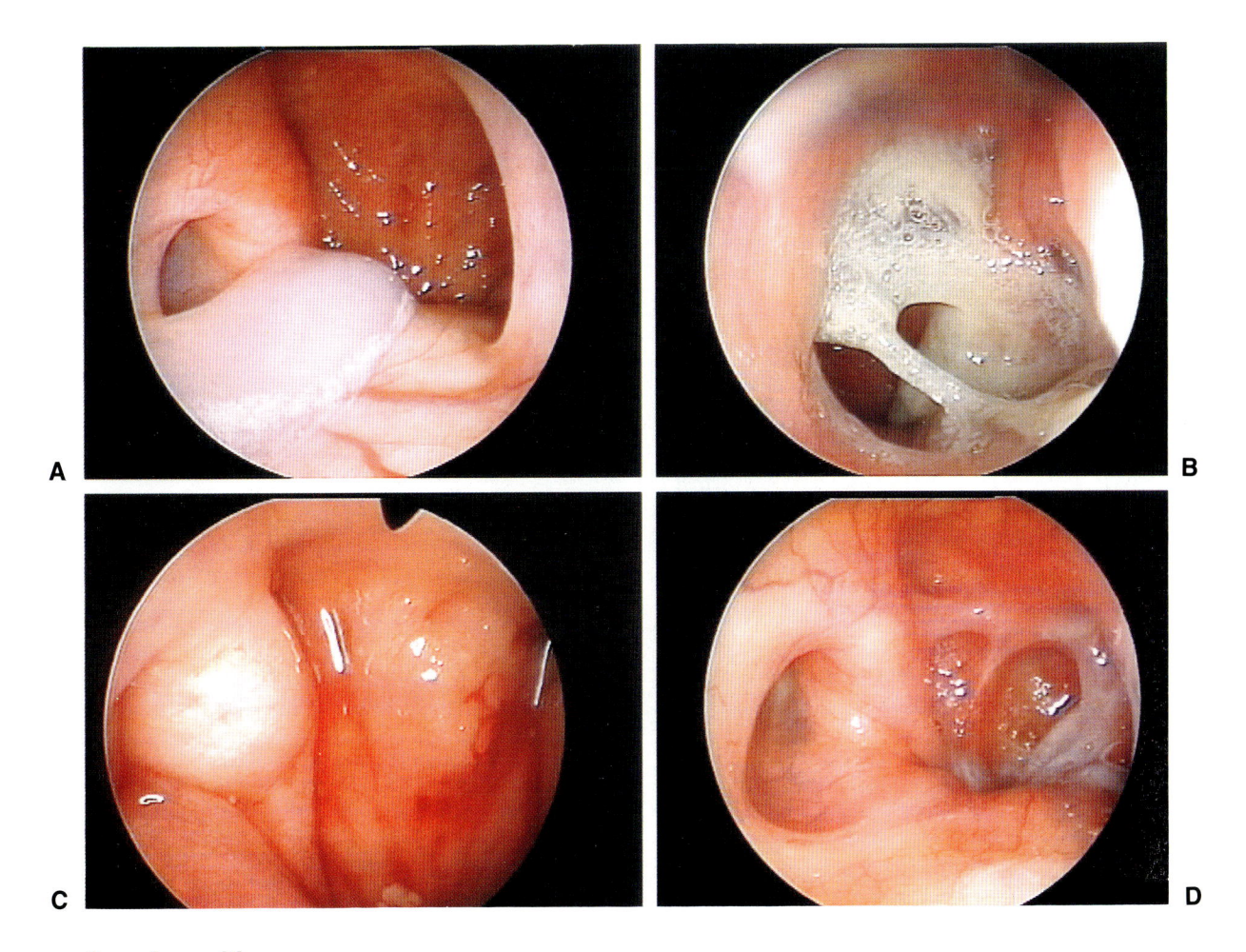

Endoscopy of the Nasopharynx (Videonasopharyngoscopy)

Nasopharyngitis

Figure 7-9A. Acute nasopharyngitis. This patient suffered from acute right maxillary sinusitis, which caused postnasal drip and right eustachian tube dysfunction. The transnasal 0-degree telescopic exam reveals a stream of mucopus flowing posteriorly, partially obstructing the right eustachian tube orifice and causing postnasal drip. Note also the inflamed posterior nasopharyngeal wall.

Figure 7-9B. Acute nasopharyngitis. Acute left maxillary sinusitis and nasopharyngitis produced adherent nasopharyngeal mucopus, causing a muffled hyponasal voice and left eustachian tube dysfunction. This transnasal 0-degree telescopic exam demonstrates the partial left choana and eustachian tube orifice obstruction with mucopus.

Figure 7-9C. Chronic nasopharyngitis. The marked edema of this patient's right torus tubarius and posterior nasopharyngeal wall, seen on transnasal 0-degree telescopic exam, obstructed the right eustachian tube (*left edge of view*), causing dysfunction and persistent serous otitis media.

Figure 7-9D. Postadenoidectomy scarring of the nasopharynx causing a patulous eustachian tube. The fibrous bands and scarred tissues of the nasopharynx due to adenoidectomy and recurrent nasopharyngitis produced a right patulous eustachian tube and autophonia. Note the widely patent right eustachian tube orifice.

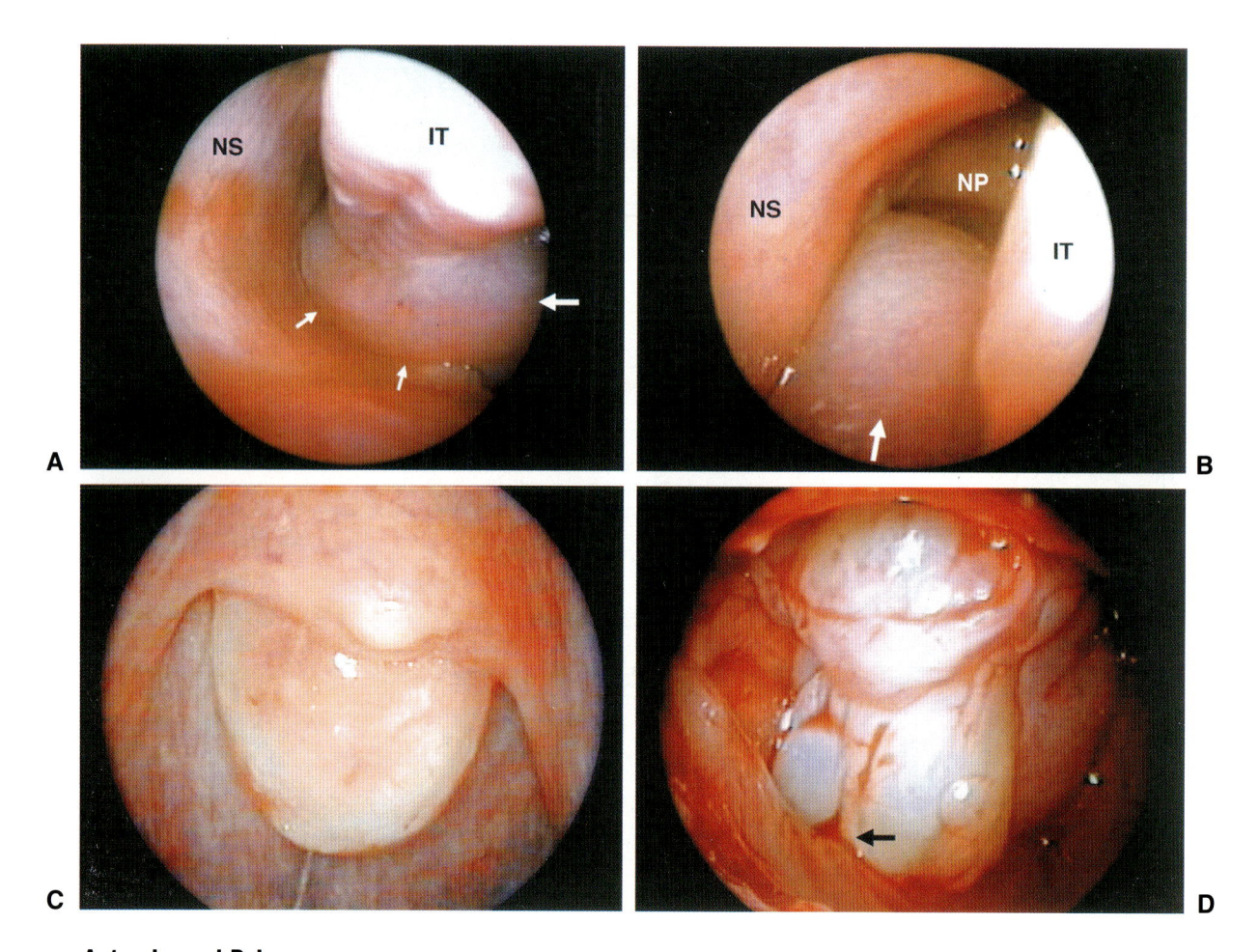

Antrochoanal Polyp

Figure 7-10A. Antrochoanal polyp. This patient presented with difficult nasal breathing and an oropharyngeal foreign body sensation 8 years after a nasal polypectomy and antrostomy. Transnasal 0-degree telescopic exam of the left nasal cavity floor demonstrates a large intranasal mass (*small arrows*) below the inferior turbinate (IT), emanating from the old inferior meatus antrostomy window (*large arrow*).

Figure 7-10B. Antrochoanal polyp. Posterior left nasal cavity 0-degree telescopic exam of the same patient reveals the intranasal mass (*arrow*) extending through the left choana into the nasopharynx (NP).

Figure 7-10C. Antrochoanal polyp. The large antrochoanal polyp of this patient extended through the nasopharynx all the way down to the oropharynx, seen here on transoral 0-degree telescopic examination.

Figure 7-10D. Antrochoanal polyp. The intra-antral view via the Caldwell–Luc approach reveals a large polypoid mass nearly filling the left maxillary sinus, originating from the antral roof and extending out the old inferior antrostomy (*arrow*). The intra-antral mass was incised at the superior base and its inferior end and removed via the Caldwell–Luc opening. The oropharyngeal mass was grasped and removed through the mouth. In this case the Caldwell–Luc approach allowed a safe and precise excision of this antrochoanal polyp.

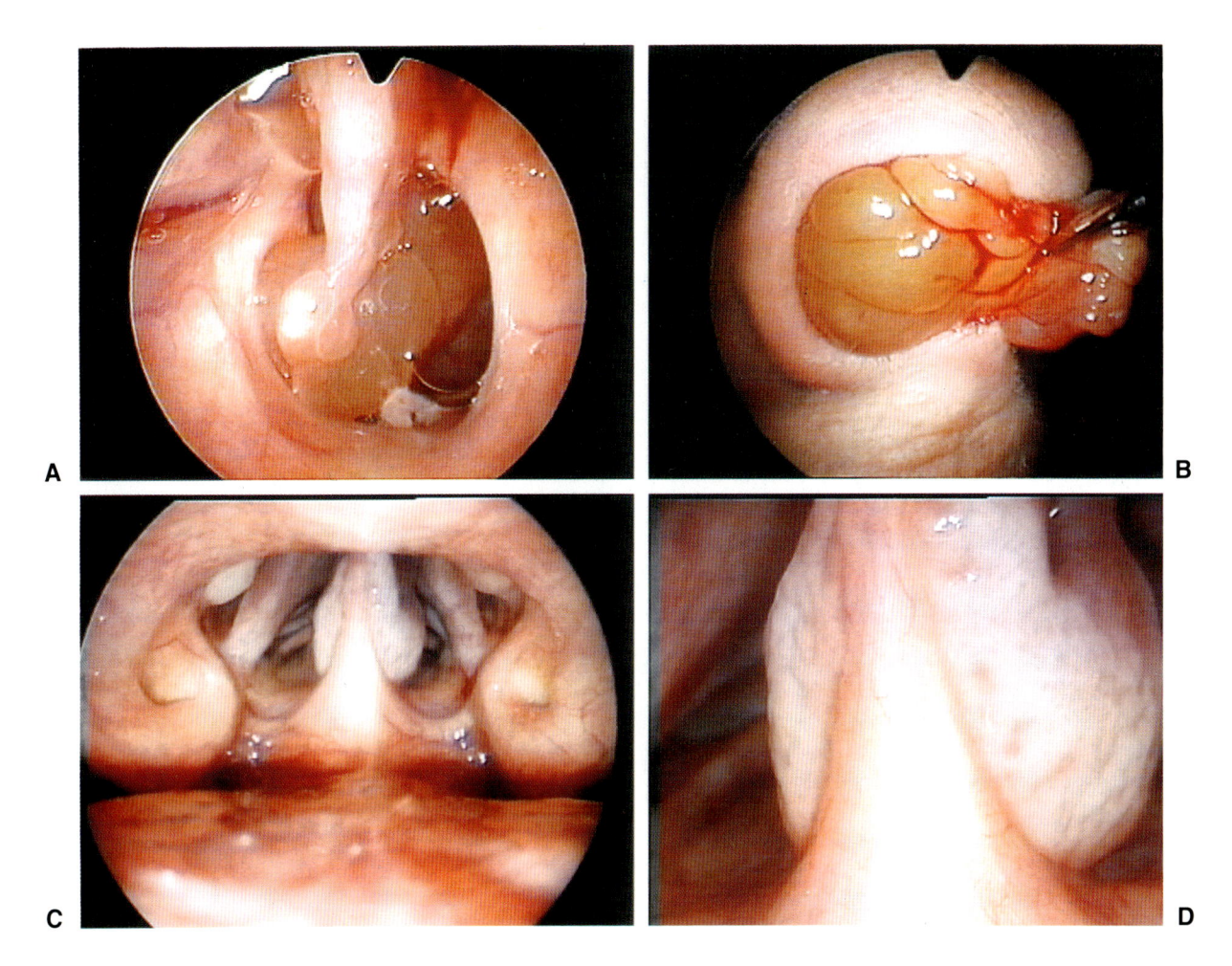

Choanal Polyp

Figure 7-11A. Choanal polyp. This transnasal 0-degree telescopic view reveals a large right choanal polyp stemming from the posterior middle turbinate and extending posteriorly into the nasopharynx.

Figure 7-11B. Choanal polyp. This polyp was removed with a transnasal snare, seen here exiting the right nostril.

Posterior Nasal Septal Hypertrophy

Figure 7-11C. Posterior nasal septal hypertrophy. The marked mucosal swelling of the posterior nasal septum on both sides is seen in the choanae of this transoral 90-degree telescopic examination of the nasopharynx. Some other terms used for this common structure include posterior tuberculum of the nasal septum, septal wings, adenomatoid hamartomas, and adenovascular body. The posterior edges of the inferior and middle turbinates are seen as well as the eustachian tube orifices, tori tubarii, and Rosenmüller's fossae.

Figure 7-11D. Posterior nasal septal hypertrophy. The posterior septal mucosal change is highlighted in this close-up view via the transoral 90-degree telescope.

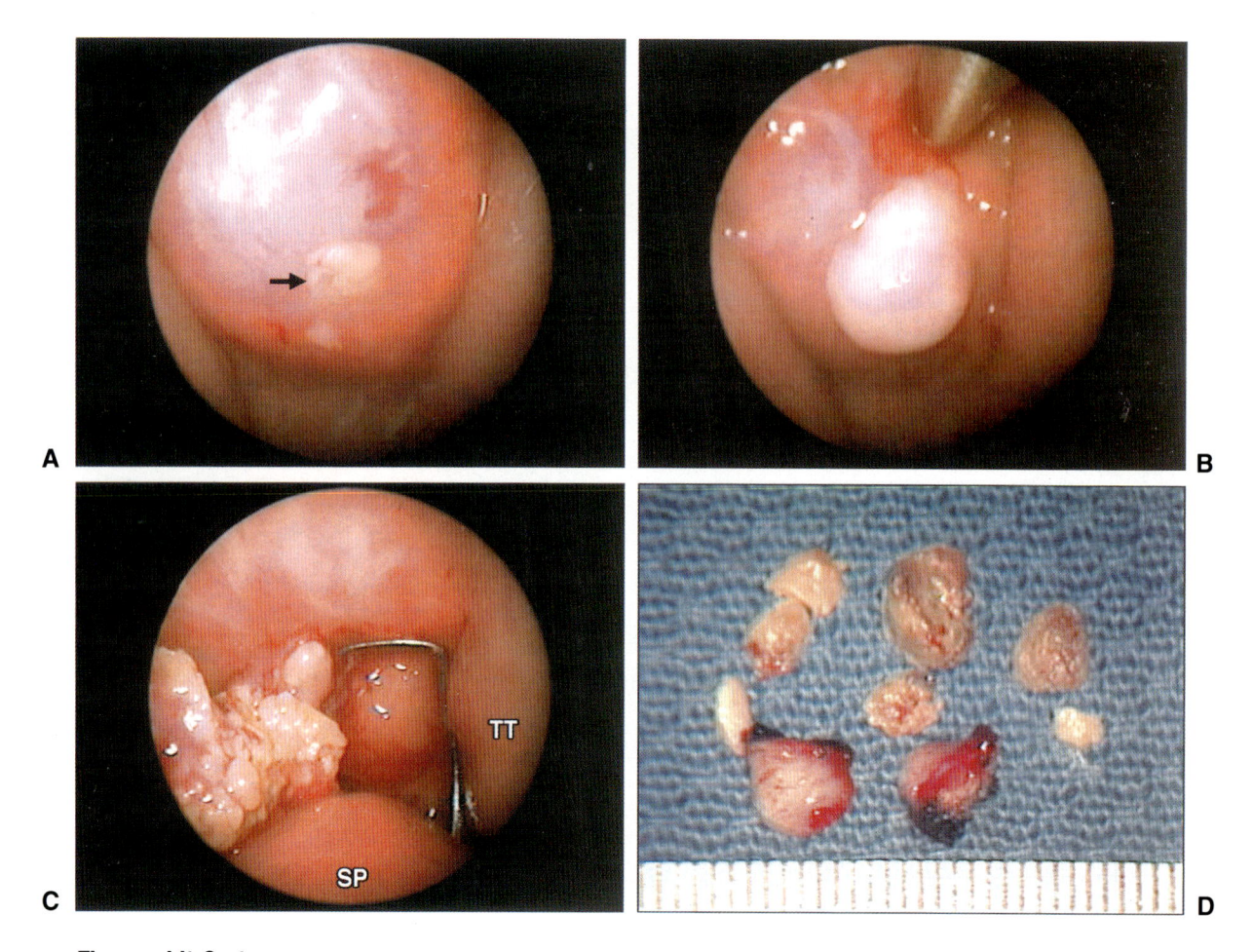

Thornwaldt Cyst

Figure 7-12A. Thornwaldt cyst. This patient complained of nasal obstruction, postnasal discharge, throat discomfort, and intermittent throat pain. This transnasal 0-degree telescopic exam of the nasopharynx reveals a large Thornwaldt cyst on the posterior wall. The cyst was covered with smooth mucosa and had a small central punctum (*arrow*).

Figure 7-12B. Thornwaldt cyst. Gentle compression on the cyst produced purulent drainage from the midline cyst opening as seen on this transnasal 0-degree telescopic view.

Figure 7-12C. Thornwaldt cyst. Firm compression on the cyst produced a cheesy discharge from the cyst opening, seen here on a transnasal 30-degree telescopic view. The cyst was widely marsupialized with no recurrence.

Figure 7-12D. Abundant material was removed from the Thornwaldt cyst.

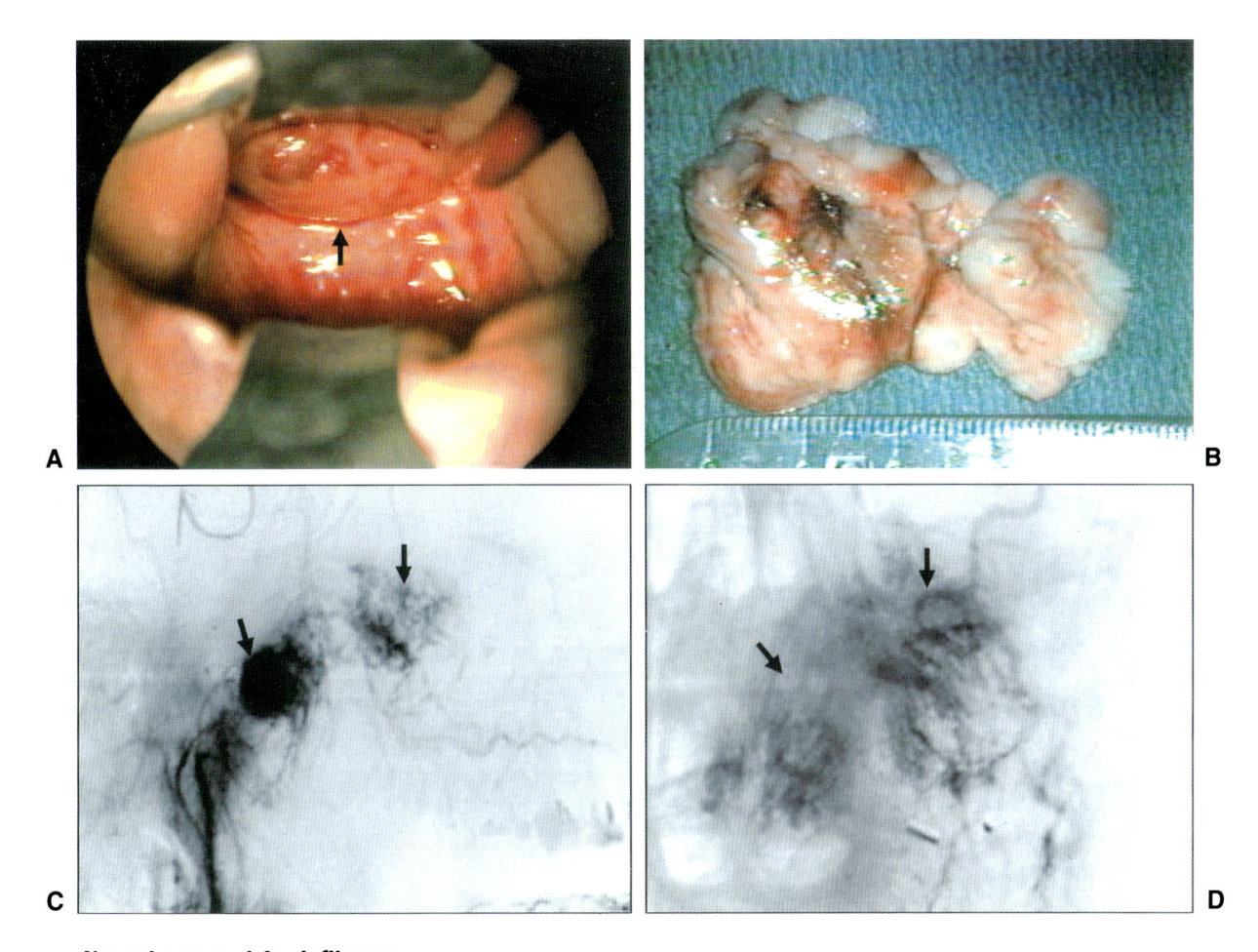

Nasopharyngeal Angiofibroma

Figure 7-13A. Nasopharyngeal angiofibroma. The transoral microscopic upright view of the oropharynx and nasophyarynx demonstrates the inferior aspect of the nasopharyngeal mass (*arrow*). The soft palate was retracted superiorly, thereby revealing the mass; the tongue was retracted inferiorly.

Figure 7-13B. Nasopharyngeal angiofibroma. The complete 4.5-cm surgical specimen had two lobes. The larger left lobe was in the left nasopharynx with the visible inferior edge at the bottom left of this picture. The smaller right lobe was in the left pterygomaxillary space.

Figure 7-13C. Nasopharyngeal angiofibroma. This preoperative lateral view angiogram demonstrates the vascular nature of this mass. Note here two lobes, the more prominent nasopharyngeal portion (*left arrow*) and the less prominent pterygomaxillary space portion (*right arrow*).

Figure 7-13D. Nasopharyngeal angiofibroma. The preoperative anteroposterior view angiogram also demonstrates both the left nasopharyngeal portion (*left arrow*) and the left pterygomaxillary space portion (*right arrow*). The nasal cavity and nasal septum are faintly visible.

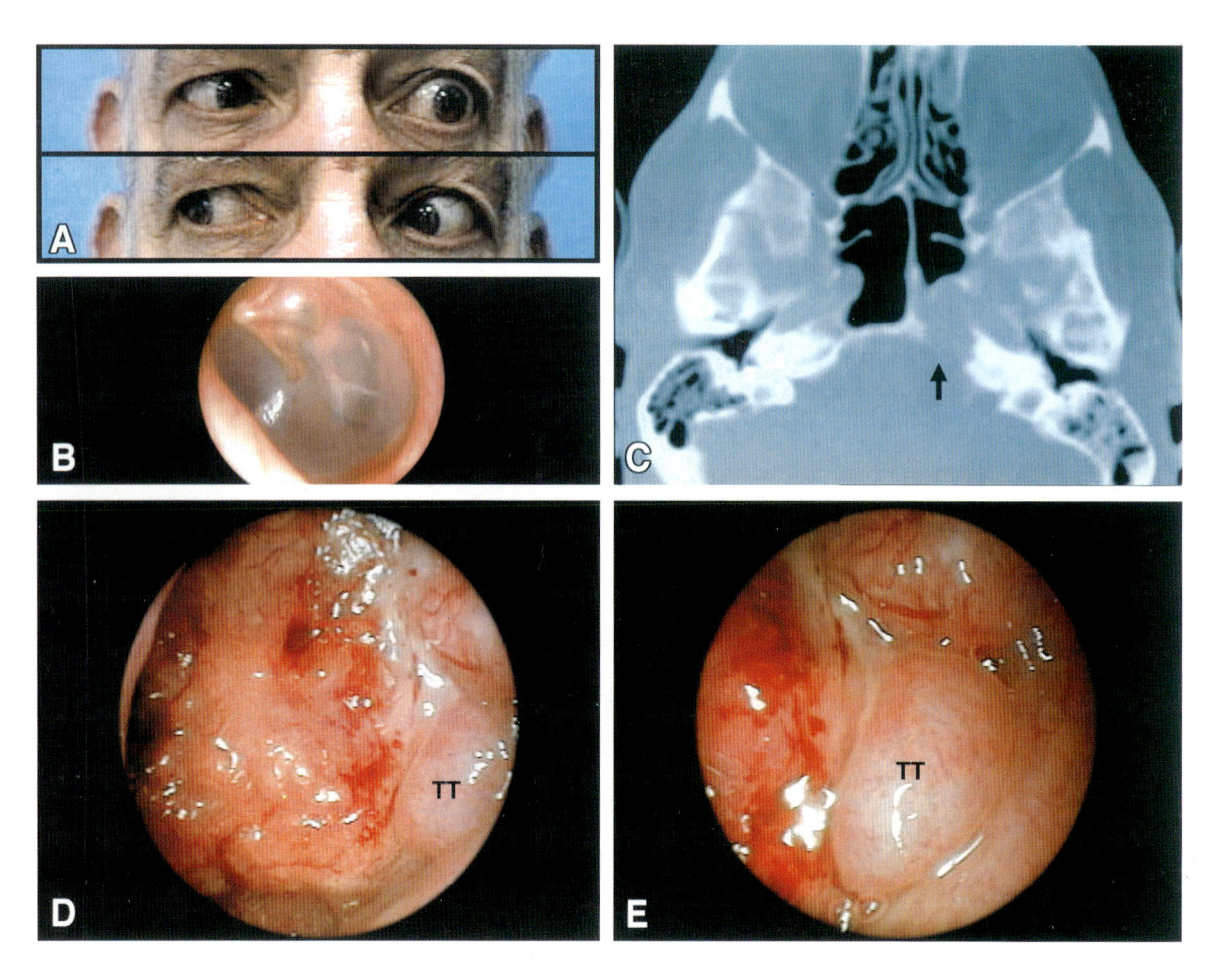

Nasopharyngeal Carcinoma

Figure 7-14A. Abducens palsy caused by nasopharyngeal carcinoma. This patient presented with complaints of recurrent left epistaxis, double vision on left gaze, progressive temporal and occipital headaches, left hearing loss, and obstructed left nasal breathing. Extraocular examination demonstrated his left CN VI palsy.

Figure 7-14B. Serous otitis media caused by nasopharyngeal carcinoma. Transaural 0-degree telescopy of the left ear demonstrates a left serous otitis media.

Figure 7-14C. Nasopharyngeal carcinoma. The axial CT scan bone window reveals a large soft tissue mass from the posterior nasopharynx extending up into the left posterior sphenoid sinus and eroding the left clivus (*arrow*).

Figure 7-14D. Nasopharyngeal carcinoma. Transnasal 0-degree telescopic exam of the naspharynx demonstrates the large exophytic tumor involving the entire nasopharynx and extending superiorly toward the sphenoid sinus. The left torus tubarius (TT) was displaced laterally. Standard treatment for this cancer consists of radiotherapy with or without chemotherapy.

Figure 7-14E. Nasopharyngeal carcinoma. A close-up view of the left torus tubarius through the transnasal 30-degree telescope shows that it was markedly swollen and displaced laterally, completely obstructing the left eustachian tube and causing this patient's left serous otitis media. The prognosis for this patient was poor.

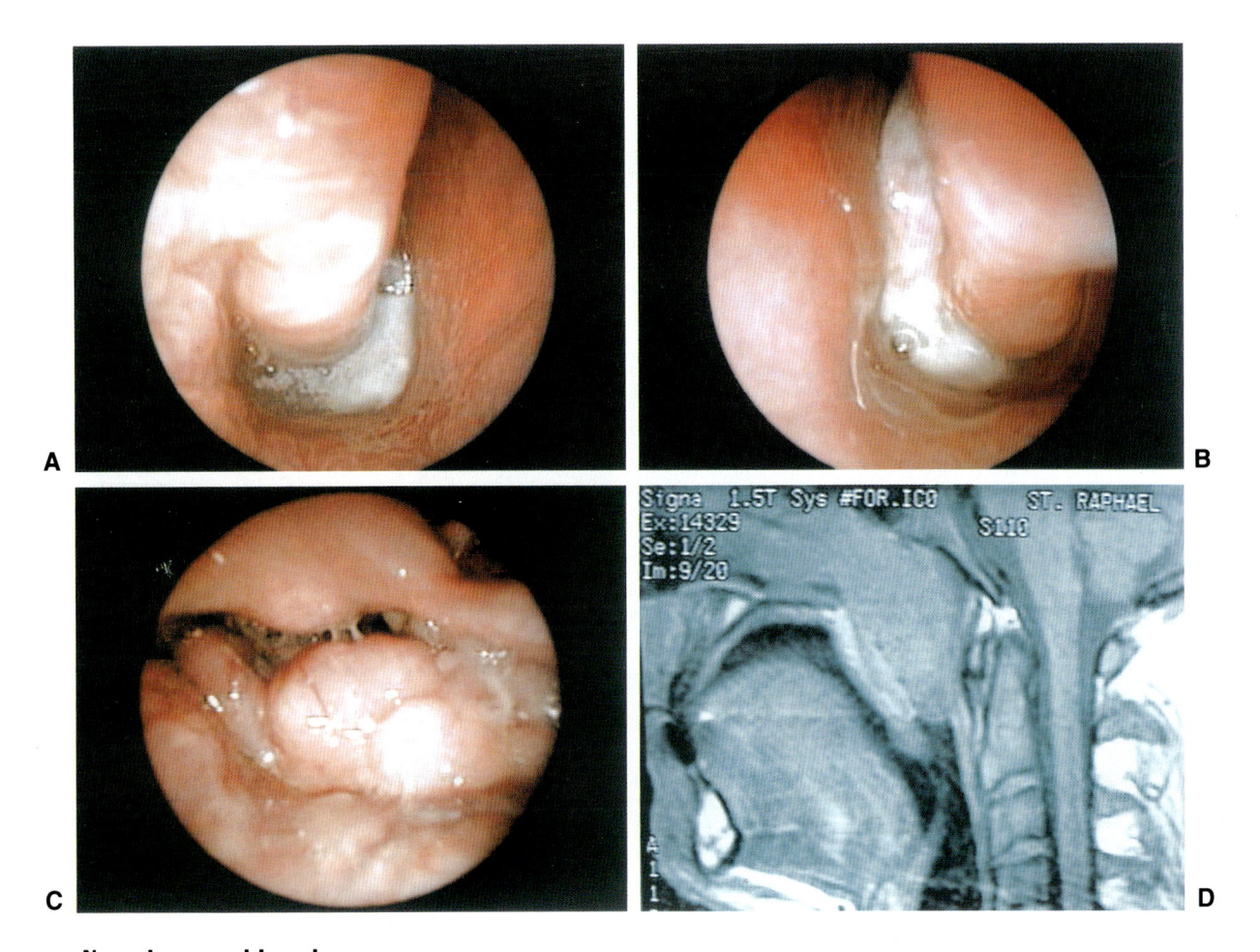

Nasopharyngeal Lymphoma

Figure 7-15A. Nasopharyngeal lymphoma. This patient presented with a complaint of nasal obstruction refractory to antibiotics and steroids. Transnasal 0-degree telescopy demonstrates right choanal obstruction.

Figure 7-15B. Nasopharyngeal lymphoma. Transnasal 0-degree telescopy demonstrates left choanal obstruction with extension of the tumor into the posterior nasal cavity.

Figure 7-15C. Nasopharyngeal lymphoma. This transoral 120-degree telescopic view shows a large irregular mass stemming from the posterior wall of the nasopharynx and almost completely obstructing the nasopharynx. Only a slit of choana was visible anterior to the mass. The uvula and soft palate are seen anteriorly (*top of view*).

Figure 7-15D. MRI of nasopharyngeal lymphoma. Sagittal T1-weighted MRI images reveal a large mass completely obliterating the nasopharynx and choanae, extending into the posterior nasal cavity. This patient was successfully treated with external beam radiotherapy and combination chemotherapy.

Chapter 8
Endoscopy of the Oropharynx (Videopharyngoscopy)*

Pharyngoscopy is the examination of the oropharynx using a transoral rigid telescope. When pharyngoscopic findings are documented with a video camera, the procedure is called *videopharyngoscopy*.

This technique provides a method of detailed examination and documentation of oropharyngeal anatomy and pathology. Important structures include the soft palate, uvula, anterior and posterior pillars, palatine tonsils, posterior wall of the oropharynx, and posterior tongue. Common pathologic conditions include tonsillar hypertrophy, tonsillitis, neoplasm, trauma, foreign body, and surgical changes.

Equipment needed for pharyngoscopy includes (1) 0-, 90-, and 120-degree rigid telescopes (4.0, 5.8, and/or 10 mm), (2) light source, and (3) oral topical anesthesia. Videopharyngoscopy also requires (1) video camera, (2) video recorder, (3) video monitor, and (4) video printer.

Pharyngoscopy provides unique views of the oropharynx, detailing anatomy and pathology that can go unappreciated on the standard oropharyngeal exam. Videopharyngoscopy can record these findings for treatment planning, pre- and postoperative comparisons, patient and student education, and medical records.

* This chapter was written in collaboration with Edward M. Weaver, M.D.

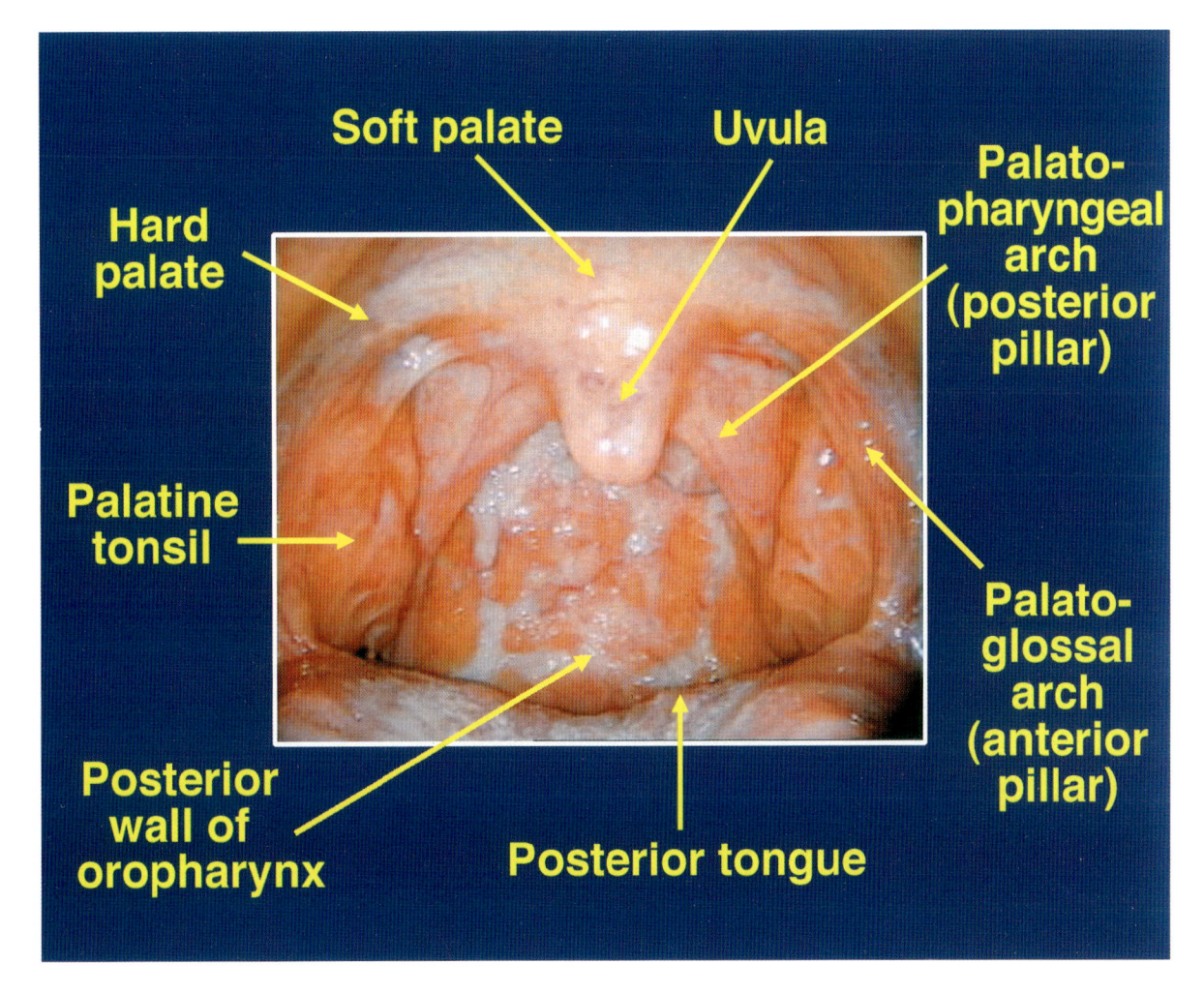

OVERVIEW OF OROPHARYNGEAL ANATOMY

Figure 8-1. Transoral 0-degree telescopic view of the oropharynx. The 10-mm 0-degree transoral telescopic exam of the normal oropharynx demonstrates most of the key structures of the pharynx including the posterior pharynegeal wall, palatine tonsils, soft palate, uvula, palatopharyngeal arch (posterior pillar), and palatoglossal arch (anterior pillar).

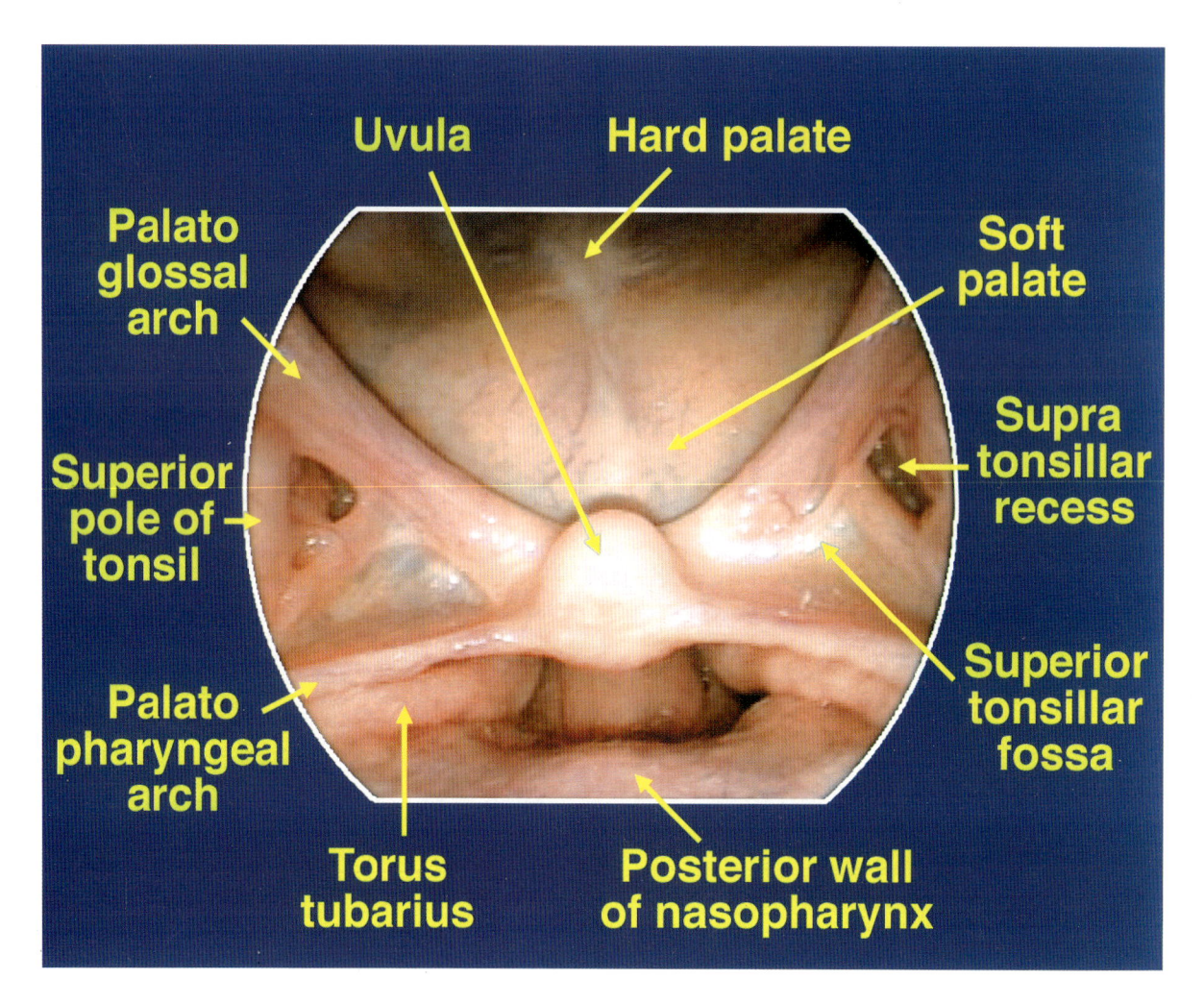

Figure 8-2. Transoral 120-degree telescopic view of the oropharynx. The 5.8-mm 120-degree transoral telescopic exam of the superior oropharynx provides a different perspective of the oropharyngeal structures. The velopharyngeal isthmus is the narrow portion of the pharynx behind the soft palate. It is not seen on 0-degree transoral telescopy but is shown in this view. The relationship between the soft palate, the anterior pillars (palatoglossal arches), the posterior pillars (palatopharyngeal arches), the velopharyngeal port, and the nasopharynx is also well-depicted in this telescopic view. The superior portion of the tonsillar fossa (superior tonsillar fossa) is clearly demonstrated here as well as on 90-degree transoral pharyngoscopy. Unique to this view are the supratonsillar recesses (the deep recesses in the superior tonsillar fossae) which extend over and lateral to the tonsil.

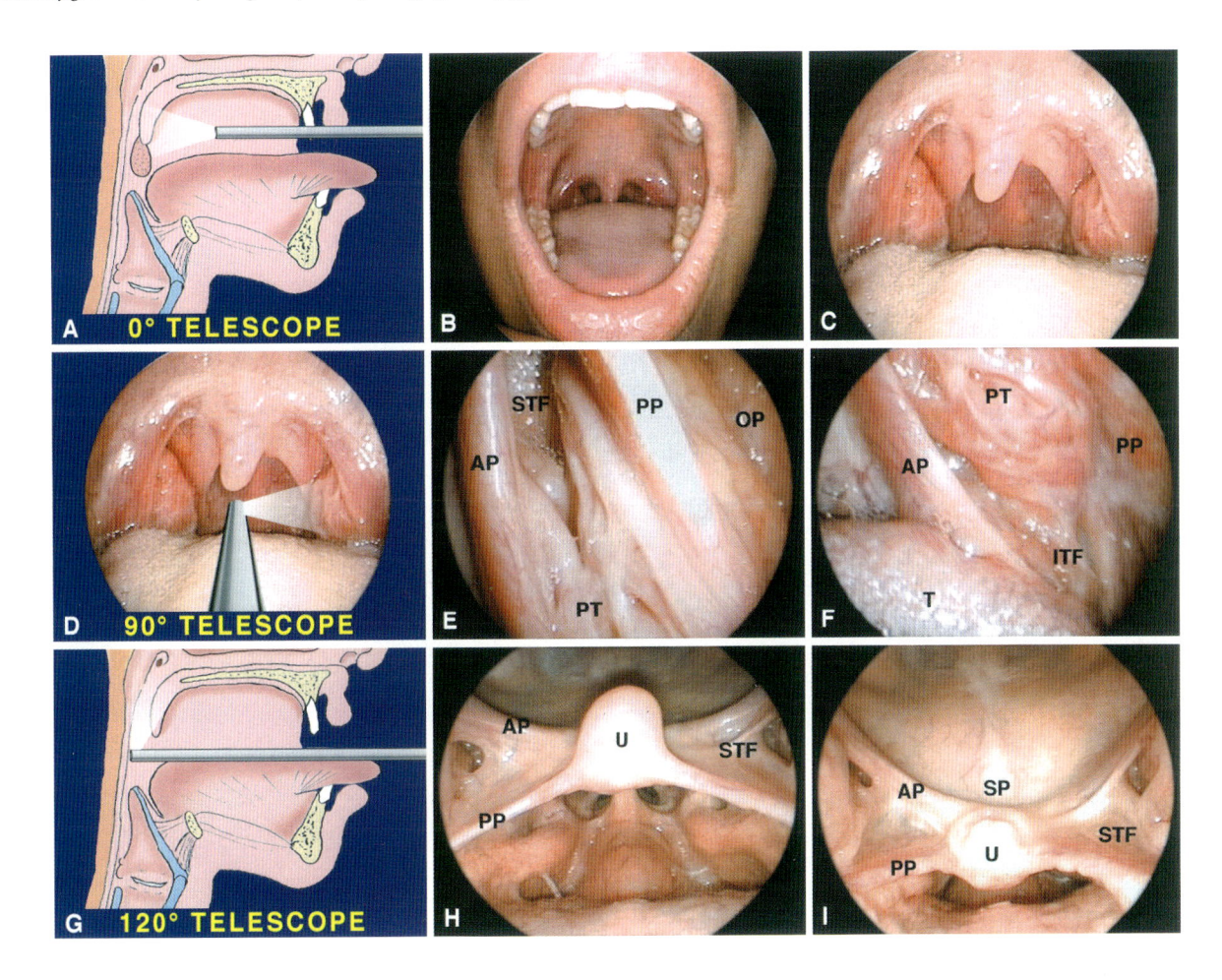

Endoscopy of the Oropharynx (Videopharyngoscopy) 105

TECHNIQUES OF PHARYNGOSCOPY

Figure 8-3. *Top row:* Zero-degree transoral pharyngoscopy. After the oropharynx is topically anesthetized, the 0-degree wide-angle telescope is passed into the oral cavity back to the oropharynx. The wide-angle lens provides a deep field of focus (Figure 8-3B). *Middle row:* 90-degree transoral pharyngoscopy. The 90-degree telescope yields a different perspective of the oropharynx. With the lens directed superiorly, one views the nasopharynx. With it directed inferiorly, the telescope displays the hypopharynx. The lens can be directed laterally to view (Figure 8-3D), for example, the medial aspect of the tonsil and the whole tonsillar fossa. Figure 8-3E shows the right anterior and posterior pillars (AP and PP) with the palatine tonsil (PT) lying between them and the superior tonsillar fossa (STF) above the tonsil. The lateral oropharyngeal wall (OP) is also in view. Figure 8-3F shows the right inferior tonsillar fossa (ITF) between the anterior and posterior pillars (AP and PP) and below the tonsil (PT). The tongue (T) is visible. *Bottom row:* 120-degree transoral pharyngoscopy. This telescope offers a unique view of pharyngeal structures. When directed anterosuperiorly the uvula (U), posterior pillars (PP), anterior pillars (AP), and superior tonsillar fossae (STF) come into clear view (Figures 8-3H and 8-3I). In Figure 8-3H the uvula (U) rests anteriorly, leaving a clear view of the nasopharynx. In Figure 8-3I the patient is saying "eeee," which moves the soft palate (SP) posteriorly and pulls the uvula (U) up.

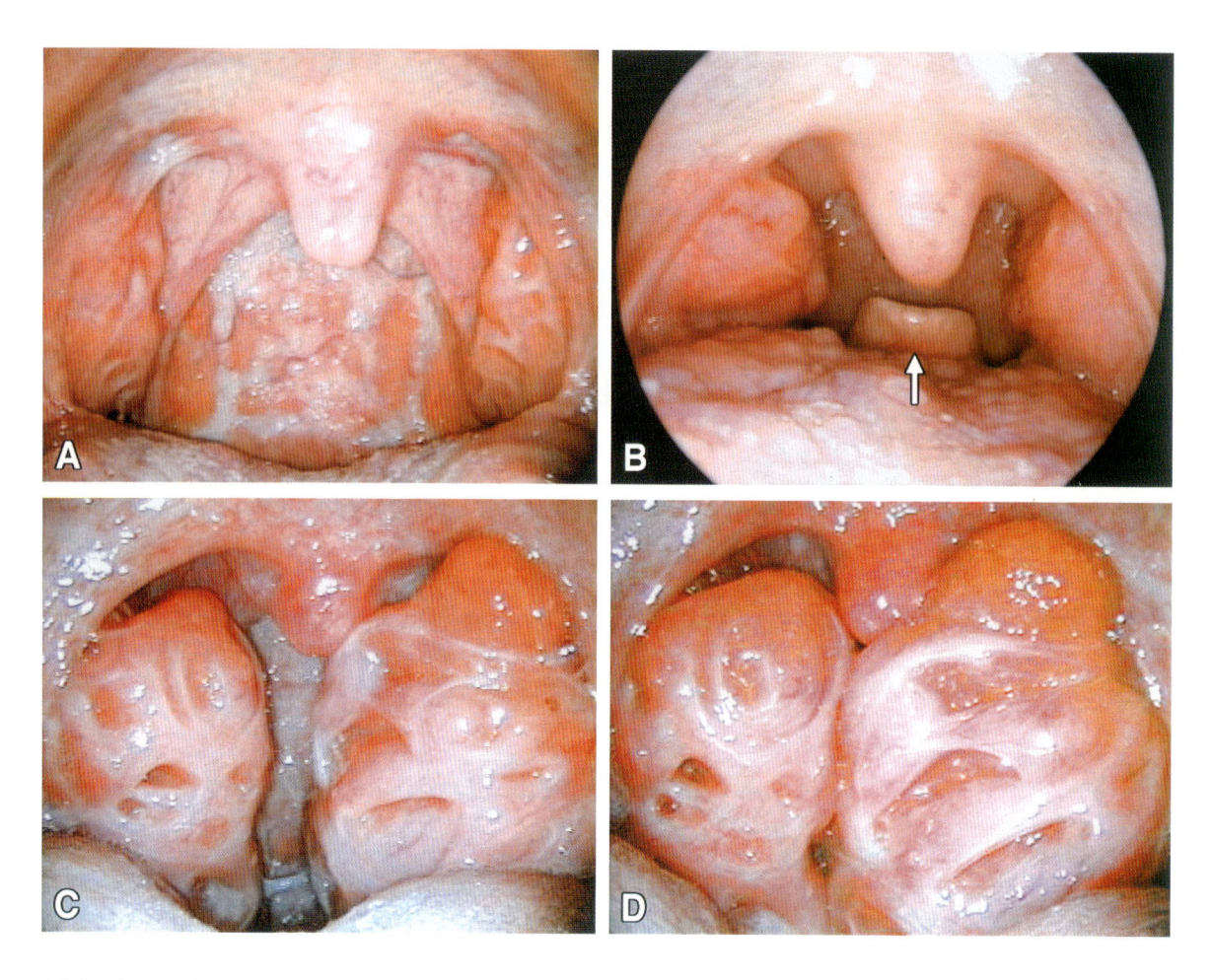

OROPHARYNGEAL ENDOSCOPIC ANATOMY

Palatine Tonsils

Figure 8-4A. Normal palatine tonsils. The 0-degree broad telescopic view of the oropharynx demonstrates normal tonsils laterally. Tonsil size is graded from +0 (no tonsil showing) to +4 (>75% of interfaucial distance filled). These tonsils are +2 (25–50% of the interfaucial distance filled by tonsils).

Figure 8-4B. Enlarged palatine tonsils and visible epiglottis. Tonsillar hypertrophy is a common condition that, in the extreme, can cause a variety of problems. These tonsils are +3 (50–75% of interfaucial distance filled). Sometimes the epiglottis (*arrow*) is visible in the oropharynx, especially in children.

Figure 8-4C. Tonsillar hypertrophy. These markedly enlarged exophytic tonsils nearly fill the oropharynx. The left tonsil touches the uvula. These tonsils are +4 (>75%).

Figure 8-4D. Kissing tonsils. When this same patient gagged, the tonsils met in the midline completely filling the oropharynx. This condition can completely obstruct the airway, especially if the adenoids are also large.

Endoscopy of the Oropharynx (Videopharyngoscopy)

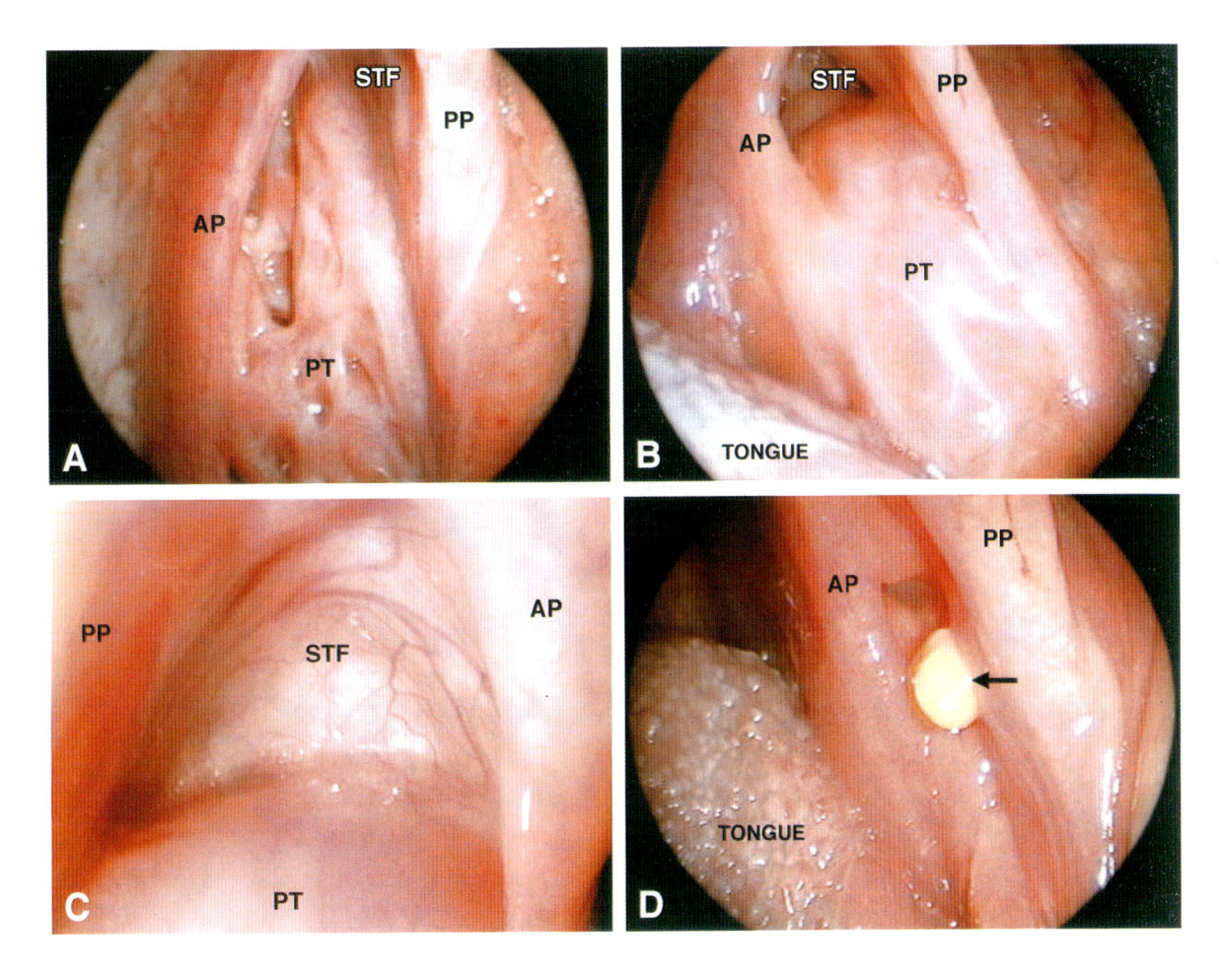

Superior Tonsillar Fossa

Figure 8-5A. Superior tonsillar fossa. This 90-degree telescopic view of the right oropharynx reveals the posterior pillar (PP), the anterior pillar (AP), the palatine tonsil (PT), and the superior tonsillar fossa (STF) above the tonsil. This space is not seen well on 0-degree telescopy or on regular oral examination.

Figure 8-5B. Superior tonsillar fossa. A similar view of another right superior tonsil fossa (STF) demonstrates also the lateral tongue (T) and lateral oral cavity just anterior to the anterior pillar (AP).

Figure 8-5C. Superior tonsillar fossa. One can appreciate the prominent blood supply to the tonsil in this 90-degree telescopic close-up view of the left superior tonsillar fossa (STF). This picture also shows why most tonsillectomies do not require sacrifice of soft palate or pillars if the dissection begins on the tonsillar capsule.

Figure 8-5D. Tonsillar plug. Tonsillar plugs are cheesy foul pearls of squamous, bacterial, and food debris packed in the crypts of chronically infected tonsils. This 90-degree pharyngoscopic view prominently displays a loose plug (*arrow*) lying in the right superior tonsillar fossa.

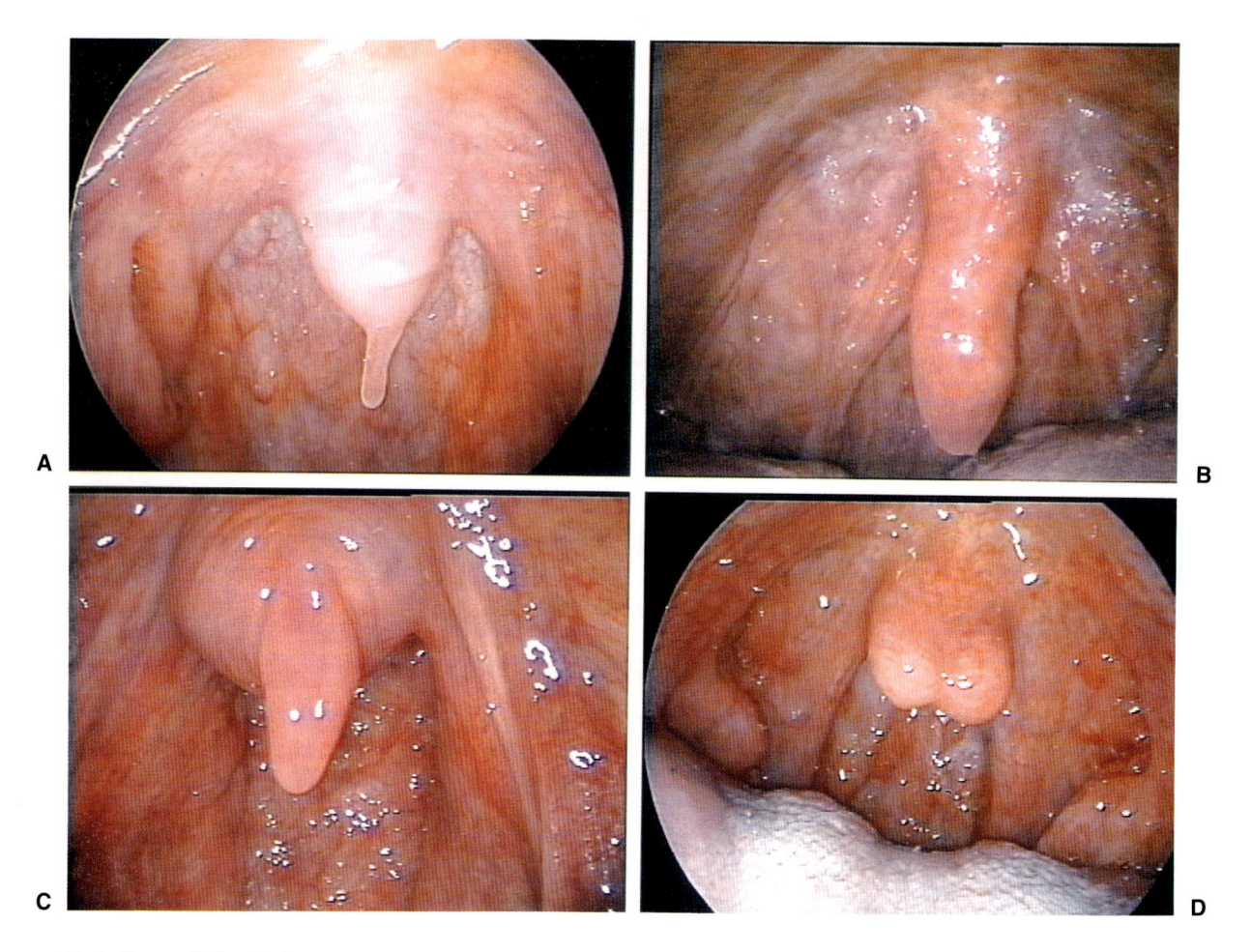

Variations of the Uvula

Figure 8-6A.   Uvula papilloma. The long strand off the tip of the uvula is a papilloma.

Figure 8-6B.   Long uvula. A long uvula like this one can cause gagging and choking when it stimulates the epiglottis. Along with the short posterior pillars that substantially narrow the velopharyngeal port, the long uvula also contributes to snoring.

Figure 8-6C.   Wide uvula. The very wide base of this uvula partially obstructed the nasopharynx.

Figure 8-6D.   Bifid uvula. The bifid uvula often accompanies a submucosal cleft of the soft palate. One should avoid an adenoidectomy in the presence of a bifid uvula because the adenoid may be crucial for sealing the nasopharynx from the oropharynx on swallowing. Hence, adenoidectomy may result in velopharyngeal insufficiency.

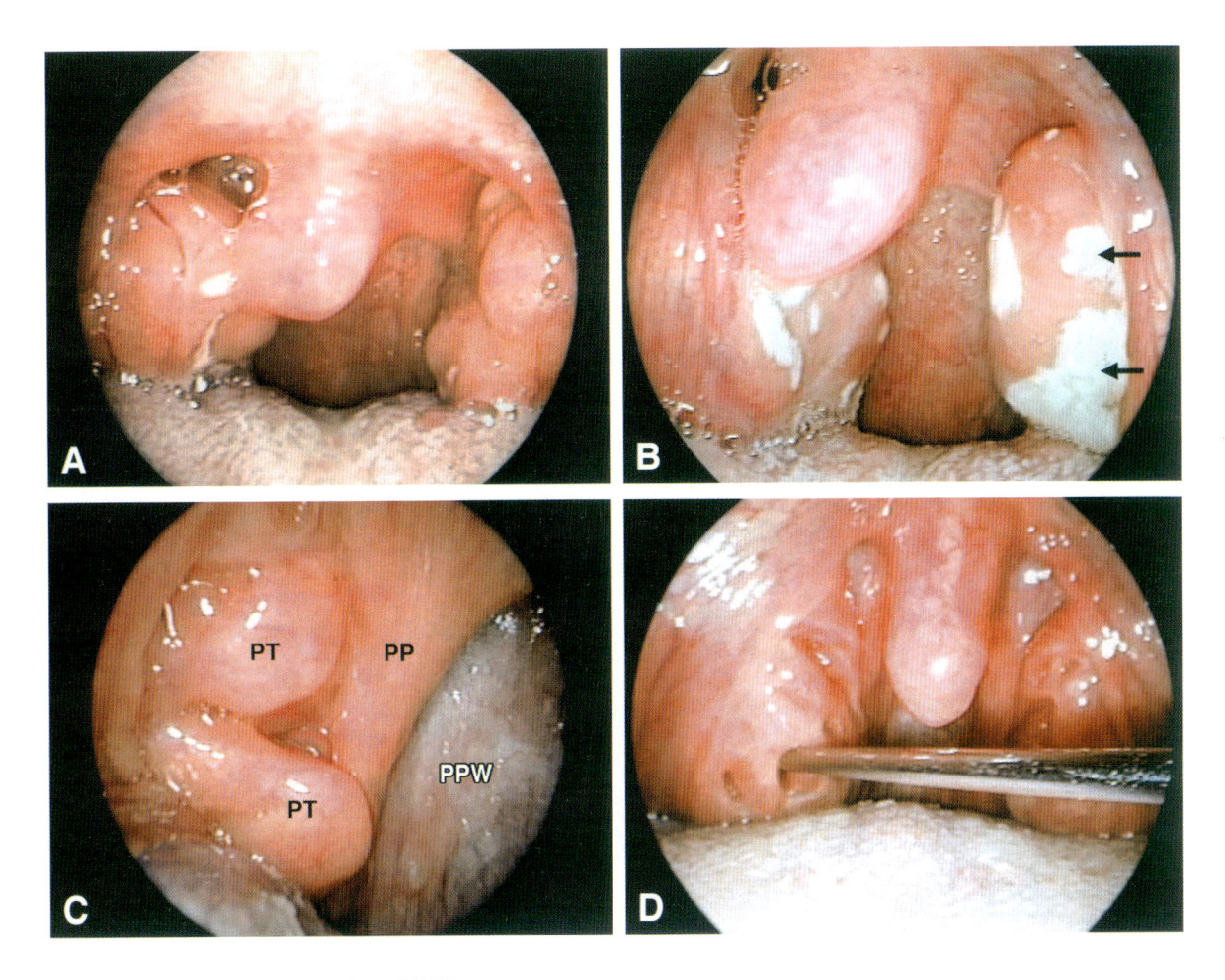

Endoscopy of the Oropharynx (Videopharyngoscopy)

DISORDERS OF THE OROPHARYNX

Tonsillitis

Figure 8-7A. Acute tonsillitis. These lobulated swollen tonsils produced white tonsillar plugs. The uvula, anterior pillars, posterior pillars, tonsils, and posterior pharynx were all inflamed. The border of the erythema ran horizontally across the soft palate.

Figure 8-7B. Infectious mononucleosis tonsillitis. These acutely infected tonsils had the classic exudative coating (*arrows*) of mononucleosis tonsillitis. These patients usually have atypical lymphocytes on a blood smear and test positive for heterophil antibodies (Monospot).

Figure 8-7C. Bilobed tonsil. This swollen chronically infected right tonsil (PT) had two distinct lobes. If one lobe were small it could be left intact accidentally during tonsillectomy and then reappear later as it hypertrophied. The posterior pillar (PP) and posterior pharyngeal wall (PPW) were also seen in this view.

Figure 8-7D. Cryptic chronic tonsillitis. Chronically infected tonsils commonly develop multiple deep crypts. Sloughed squamous debris, food debris, and bacteria pack into these crypts and form pearls of white cheesy foul material that causes halitosis and distresses the patient. The depth of the crypts in these infected tonsils is demonstrated with the probe.

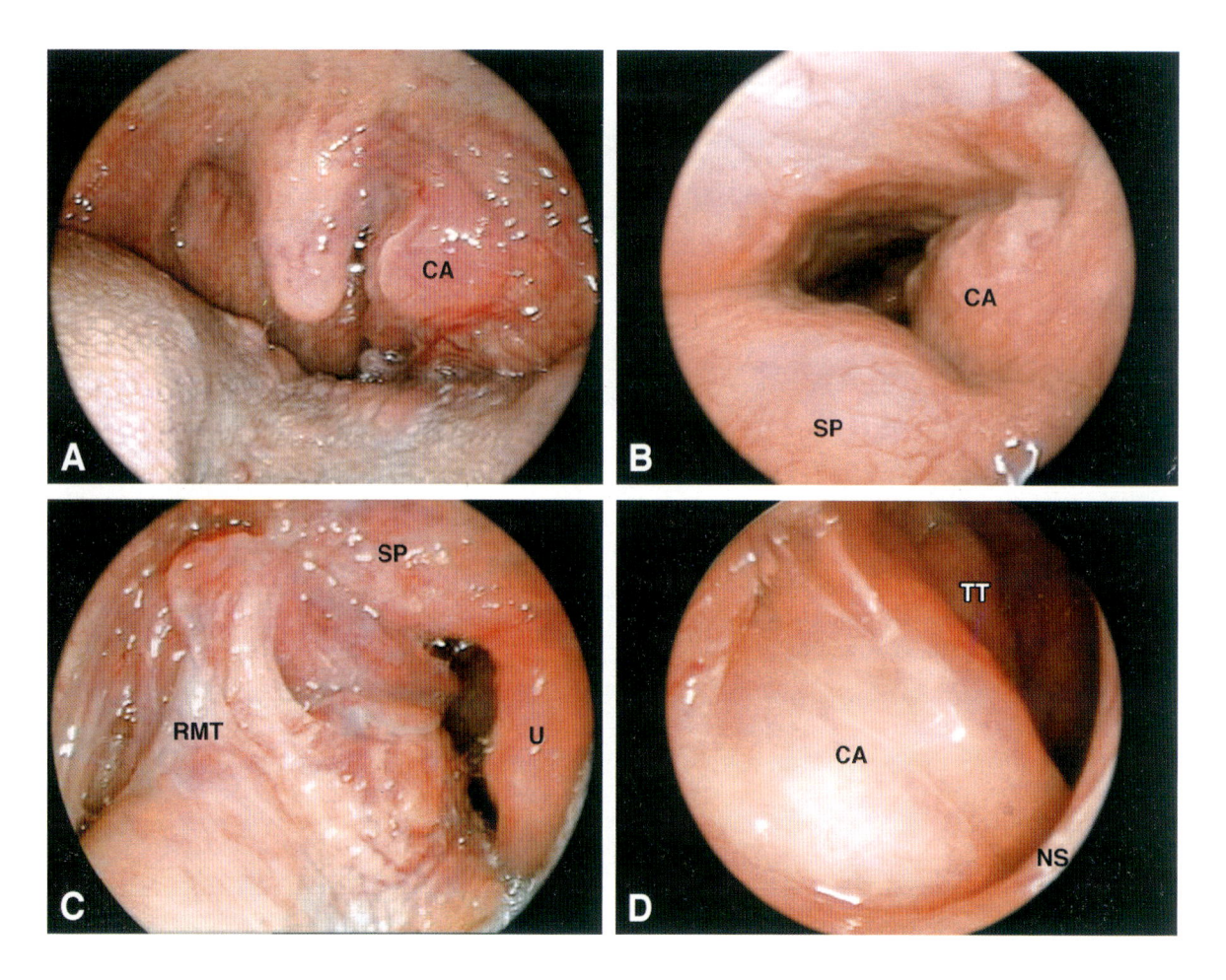

Squamous Cell Carcinoma of the Tonsil

Figure 8-8A. Squamous cell carcinoma of the left tonsil. The carcinoma (CA) created a ragged irregular swollen surface compared to the normal right tonsil. The full extent of this cancer was not appreciated on the 0-degree transoral telescopic exam.

Figure 8-8B. Squamous cell carcinoma of the left tonsil. This 90-degree transoral telescopic view of the nasopharynx in the same patient reveals the tumor (CA) pushing up on the soft palate (SP). The irregular ragged character of the cancer was seen under the overlying mucosa.

Figure 8-8C. Squamous cell carcinoma of the right tonsil. This patient refused treatment for his right tonsillar squamous cell carcinoma. The cancer spread extensively: superiorly onto the soft palate (SP), laterally to the buccal mucosa, medially to the lateral tongue, and anteriorly to the retromolar trigone (RMT). The uvula (U) and tongue were seen at the far right of this view. The right soft palate was paralyzed and the right vocal cord was densely paretic, suggesting extension of the cancer to the base of skull with right vagus nerve compromise.

Figure 8-8D. Squamous cell carcinoma of the right tonsil. This 0-degree transnasal telescopic view of the right nasopharynx reveals that this same tumor (CA) is pushing the swollen soft palate up, apparently extending to the base of the skull laterally. The torus tubarius (TT) appears infiltrated and is markedly displaced posteriorly by the tumor. The right eustachian tube orifice, not seen on this view, is completely obstructed, resulting in a chronic serous otitis media.

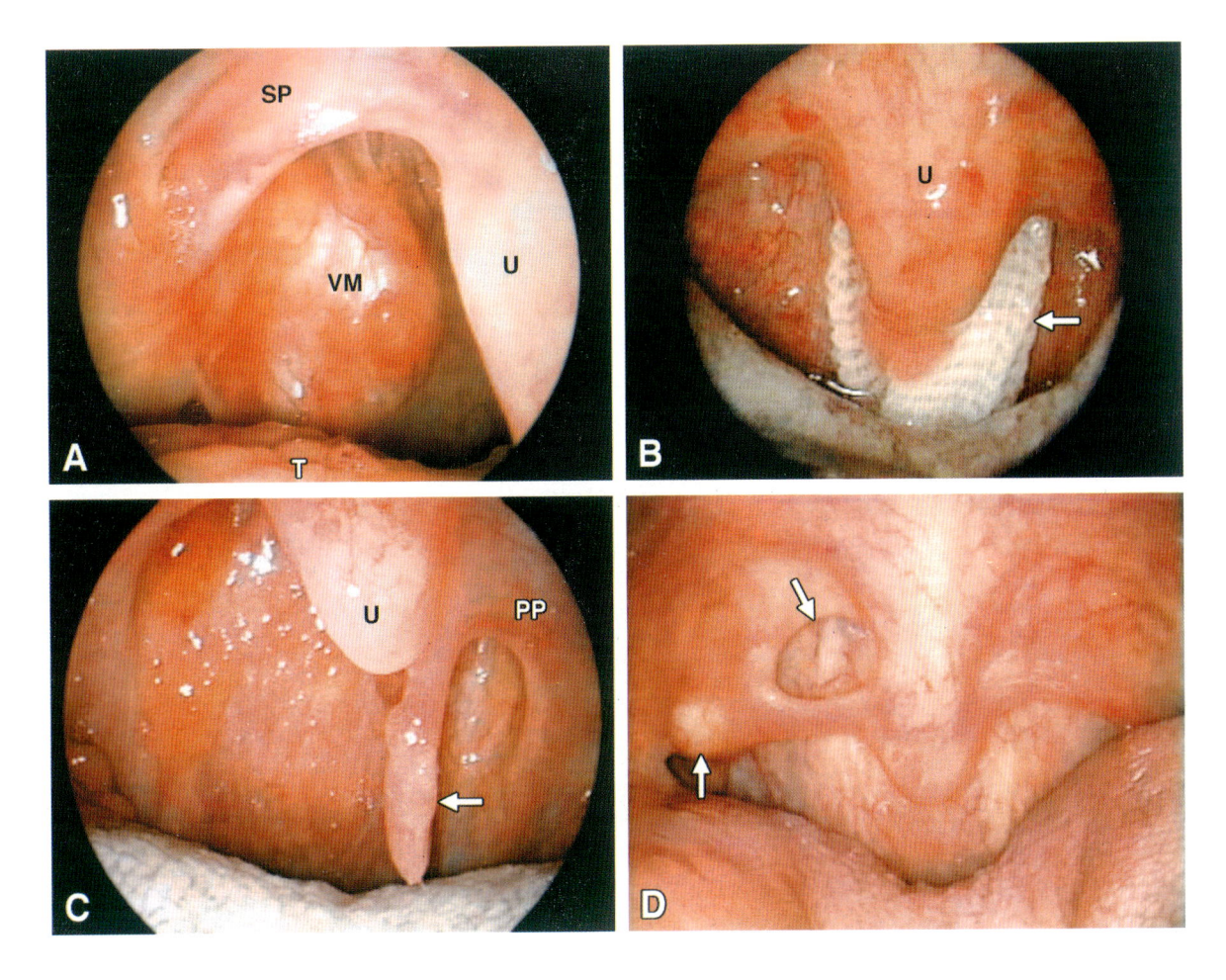

Miscellaneous Oropharyngeal Findings

Figure 8-9A. Anomalous pharyngeal carotid artery. The right posterolateral pulsating pharyngeal vascular mass (VM) in this 0-degree transoral telescopic view is an anomalous carotid artery on MRI. Do not biopsy this lesion!

Figure 8-9B. Pharyngeal foreign body. This patient complained of a foreign body sensation in the throat two days after septorhinoplasty, followed by recurrent episodes of choking spells. He was taken to the emergency room where the examination revealed the nasal gauze packing (*arrow*) in the posterior portion of the oropharynx which appeared to extend down into the laryngeal area. Removal of the packing immediately resolved this patient's complaints of respiratory difficulties.

Figure 8-9C. Uvulopalatal web. Although this patient denied previous surgery, it appeared that he had a previous tonsillectomy with residual scarring of the left posterior pillar (PP) to the uvula (U). There was also a remnant of soft tissue hanging freely (*arrow*). The patient wanted no corrective surgery because he was asymptomatic and liked the unique appearance.

Figure 8-9D. Soft palate defect. This patient presented with a hole in the right soft palate (*angled arrow*) with a long history of liquid and food reflux into the nasopharynx on swallowing. The defect probably was the result of trauma, although there was no clear history. Repair options included either primary closure or a mucosal flap. Note the round cream-colored mucus retention cyst (*vertical arrow*) along the right posterior pillar.

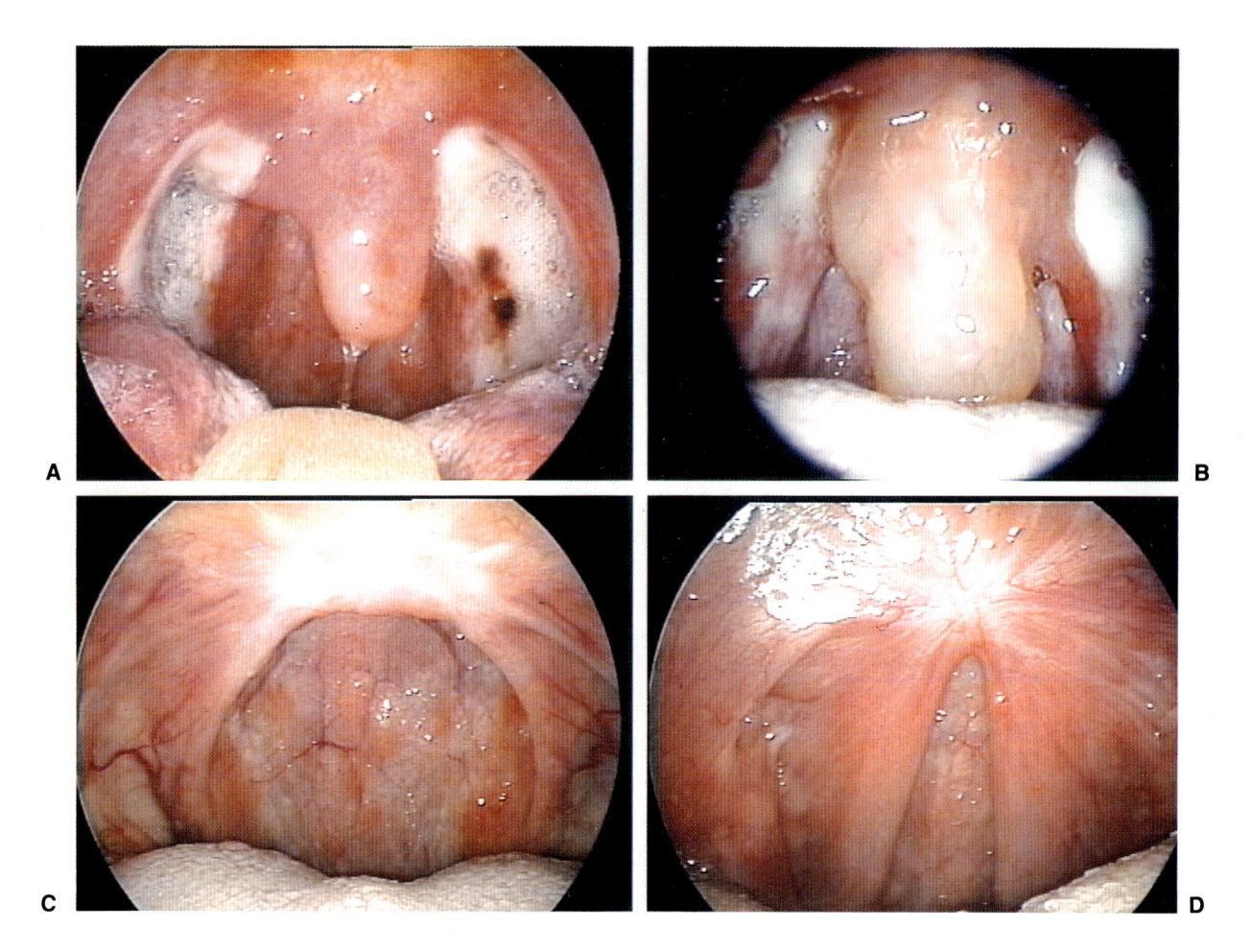

Postoperative Findings

Figure 8-10A. Postoperative tonsillectomy findings. The white fibrinous eschar covers the tonsillar fossae for 7–10 days following a tonsillectomy.

Figure 8-10B. Postoperative tonsillectomy findings. The marked uvular edema one week after tonsillectomy was due to the compromise of uvula lymphatic drainage by a high periuvular dissection with the electrocautery. Periuvular eschar was seen bilaterally. Care must be taken during tonsillectomy not to cauterize too closely to the uvula.

Figure 8-10C. Postoperative uvulopalatopharyngoplasty (UPPP) findings. The oropharynx was wide open after this UPPP. Notice the soft palate scar where the uvula and part of the soft palate were excised. Contraction of this scar helped open the airway to decrease snoring and obstructive sleep apnea.

Figure 8-10D. Postoperative UPPP findings. This patient had a very narrow oropharynx even after excision of the uvula and some of the soft palate. Despite very similar procedures, UPPP results can vary greatly.

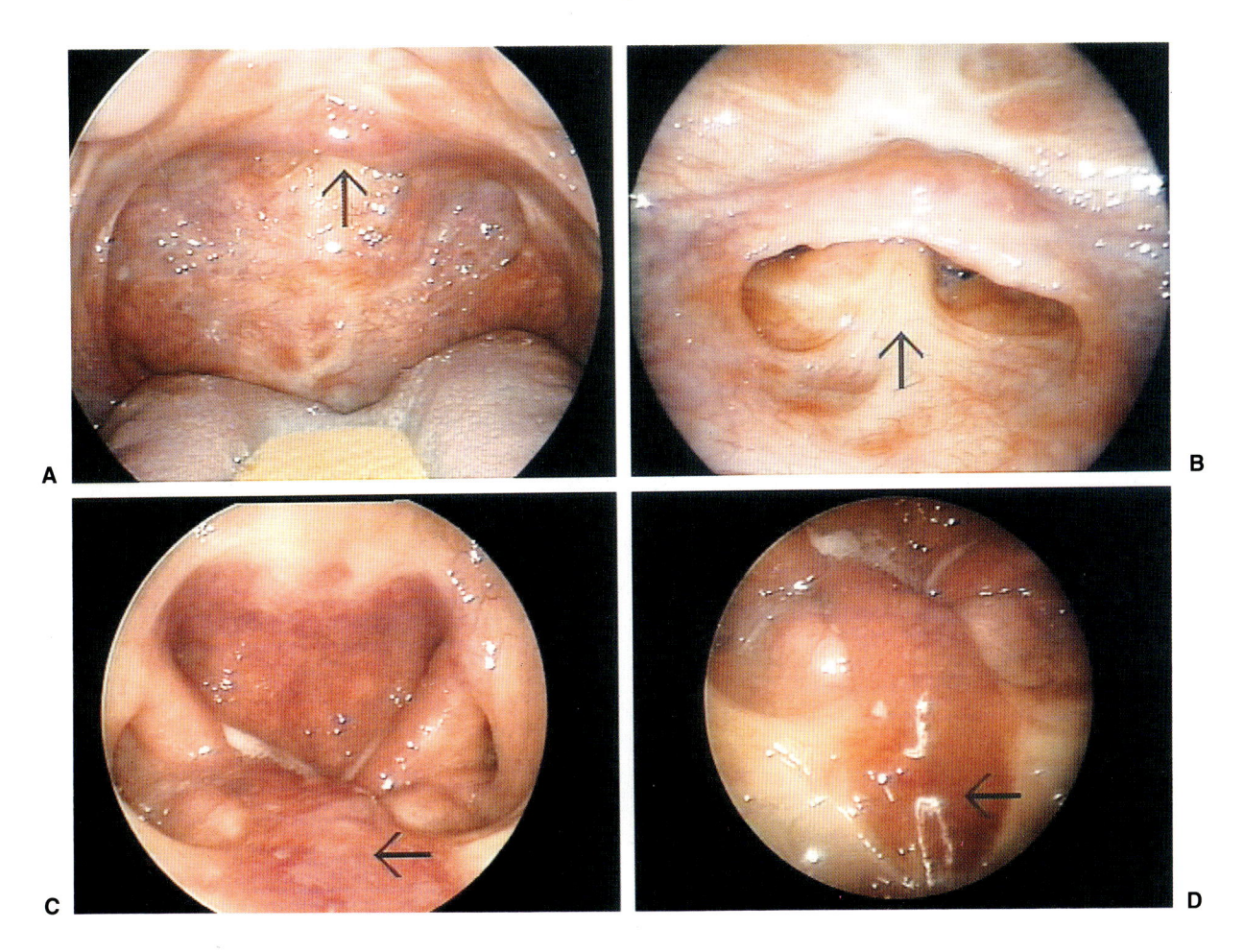

Endoscopy of the Oropharynx (Videopharyngoscopy)

Postoperative Pharyngeal Flap Findings

Figure 8-11A. Pharyngeal flap. This patient had a cleft palate repair with a superiorly based pharyngeal flap for velopharyngeal insufficiency. The 0-degree transoral telescopic exam of the oropharynx displays the base of the pharyngeal flap (*arrow*) as well as the midline soft palate scar.

Figure 8-11B. Pharyngeal flap. This 90-degree transoral telescopic view of the pharynx best shows the effect of this flap (*arrow*). The flap attached the posterior pharynx to the roof of the soft palate to pull the soft palate posteriorly in the midline. The velopharyngeal port was divided into two small ports by the flap. The combined area of the velopharyngeal ports should be 20 mm^2 or less for adequate velopharyngeal competence. However, realize that the smaller the ports are, the worse the postoperative nasal obstruction will be. Note also the midline soft palate scar from the cleft palate repair.

Figure 8-11C. Pharyngeal flap. The 30-degree transnasal telescopic view of the nasopharynx demonstrates the well-healed pharyngeal flap (*arrow*) that attached the posterior pharyngeal wall to the roof of the soft palate. This flap partially closed the velopharyngeal port. Also seen in this view were the tori tubarii, eustachian tube orifices, and fossae of Rosenmüller. Notice the eustachian tube orifices were low set which may have contributed to this patient's severe eustachian tube dysfunction.

Figure 8-11D. Pharyngeal flap. This 70-degree transnasal nasopharyngoscopic view clearly displays the well-healed pink flap (*arrow*) on the roof of the soft palate. The pharyngeal component of this flap contains mucosa, submucosa, and superior pharyngeal constrictor muscle.

Chapter 9
Endoscopy of the Larynx (Videolaryngoscopy)

Laryngoscopy is the examination of the larynx using a rigid telescope, flexible fiberscope, or direct laryngoscope. When laryngoscopic findings are documented with a video camera, the procedure is called *videolaryngoscopy*.

Videolaryngoscopy is an excellent method of examining and documenting laryngeal anatomy, pathology, and function. Important anatomical structures include the vallecula, epiglottis, arytenoids, false vocal folds, ventricles, and true vocal folds.

The larynx can be examined in the office with a transoral rigid telescope (70- or 90-degree) or a transnasal flexible fiberscope. The telescopic views are sharper and clearer, but the fiberscope is easier to use and tolerated better by patients. The larynx can also be examined in the operating room with direct laryngoscopes with or without a microscope or telescope to magnify the larynx image.

Equipment required for office laryngoscopy includes (1) 5.8-mm 70- and 90-degree telescopes, (2) flexible fiberscope, (3) light source, and (4) topical oral and nasal anesthetic and nasal decongestant. Equipment required for intraoperative laryngoscopy includes (1) direct laryngoscopes, (2) telescopes, (3) microscope, (4) light source, and (5) suspension system. Videolaryngoscopy also requires (1) video camera, (2) video recorder, (3) video monitor, and (4) video printer.

Videolaryngoscopy provides objective documentation of laryngeal anatomy, anomalies, pathologies, and physiology by a variety of techniques. These techniques are useful for diagnosis, teaching, patient counseling, medical recording, and pre- and postoperative comparison.

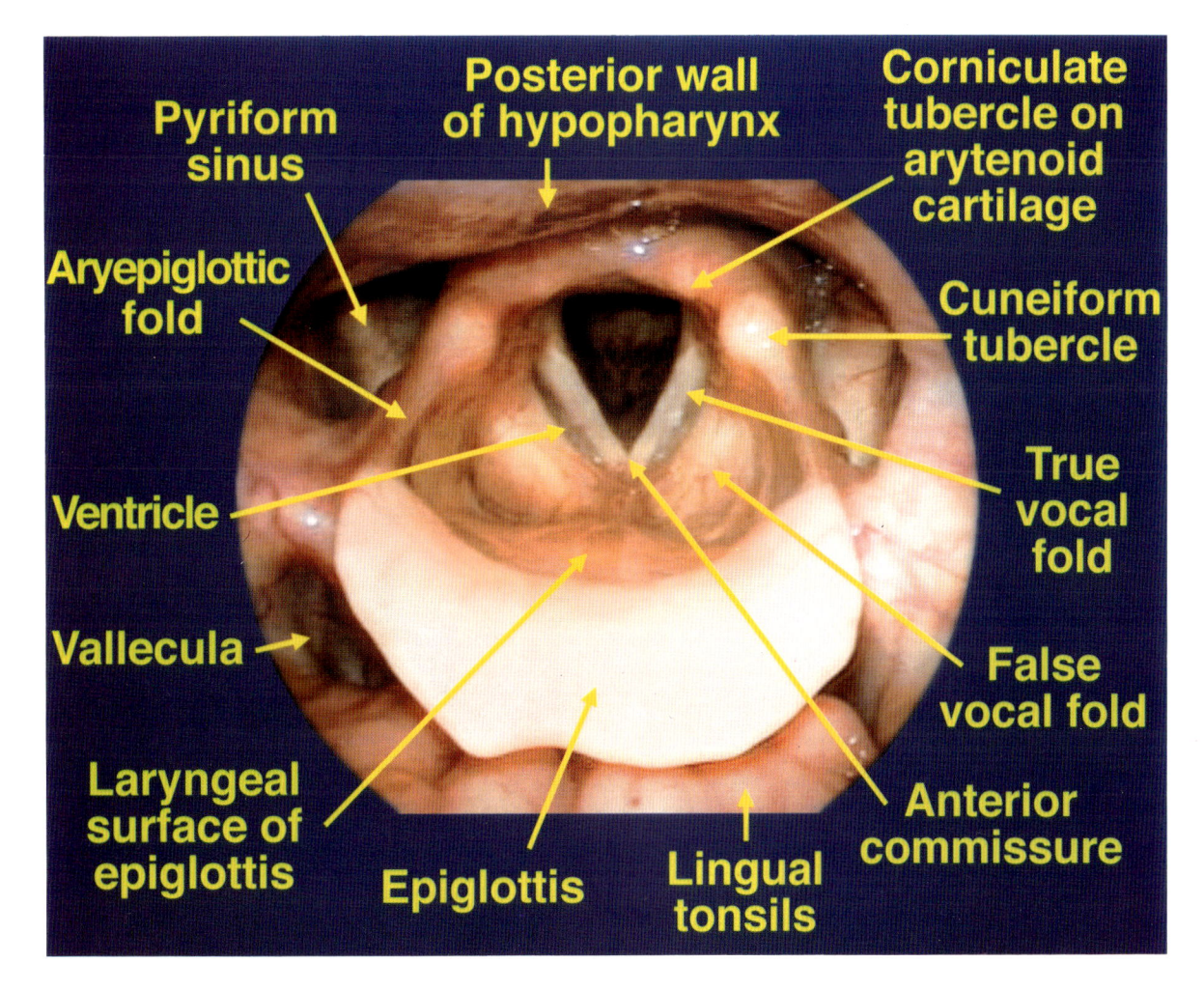

Endoscopy of the Larynx (Videolaryngoscopy) 115

OVERVIEW OF LARYNGEAL ANATOMY

Figure 9-1. Ninety-degree telescopic view of the larynx. This panoramic view of the larynx details the normal structures of the larynx and hypopharynx. The top of the view is posterior and the bottom is anterior as seen through the telescope. Note the ventricle, the space between the true and false vocal folds, typically is obscured by the false vocal fold and thus is very difficult to see from above. While the true vocal folds are sometimes simply called the vocal folds, the false vocal folds are sometimes called the ventricular folds. The pyriform sinuses slope down into the esophageal inlet, which is a transverse slit posterior to the arytenoids in the "postcricoid" area. The bridge of mucosa between the lateral epiglottis and pharyngeal wall is the pharyngoepiglottic fold (unlabled).

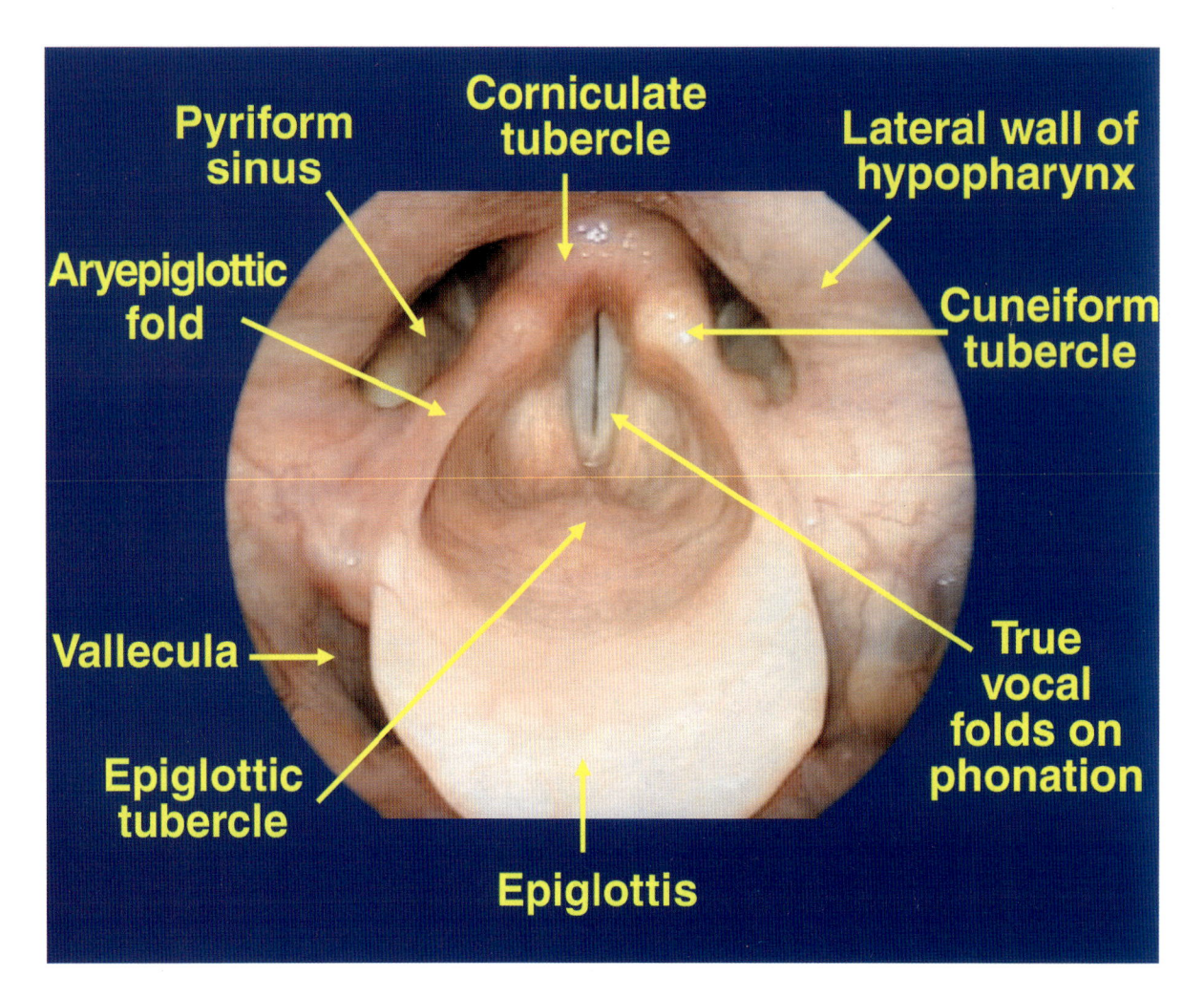

Figure 9-2. Ninety-degree telescopic view of the larynx on phonation. This panoramic view displays the normal laryngeal anatomy on phonation. The true vocal folds are tightly apposed, and the arytenoid cartilages (including the corniculate and cuneiform tubercles, also known as cartilages of Santorini and Wrisberg, respectively) are medialized. The vocal folds, formerly termed *vocal cords,* are folds of mucosa over soft tissues. The true vocal folds overlie a layered submucosal and muscular structure that is important in the physiology of phonation (see Figure 10-1).

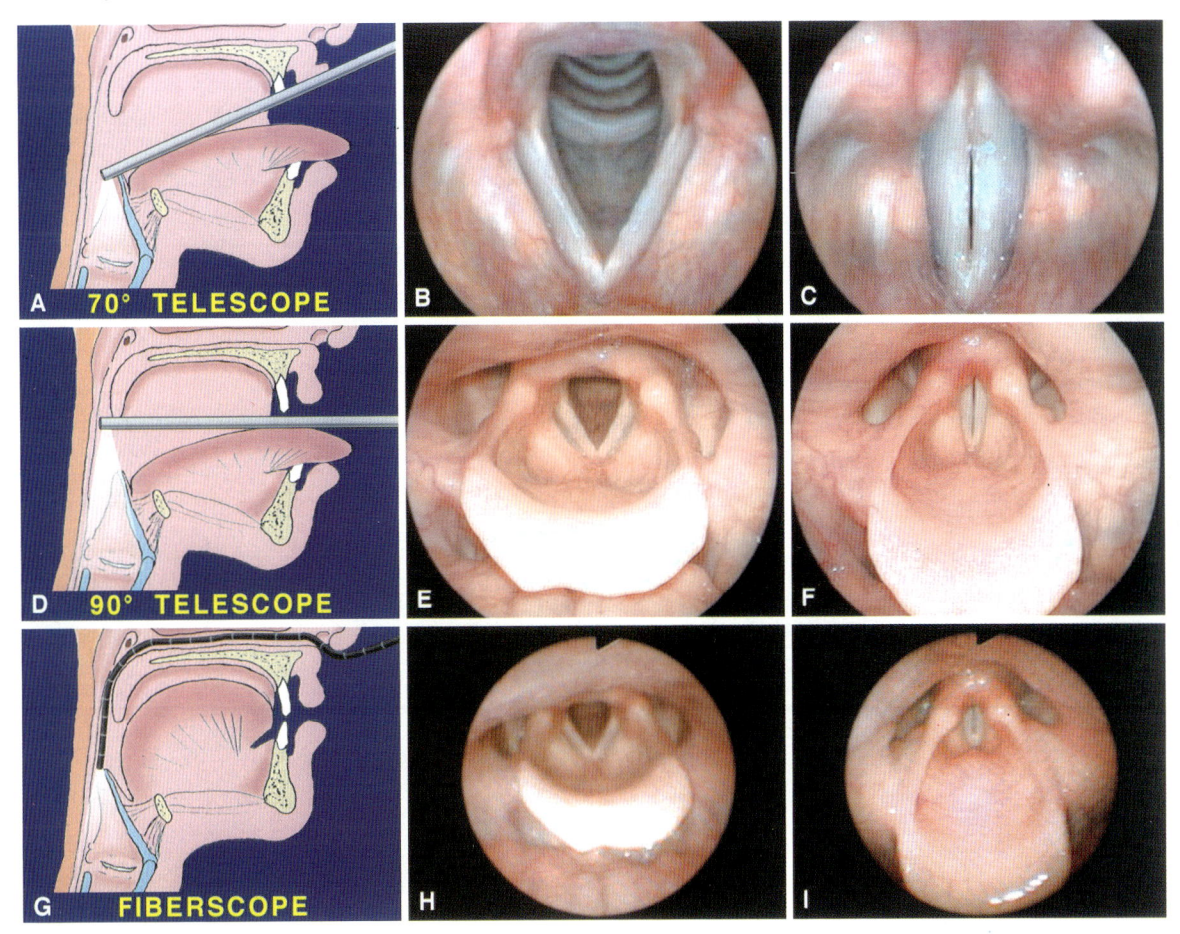

TECHNIQUES OF LARYNGEAL ENDOSCOPY

Office Techniques

Figure 9-3. The larynx views seen with these office techniques orient the anterior structures at the bottom of the view and the posterior structures at the top of the view, unlike the operating room techniques that are oriented the opposite way. *Top row:* 70-degree transoral telescopic laryngoscopy. After the oropharynx is topically anesthetized, the tongue is grasped with a gauze and the 70-degree rigid telescope is passed into the pharynx with a downward tilt of approximately 20 degrees (Figure 9-3A). The anatomical structures and pathological conditions of the larynx are then examined during normal respiration (Figure 9-3B) and during phonation (Figure 9-3C). The tilt of the scope brings it near the larynx, providing good light and a large close-up view that includes both the anterior and posterior commissures. The tracheal rings are even visible in Figure 9-3B. This technique is the best for the stroboscopic laryngeal exam. This technique is difficult, however, in patients with a sensitive gag reflex. *Middle row:* 90-degree transoral telescopic laryngoscopy. The oropharynx is topically anesthetized. The tongue is grasped and retracted anteriorly while the scope is passed straight back to the oropharynx with the distal lens directed inferiorly (Figure 9-3D). The larynx and hypopharynx are examined during normal respiration (Figure 9-3E) and phonation (Figure 9-3F). This technique stimulates less of a gag response than with the 70-degree scope. The scope is further from the larynx with this technique compared to the 70-degree scope. This technique therefore provides a panoramic view of the larynx and hypopharynx where the pyriform sinuses and epiglottis are seen in addition to the glottis. However, the lighting of the larynx is not quite as good. Because of the angle of view with the 90-degree scope it is usually difficult to see the posterior commissure with this technique. In order to get a closer view of the larynx the whole scope can be moved inferiorly pushing down on the tongue as tolerated. *Bottom row:* Transnasal fiberscopic laryngoscopy. The wider nasal passage is topically decongested and anesthetized. Then the fiberscope is passed along the floor of this nasal passage to the nasopharynx. The patient is asked to sniff, which opens the velopharyngeal inlet and thereby allows easy passage to the oropharynx and hypopharynx (Figure 9-3G). It provides a wide-angle view, and the tip bends 90 degrees in either direction. The fiberscope is the easiest scope to position and is best tolerated among patients. The larynx is examined during respiration (Figure 9-3H) and phonation (Figure 9-3I). The fiberscope, however, produces grainy images, and the wide-angle lens distorts the image.

118

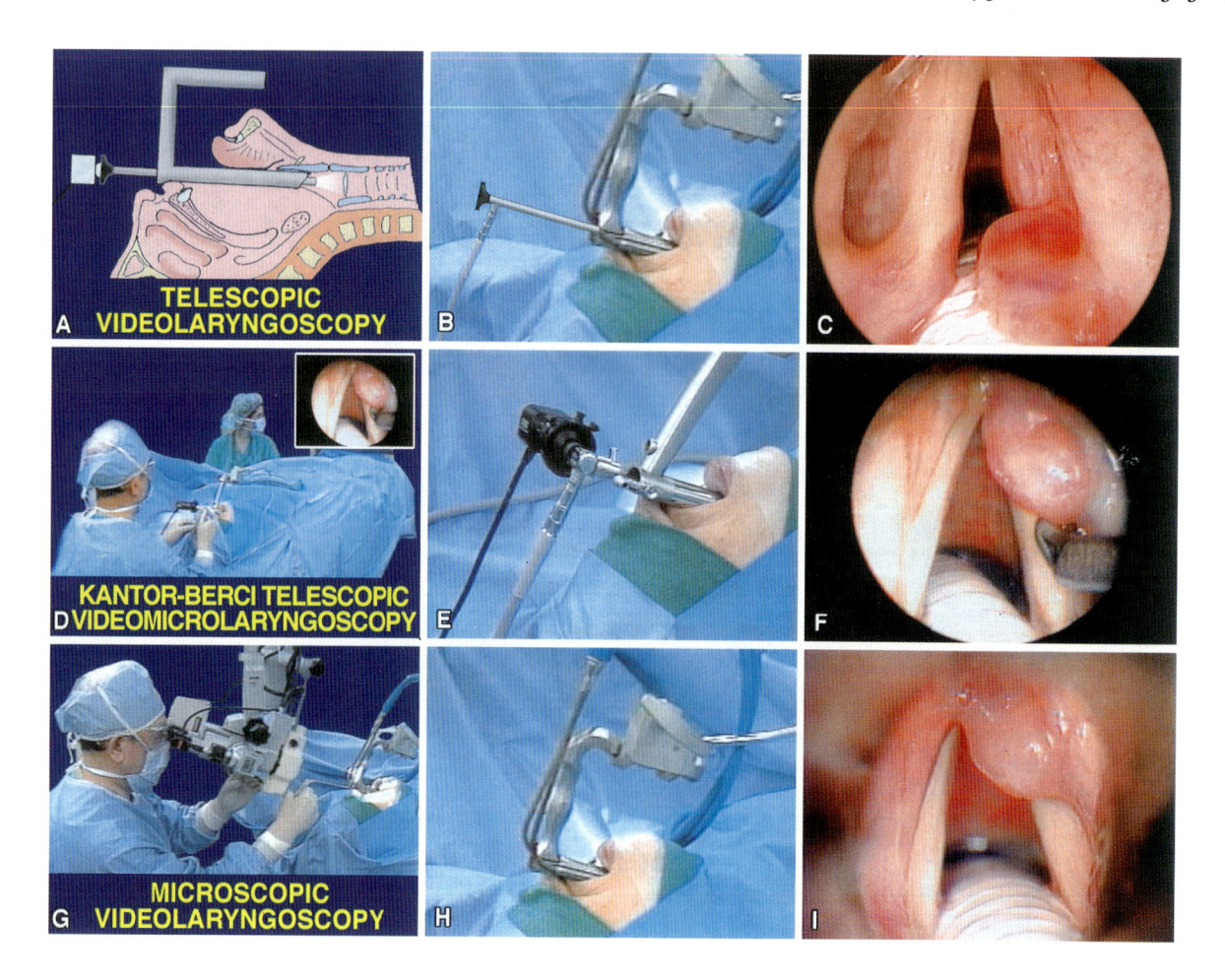

A TELESCOPIC VIDEOLARYNGOSCOPY

B

C

D KANTOR-BERCI TELESCOPIC VIDEOMICROLARYNGOSCOPY

E

F

G MICROSCOPIC VIDEOLARYNGOSCOPY

H

I

Endoscopy in Otorhinolaryngology

Endoscopy of the Larynx (Videolaryngoscopy)

Operating Room Diagnostic Techniques

Figure 9-4. These techniques all require suspension laryngoscopy in the intubated anesthetized patient. The operating room technique orients the larynx differently in the scope than the office techniques. In the office the anterior larynx is in the bottom of the view, whereas in the operating room (where the patient is lying supine) the posterior larynx and the endotracheal tube are in the bottom of the view. *Top row:* Telescopic videolaryngoscopy. First the patient is placed under general anesthesia and intubated. Then the larynx and hypopharynx are examined as the direct laryngoscope is passed to just above the true vocal folds and suspended. A rigid telescope is passed through the laryngoscope to view and record the anatomical structures and pathologic conditions of the larynx (Figures 9-4A and 9-4B). Figure 9-4C shows a large right true vocal fold granuloma as seen by telescopic videolaryngoscopy. Note also the clear view of the left ventricle. The endotracheal tube is visible at the bottom of the view. *Middle row:* Telescopic videomicrolaryngoscopy (Kantor–Berci technique). The Kantor–Berci videomicrolaryngoscope is an adapted direct laryngoscope with an attached magnifying rigid telescope and video camera. It is placed and suspended as described above. This technique provides magnified laryngeal images without the bulky microscope while freeing both hands. Figure 9-4F demonstrates a right supraglottic fibroma seen through Kantor–Berci telescopic microlaryngoscopy. *Bottom row:* Microscopic videolaryngoscopy. The Dedo microlaryngoscope is positioned as described above (Figure 9-4H). The microscope with a 400-mm focal length lens and an attached video camera is positioned to view the larynx at various magnifications (Figure 9-4G). Figure 9-4I shows the same right supraglottic fibroma as in Figure 9-4F.

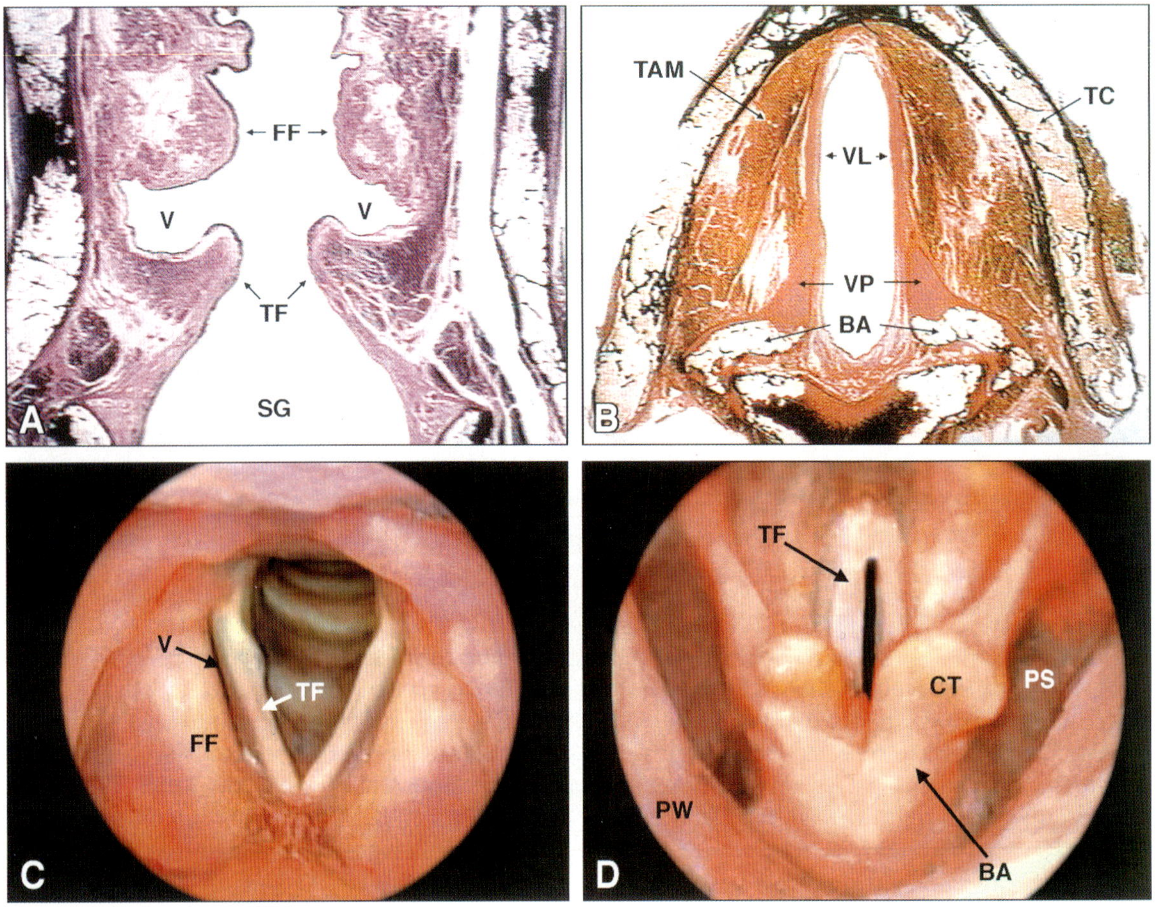
FF
V
V
TF
SG
A
TAM
TC
VL
VP
BA
B
V
TF
FF
C
TF
CT
PS
PW
BA
D

LARYNGEAL ENDOSCOPIC ANATOMY

Glottis

Figure 9-5A. Coronal section of the larynx. The vocal folds have certain important features that are revealed on this coronal section through the membranous vocal folds and not appreciated on the more common endoscopic view of the vocal folds. First, the true vocal folds (TF) are in fact *folds* and not *cords* of mucosa and superficial lamina propria over the vocal ligament and vocalis muscle. Second, the false vocal folds (FF) and true vocal folds are separated by a sulcus called the *ventricle* (V). The depth of the ventricles is impossible to appreciate on a superior view of the glottis. The ventricles represent an important oncologic boundary. They are also the location of laryngoceles and saccular cysts. Third, the false vocal folds angle inferiorly while the true vocal folds angle superiorly. This orientation optimizes the function of each: False vocal fold closure allows one to build high subglottic (SG) pressure for a cough (see Figure 11-5), and true vocal fold closure protects the airway from foreign material from above. (Courtesy of John A. Kirchner, M.D., Yale University, New Haven, CT.)

Figure 9-5B. Axial section through the glottis. This specimen displays the underlying structures of the larynx not seen through the endoscope. The top of the view is anterior and the bottom is posterior. The thyroid cartilage (TC) protects and supports the larynx. The thyroarytenoid muscle (TAM) is a strong adductor and also shortens the true vocal folds. The true vocal folds and the space between them make up the glottis. The space alone is called the rima glottidis or sometimes the "true glottis." The vocal ligament (VL) attaches to the arytenoid vocal process (VP) posteriorly and to the thyroid cartilage anteriorly. It represents the membranous, or vocal, portion of the vocal folds and constitutes approximately three-fifths of the vocal fold length. The vocal process (VP) of the arytenoid cartilage represents the cartilaginous, or respiratory, portion of the vocal folds and constitutes two-fifths of the length. The body of the arytenoid cartilage (BA) articulates with the posterior superior cricoid cartilage. (Courtesy of John A. Kirchner, M.D., Yale University, New Haven, CT.)

Figure 9-5C. A 70-degree transoral telescopic view of the glottis. It is important to correlate this view from above to the coronal view in Figure 9-5A. The ventricle (V) appears as a slit between the true vocal fold (TF) and false vocal fold (FF).

Figure 9-5D. A 70-degree transoral telescopic view of the larynx. One should correlate this view with the underlying structures of the larynx as displayed above in Figure 9-5B. The vocal ligament lies underneath the mucosa of the true vocal fold (TF). The corniculate tubercle (corniculate cartilage or cartilage of Santorini) (CT) rests on top of the body of the arytenoid cartilage (BA). The pyriform sinuses (PS), bounded medially by the aryepiglottic folds and laterally by the pharyngeal wall (PW), lead to the postcricoid area and esophageal inlet.

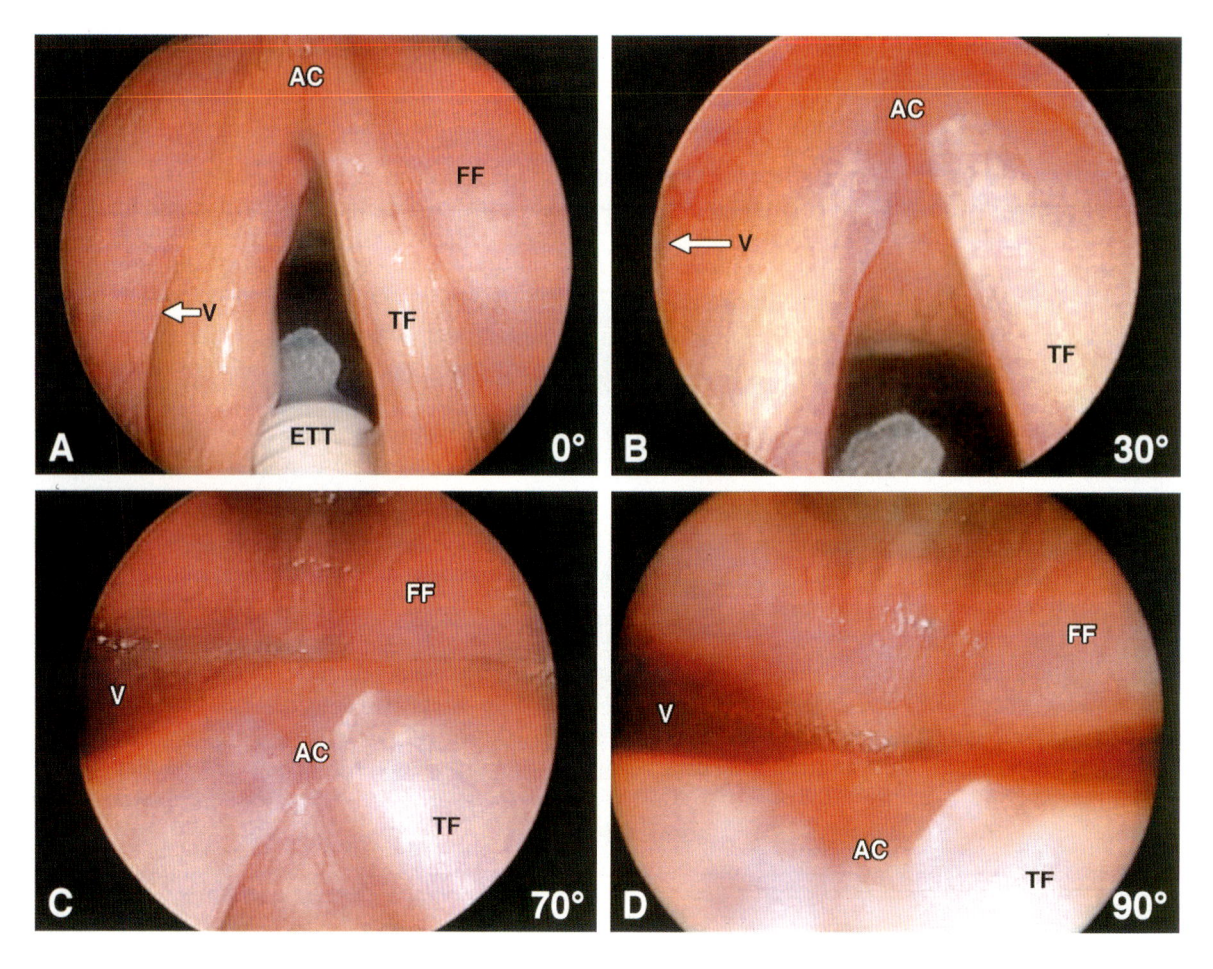

Anterior Views of the Glottis

Figure 9-6A. Intraoperative diagnostic 0-degree telescopic view of the glottis. The 0-degree telescope displays the true vocal folds (TF), false vocal folds (FF), and anterior commissure (AC). The ventricle (V) appears as a fine slit between the true and false folds. The endotracheal tube (ETT) is seen in the posterior glottis. The saline-filled cuff is in the subglottis with an air bubble visible within it. There is a small left anterior true vocal fold sessile polyp.

Figure 9-6B. Anterior 30-degree telescopic view of the glottis. This close-up view of the anterior glottis shows the true vocal fold (TF) and anterior commissure (AC). The edge of the ventricle (V) is also seen.

Figure 9-6C. Anterior 70-degree telescopic view of the glottis. One gets a nearly direct view of the anterior commissure (AC) and the anterior portion of the ventricles (V). One can begin to appreciate the depth of the ventricles on this view.

Figure 9-6D. Anterior 90-degree telescopic view of the glottis. This direct view of the anterior glottis clearly shows the convergence of the true vocal folds (TF) at the anterior commissure (AC). The depth of the ventricle (V) is now obvious.

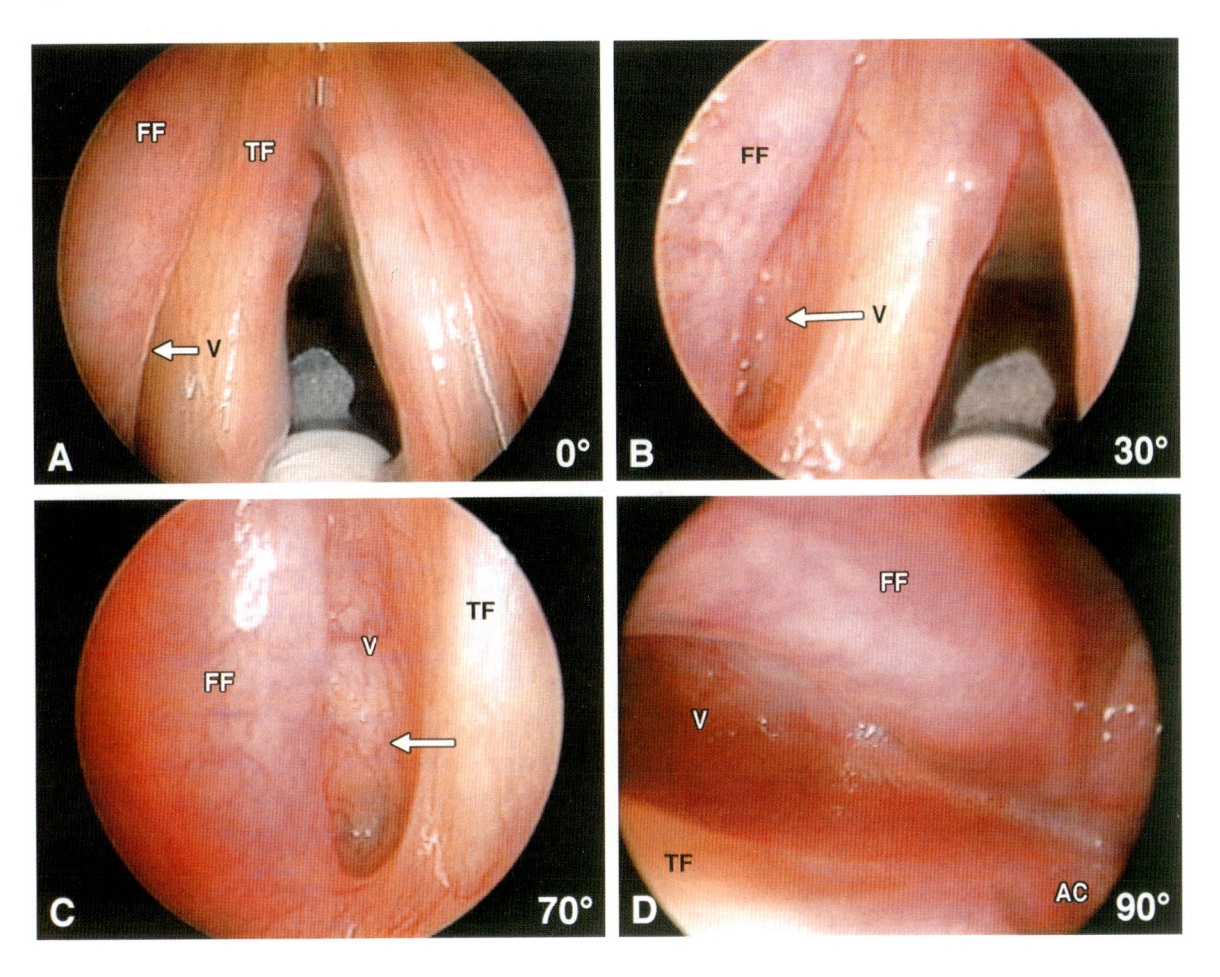

Endoscopy of the Larynx (Videolaryngoscopy) 123

Lateral View of the Ventricle

Figure 9-7A. Intraoperative diagnostic 0-degree telescopic view of the glottis. The ventricle (V) appears to be only a slit between the false and true vocal folds.

Figure 9-7B. Lateral 30-degree telescopic view of the left glottis and ventricle. The ventricle (V) begins to come into view from this angle.

Figure 9-7C. Lateral 70-degree telescopic view of the left ventricle. The ventricle (V) is in full view in this unusual endoscopic view. Clearly the ventricle is more than just a slit.

Figure 9-7D. Lateral 90-degree telescopic view of the left ventricle. Again, the ventricle (V) is of significant depth and width between the false and true vocal folds. The anterior commissure (AC) is barely seen in this view.

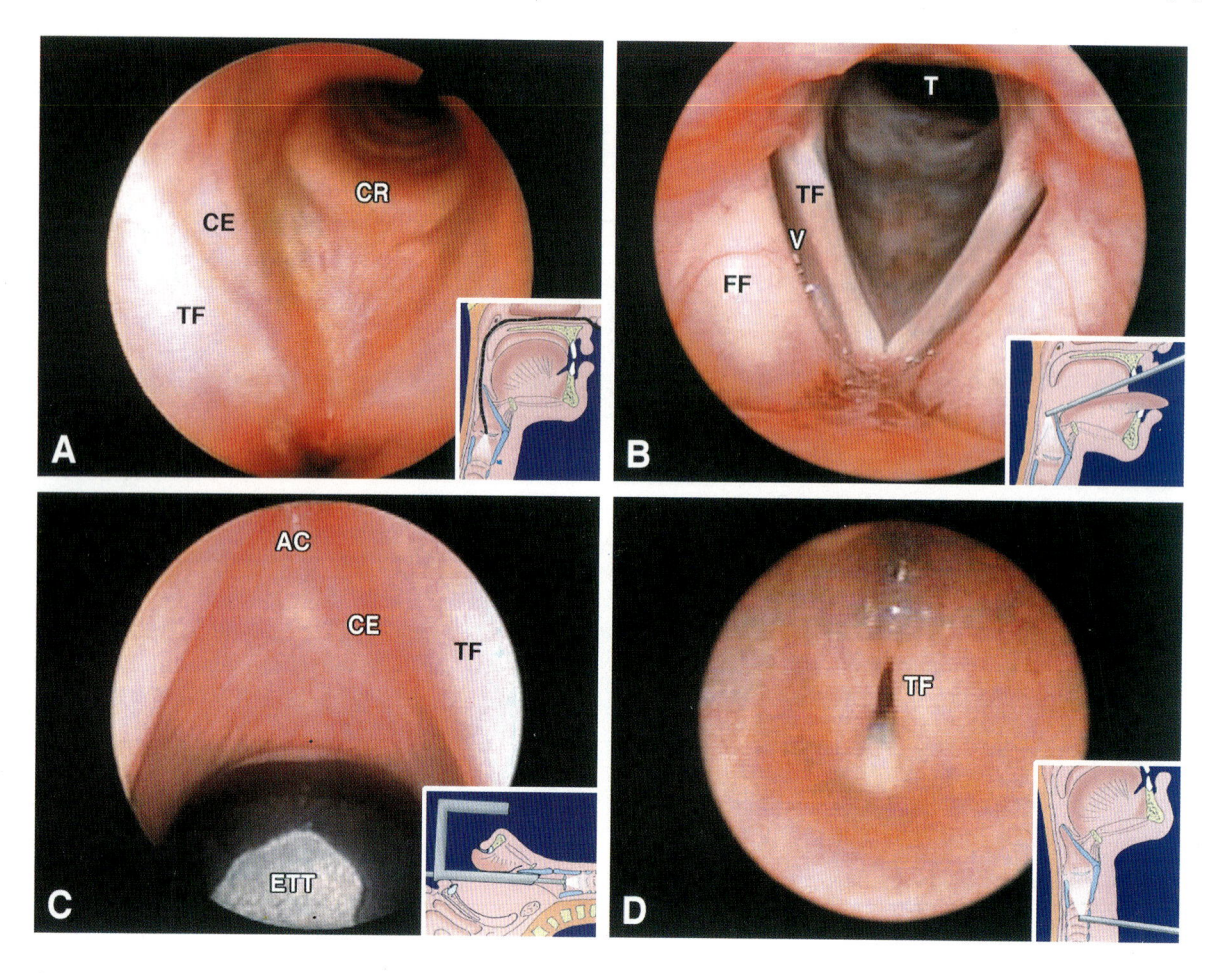

Subglottis

Figure 9-8A. Transnasal fiberscopic view of the subglottis. The subglottis extends from the glottis (true vocal folds) down to the lower border of the cricoid cartilage (CR). The conus elasticus (CE) is a strong elastic tissue layer that extends from the superior edge of the cricoid cartilage up to the vocal ligaments laterally, the inner surface of the thyroid cartilage anteriorly, and the arytenoid cartilages posteriorly. This view of the subglottis is obtained by passing the fiberscope wide-angle lens to the level of the true vocal folds (*inset*).

Figure 9-8B. Transoral 70-degree telescopic view of the subglottis. This laryngoscopic view demonstrates the true and false folds (TF, FF) and a prominent ventricle (V). The subglottis is seen leading down to the trachea (T).

Figure 9-8C. Translaryngoscopic 30-degree telescopic view of the subglottis. The intraoperative view is obtained by passing the 30-degree rigid telescope through the direct laryngoscope down to the glottis (*inset*). The anterior commissure (AC), true vocal folds (TF), conus elasticus (CE), and endotracheal tube cuff (ETT) are all seen in this view of the upper portion of the anterior subglottis.

Figure 9-8D. Transtracheotomy 70-degree telescopic view of the subglottis. The 70-degree telescope is passed through the tracheotomy and the lens is directed upward to obtain this unusual view of the subglottis from below (*inset*). The undersurface of the true vocal folds (TF) is clearly seen.

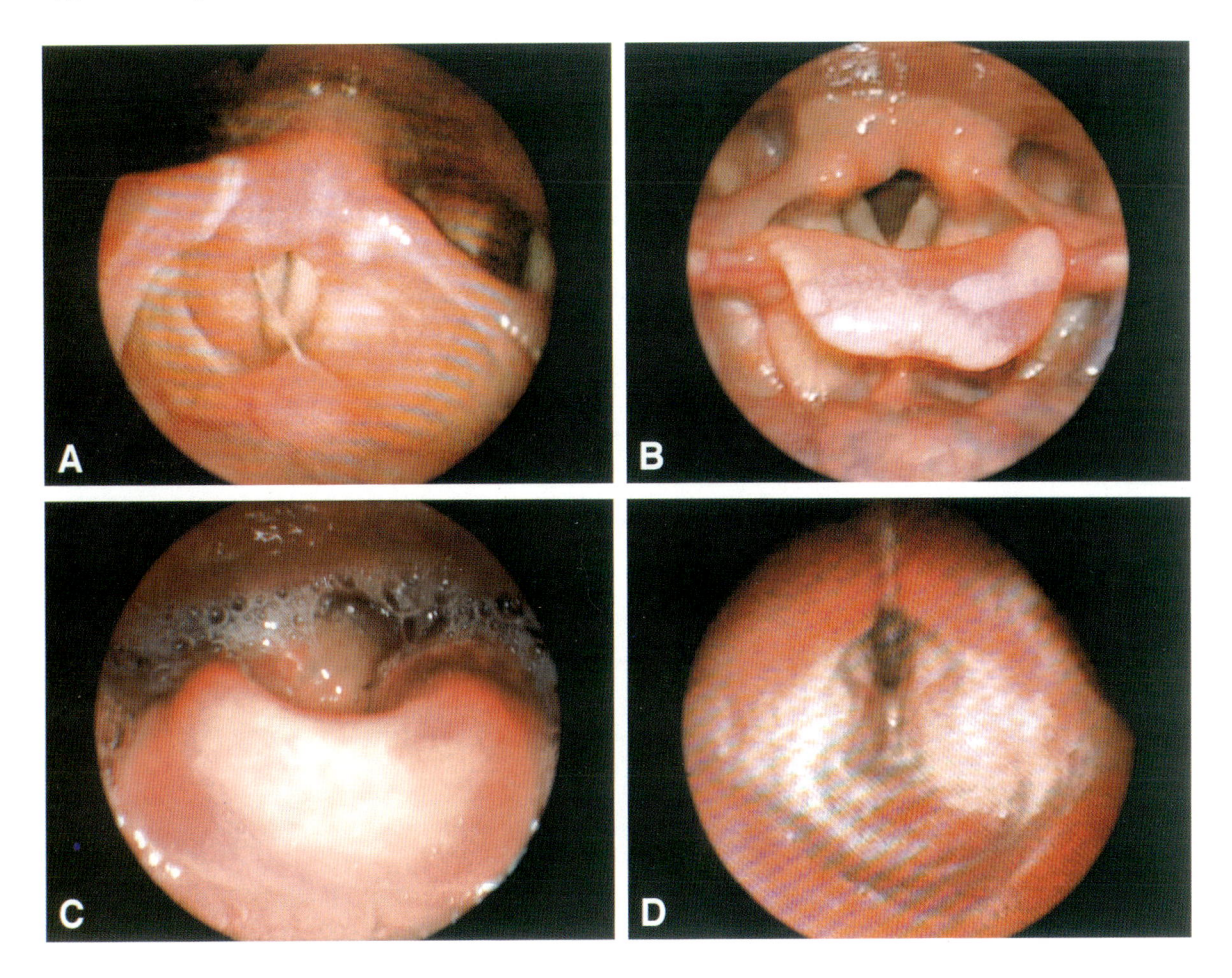

DISORDERS OF THE LARYNX

Acute Laryngitis

Figure 9-9A. Acute laryngitis and supraglottitis. This transnasal fiberscopic view displays pus streaming over the inflamed right aryepiglottic fold and a strand of mucus stretching between the arytenoid and the epiglottic tubercle. The true vocal folds are edematous and the arytenoids are inflamed.

Figure 9-9B. The 90-degree transoral telescopic exam shows marked postcricoid edema as well as a large shallow ulcer on the left laryngeal surface of the epiglottis with surrounding erythema. These findings are consistent with an acute viral laryngitis. Note this view clearly demonstrates normal pharyngoepiglottic folds.

Figure 9-9C. Acute epiglottitis. This young man presented with acute rapidly progressive odynophagia and malaise. The patient was breathing comfortably. He was successfully treated with intravenous antibiotics, steroids, and oxygen mist in the ICU. Note the very swollen epiglottis and pooling of secretions. The glottis was not visible in this view.

Figure 9-9D. Acute supraglottitis. This patient also presented with acute progressive odynophagia and malaise. The transnasal fiberscopic examination reveals inflamed arytenoids and aryepiglottic folds as well as a left posterior epiglottic and left hypopharyngeal submucosal hemorrhage due to coughing. The patient was treated successfully with IV antibiotics, steroids, oxygen mist, and racemic epinephrine in the ICU.

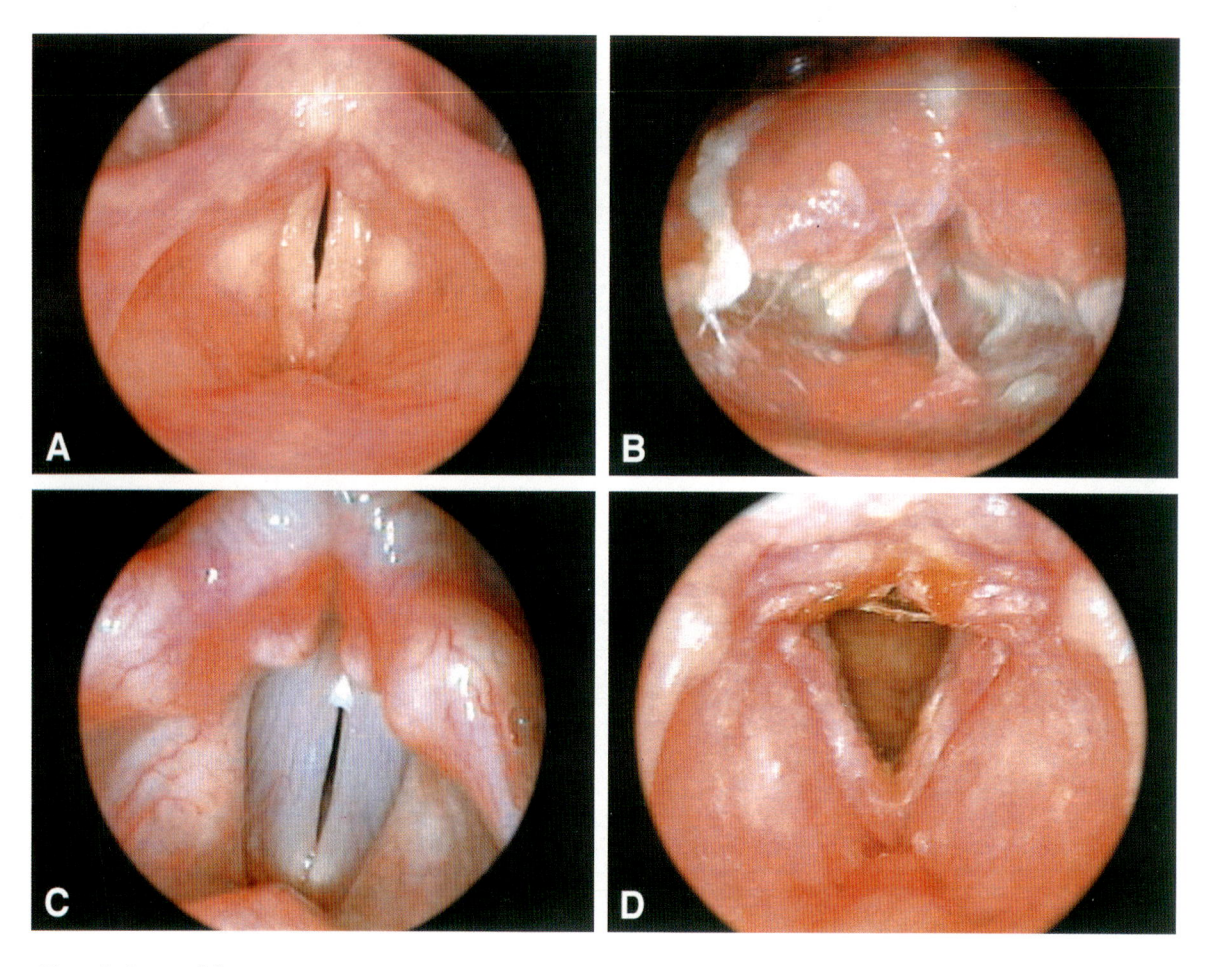

Chronic Laryngitis

Figure 9-10A. Chronic Laryngitis. The 70-degree telescopic exam of this patient with chronic hoarseness reveals bilateral irregular polypoid true vocal fold mucosa.

Figure 9-10B. Radiation-induced chronic laryngitis. This patient received external beam radiation treatments to the larynx for a $T_1N_1M_0$ laryngeal carcinoma. There was no evidence of recurrent cancer, but the patient did have chronically inflamed and dry laryngeal mucosa with dry tenacious secretions as seen on this 90-degree transoral telescopic exam. The patient was treated with aggressive oral hydration and humidified air.

Figure 9-10C. Chronic reflux laryngitis. This patient suffered from chronic hoarseness and throat-clearing. He also had gastroesophageal reflux disease (GERD). The 70-degree transoral telescopic exam of the glottis reveals persistent posterior commissure erythema and arytenoid swelling. The patient improved on an antireflux regimen (head of bed elevation, NPO for 3 hours before bed, and H_2-blocker therapy).

Figure 9-10D. Chronic laryngitis sicca. This patient's chronic hoarseness and cough were due to laryngitis sicca with its attendant dry mucosa and crusty, gluey secretions. The true vocal folds have an irregular appearance on this 90-degree transoral telescopic exam. The patient also had atrophic rhinitis.

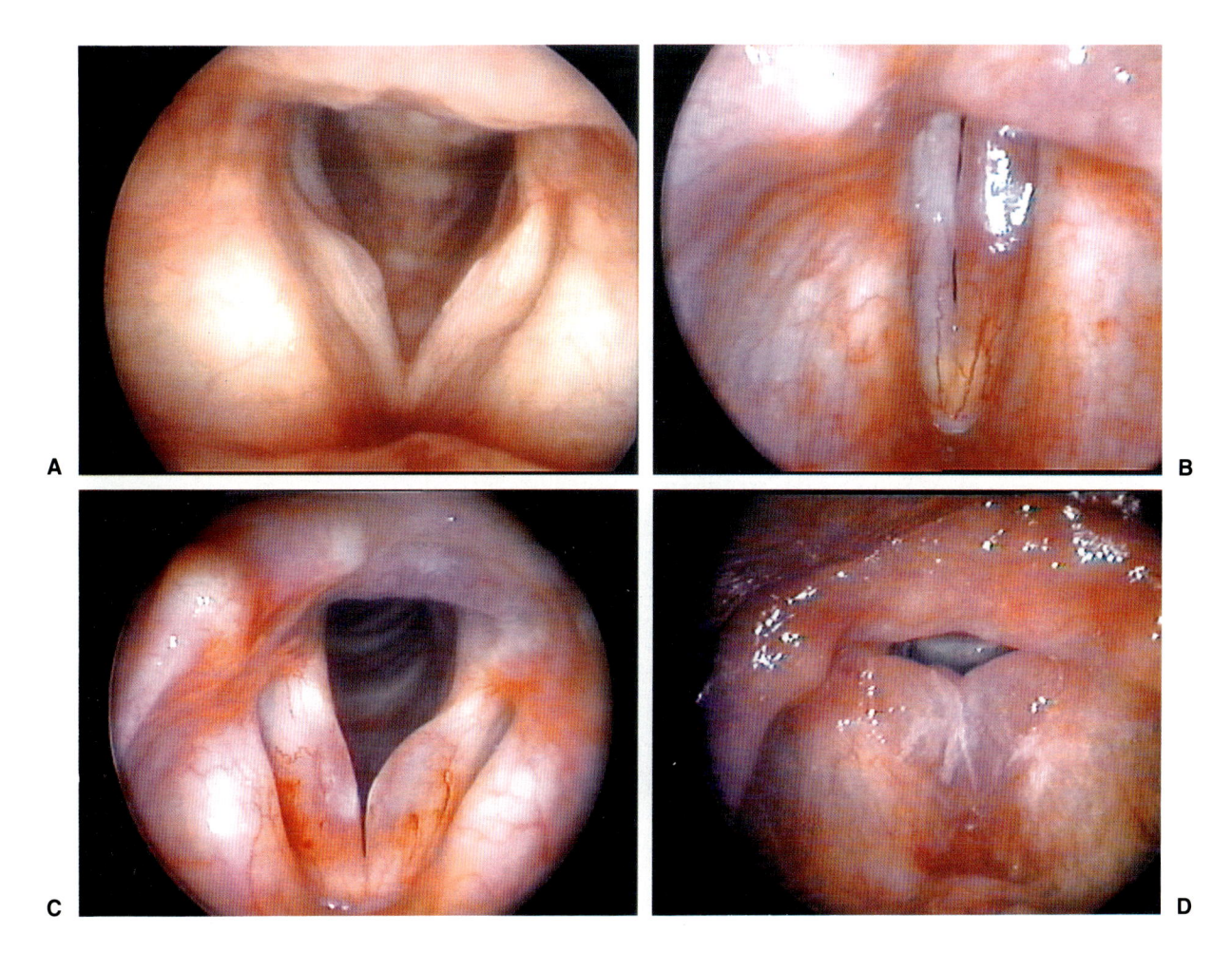

Reinke's Edema

Figure 9-11A. Reinke's edema. The true vocal fold is a layered structure consisting of squamous epithelium, a loose connective tissue layer (superficial layer of the lamina propria also called *Reinke's space*), an elastic fiber layer (vocal ligament), a collagenous fiber layer (vocal ligament), and the vocalis muscle (see Figure 10-1). Since Reinke's space is made up of loose connective tissue, edema fluid can accumulate in this space and is called *Reinke's edema*. Reinke's edema can be unilateral or bilateral and is caused by voice abuse, chronic laryngeal irritation, reflux laryngitis, and smoking. This patient had chronic hoarseness with a deepened voice. This 70-degree transoral telescopic view shows bilateral Reinke's edema that added mass to the true vocal folds.

Figure 9-11B. Unilateral Reinke's edema. This patient's hoarse heavy voice was due to the marked left Reinke's edema. The clear edema highlighted surface vessels on the true vocal folds. The right true vocal fold had mild edema.

Figure 9-11C. Bilateral Reinke's edema. Reinke's space extends along the full length of the true vocal folds. Reinke's edema can involve part or all of this space. This 70-degree telescopic view displays Reinke's edema of the whole right true vocal fold and anterior half of the left true vocal fold. It is most prominent bilaterally one-third back from the anterior commissure where there also is erythema.

Figure 9-11D. Advanced bilateral Reinke's edema. The severe Reinke's edema of these true vocal folds renders them almost unrecognizable. Reinke's edema is also called *polypoid corditis*. Reinke's edema can be treated with true vocal fold mucosal incision to release the fluid.

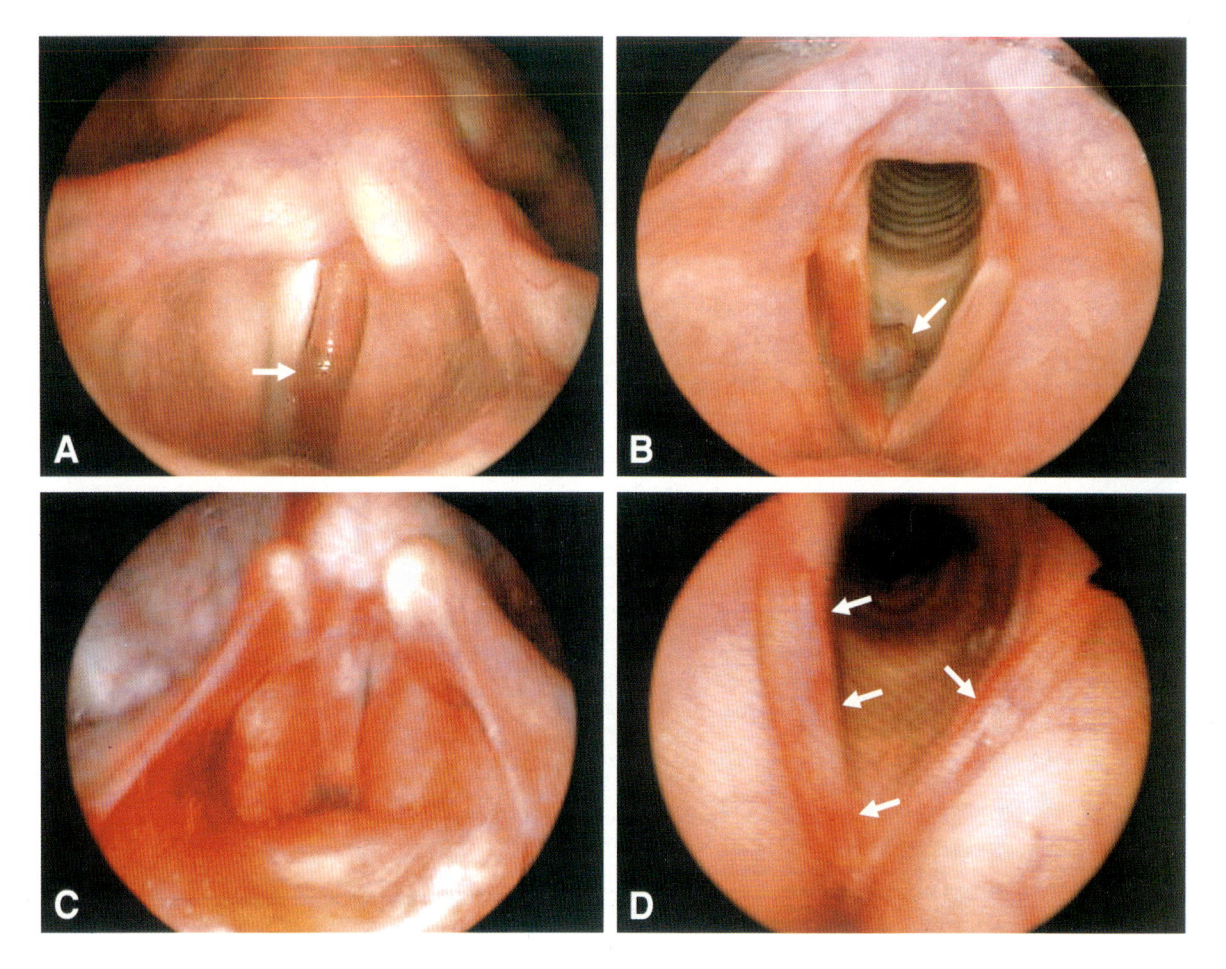

Submucosal Hemorrhage

Figure 9-12A. Vocal fold hemorrhage. This experienced singer developed sudden hoarseness while singing. Her hoarseness persisted. This 70-degree transoral telescopic laryngoscopy reveals a left true vocal fold submucosal hemorrhage with a bubble-like enlargement (*arrow*) in its midportion involving the vibratory margin. Vocal fold hemorrhage adds mass and irregularity to the vocal fold and later promotes fibrosis and stiffness, all of which create hoarseness. Stroboscopic videolaryngoscopy is used to evaluate functional deficits in true vocal fold function. Treatment consists of voice rest acutely, along with voice therapy and training chronically. Surgery can be used to remove a persistent hemorrhagic fibrotic vocal fold mass. This patient improved with voice rest and training.

Figure 9-12B. Vocal fold hemorrhage and polyp. This patient developed persistent hoarseness following an acute episode of voice abuse. The 70-degree transoral telescopic exam reveals a right true vocal fold hemorrhage and a medium-sized hemorrhagic polyp (*arrow*). Medical management, voice rest, and voice therapy should be implemented, but surgical removal of the mass is often required.

Figure 9-12C. Laryngeal hemorrhage. This HHT (hereditary hemorrhagic telangiectasias) patient presented with hemoptysis. The 90-degree laryngoscopic exam reveals fresh blood from laryngeal telangiectasias. The bleeding stopped spontaneously while the patient was supported with humidified oxygen. The patient successfully cleared her airway to prevent aspiration.

Figure 9-12D. HHT laryngeal telangiectasias. This same patient had many laryngeal telangiectasias (*arrows*), as seen on this 70-degree transoral telescopic laryngoscopic exam at a later date after no further hemorrhage.

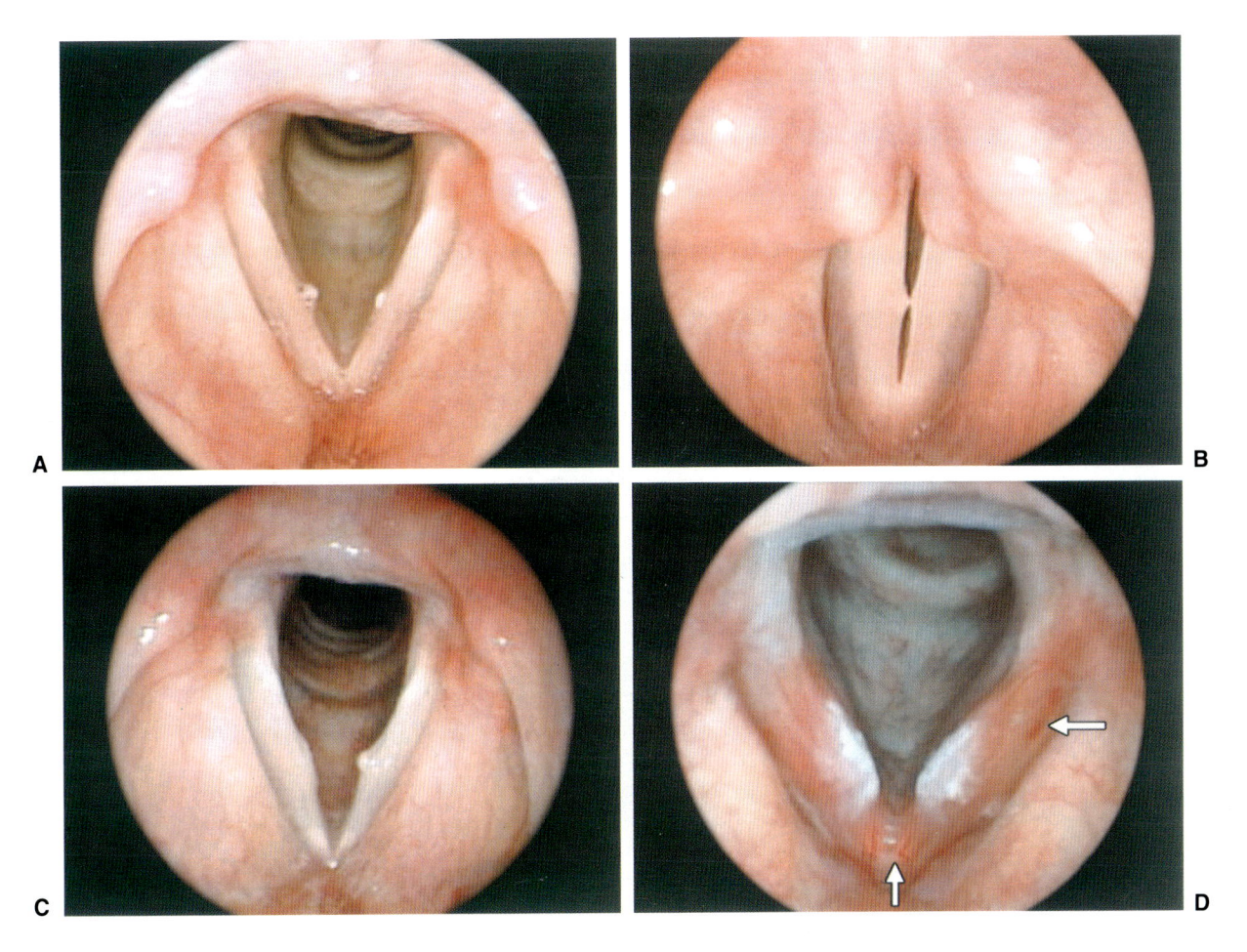

Endoscopy of the Larynx (Videolaryngoscopy)

Vocal Fold Nodules

Figure 9-13A. Vocal fold nodules. This 70-degree telescopic laryngoscopic exam reveals the classic findings of vocal fold nodules: bilateral, anterior third of vibratory vocal fold surface, small callous-like masses. These lesions are due to mucosal reactive changes to chronic voice abuse. The treatment consists of voice rest and therapy. Topical steroid spray may also benefit.

Figure 9-13B. Vocal fold nodules. This singer's vocal fold nodules were very small and visible only on stroboscopic videolaryngoscopy (see Figure 10-8) when incomplete glottic closure was observed due to these small nodules. This patient's inability to reach high registers and maintain phonation improved with conservative treatment.

Figure 9-13C. Vocal fold nodule. This left unilateral vocal fold nodule caused reactive swelling at the contact point of the right vocal fold.

Figure 9-13D. Vocal fold nodules. These large thick hyperkeratotic bilateral vocal fold lesions were due to chronic excessive untreated voice abuse with resultant marked reactive changes. Note also the erythema bilaterally, the small submucosal hemorrhage of the left vocal fold (*long arrow*), and the dilated prominent varicose vessels of the anterior vocal folds (*short arrow*).

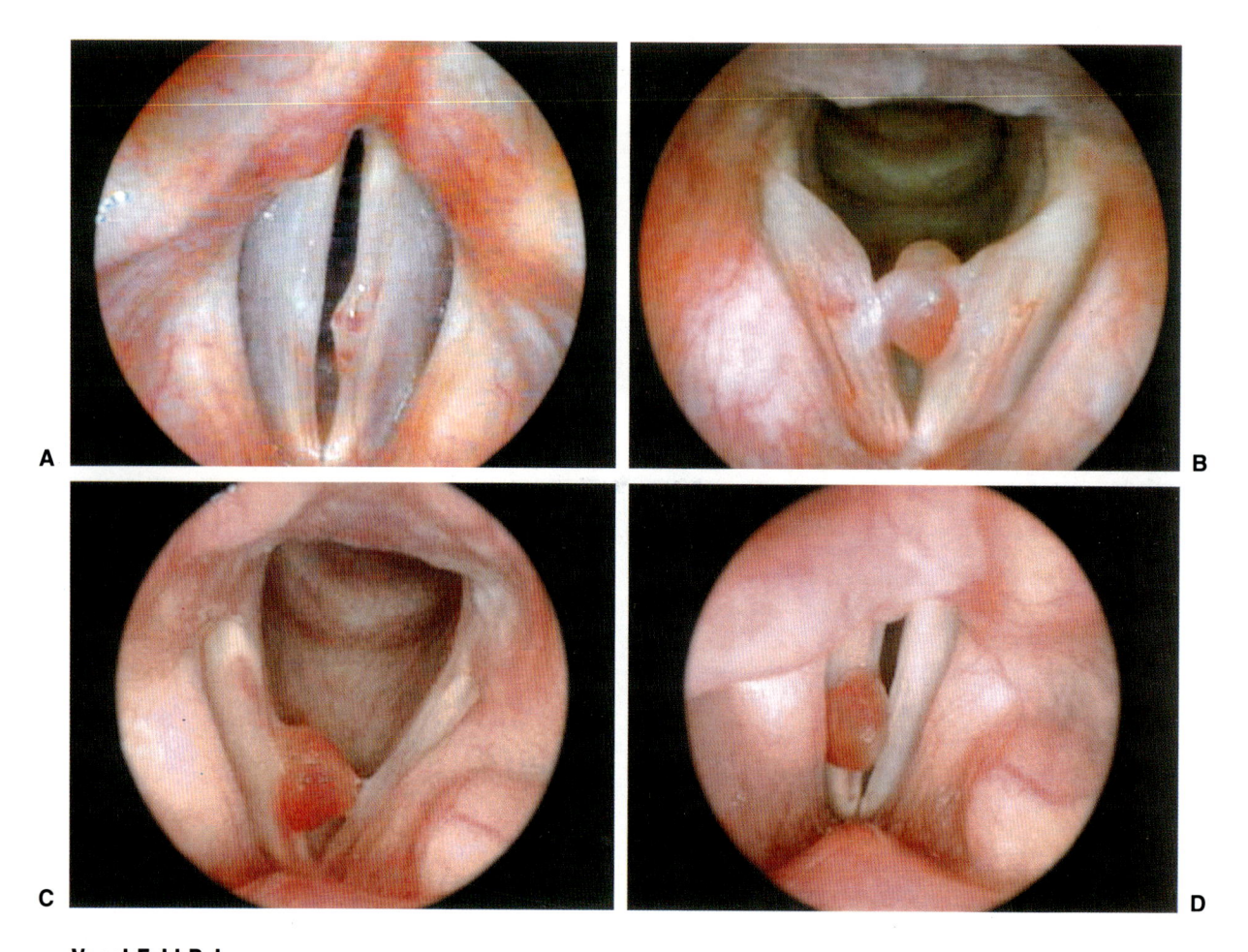

Vocal Fold Polyps

Figure 9-14A. Small vocal fold polyps. Vocal fold polyps may be sessile or pedunculated, are usually unilateral, typically arise acutely due to voice abuse causing hoarseness, and often require surgical removal for voice improvement. This 70-degree telescopic laryngoscopic exam reveals a small sessile polyp of the vibratory surface of the left true vocal fold with minor submucosal hemorrhages. Mild thickening of the contact point of the contralateral vocal fold is seen. Note also arytenoid and interarytenoid erythema consistent with reflux laryngitis.

Figure 9-14B. Medium vocal fold polyps. These two medium-sized pedunculated left vocal fold polyps caused hoarseness and required surgical removal with the microspot CO_2 laser, maximally preserving mucosa of the vibrating free edge.

Figure 9-14C. Medium pedunculated vocal fold polyp. This is a typical medium-sized pedunculated vocal fold polyp. Mid-sized polyps usually cause hoarseness.

Figure 9-14D. Medium pedunculated vocal fold polyp. This same patient, however, did not have hoarseness. As seen in this 70-degree laryngoscopic exam the pedunculated polyp flipped superiorly during phonation and did not disrupt glottic closure or the vibratory mucosal surface.

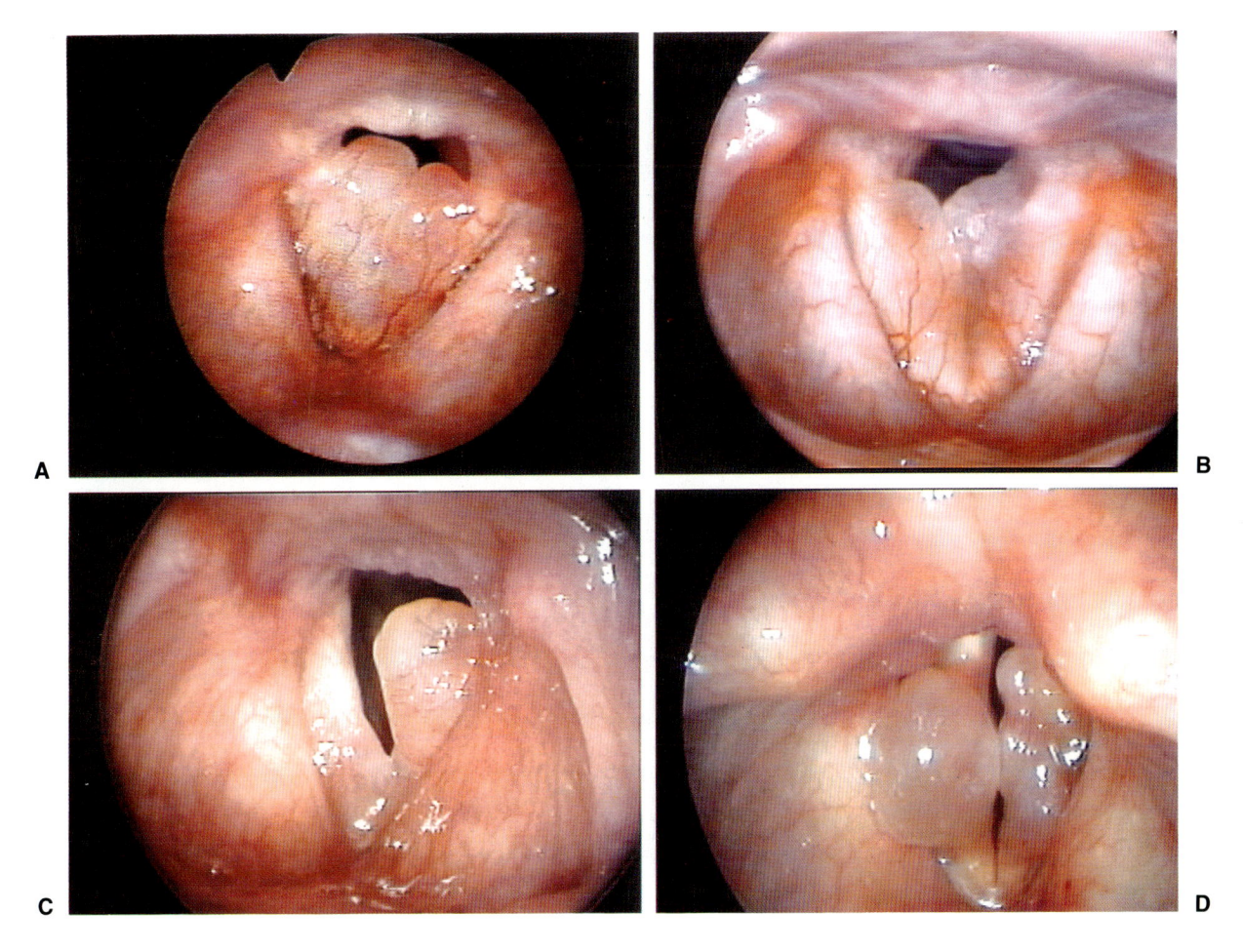

Large Vocal Fold Polyps

Figure 9-15A. Large vocal fold polyps. This patient had a markedly hoarse voice and shortness of breath due to the large vocal fold polyps that obscured the vocal folds themselves. Note the compromised airway where only a slit of posterior glottis remained. Surgical excision may be accomplished with a microspot CO_2 laser or with endoscopic laryngeal scissors. Maximal mucosal preservation is sought.

Figure 9-15B. Large vocal fold polyps. This was another patient who had partial airway compromise and hoarseness due to large vocal fold sessile polyps requiring surgical removal.

Figure 9-15C. Large left vocal fold polyp. This patient had a recurrent large left sessile vocal fold polyp and right polypoid change status post multiple previous polyp excisions. She suffered a husky hoarseness.

Figure 9-15D. Large vocal fold polyps. These large vocal fold polyps caused choking but not hoarseness as the polyps were displaced superiorly on phonation.

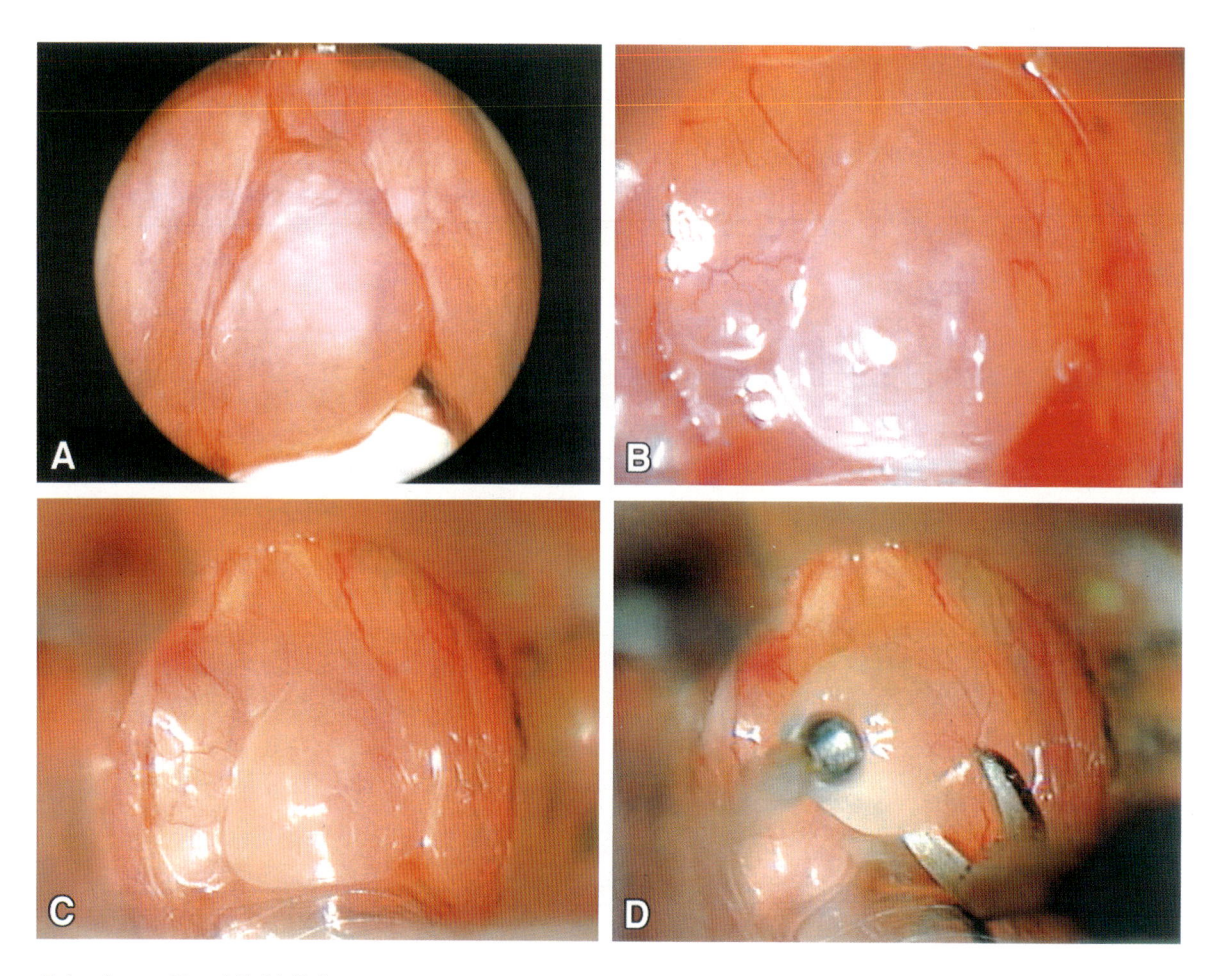

Extra Large Vocal Fold Polyps

Figure 9-16A. Extra large left true vocal fold polyp. This sessile left vocal fold polyp almost completely occluded the airway. The endotracheal tube was visible at the bottom of this intraoperative view.

Figure 9-16B. Extra large polyps. These polyps caused upper airway obstruction. On this operative view there was almost no visible airway. When the patient was awake the polyps would move with air movement so the patient could breathe.

Figure 9-16C. Extra large polyps. More extra large obstructing polyps are shown in this intraoperative laryngoscopic view. The ETT is visible inferiorly.

Figure 9-16D. Polyp excision. Polyps can be removed with a CO_2 laser or, as in this intraoperative view of the same patient, the endoscopic scissors. The suction was used to retract the bulk of the polyp so the scissors could cut it at the base.

Endoscopy of the Larynx (Videolaryngoscopy)

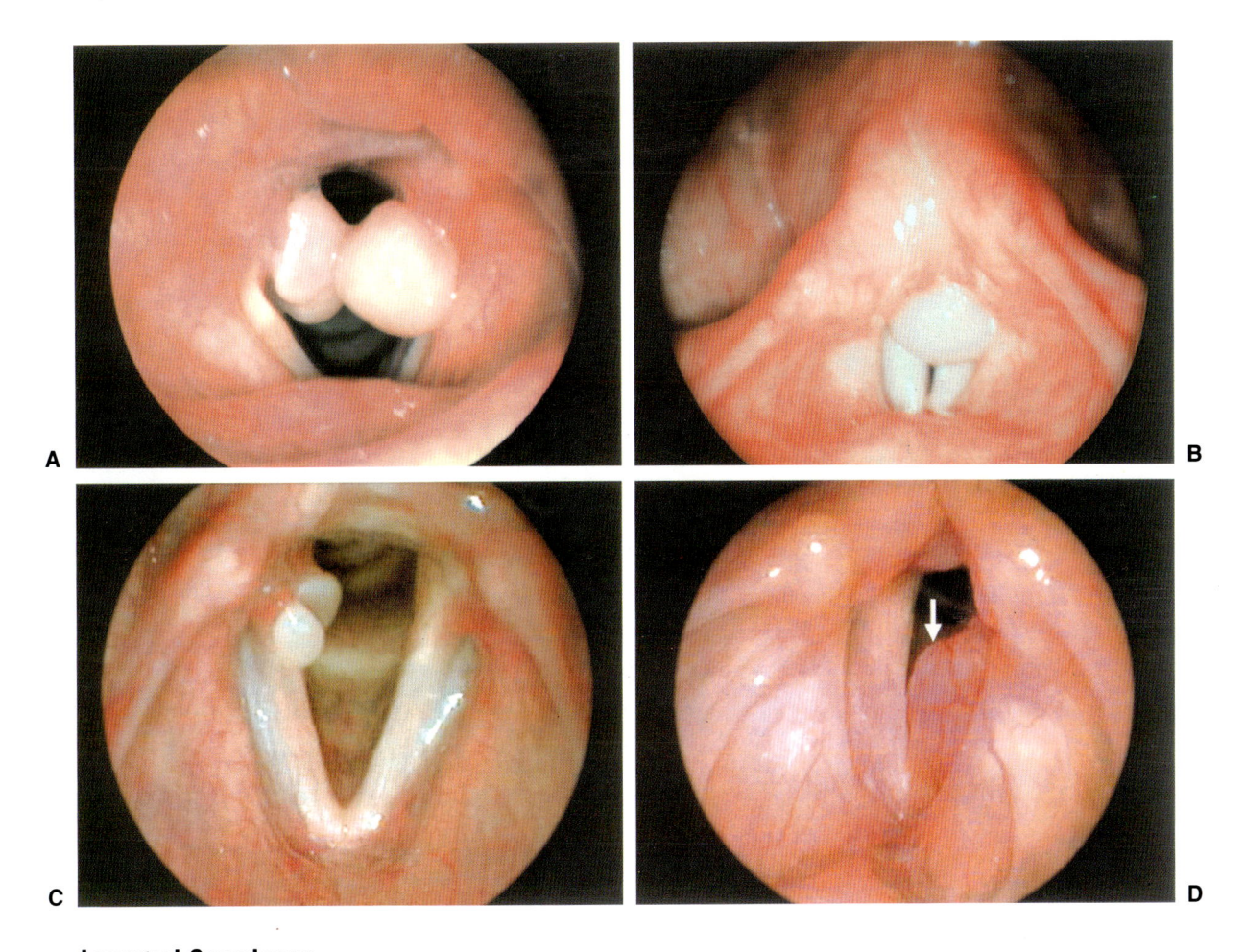

Laryngeal Granulomas

Figure 9-17A. Bilateral granulomas. This patient developed minimal hoarseness weeks after a prolonged open heart surgery. This 70-degree telescopic laryngeal exam reveals three large granulomas of the bilateral medial arytenoids. Laryngeal granulomas most commonly occur along the vocal process or medial arytenoids. The most common cause is intubation injury exacerbated by local infection or reflux laryngitis.

Figure 9-17B. Laryngeal granulomas. This same patient experienced only minimal hoarseness because on glottic closure the left granuloma moved above the vocal folds and the right granulomas moved below. The vibratory surfaces of the vocal folds met appropriately.

Figure 9-17C. Vocal fold granulomas. This patient had hoarseness after developing these right vocal process granulomas from an intubation injury. Contact irritation was seen at the contralateral vocal process.

Figure 9-17D. Teflon granuloma. This patient suffered a left vocal fold paralysis due to a football injury. He had a left vocal fold Teflon injection to medialize the paralyzed vocal fold. Subsequently he developed a large granuloma (*arrow*) overlying the Teflon.

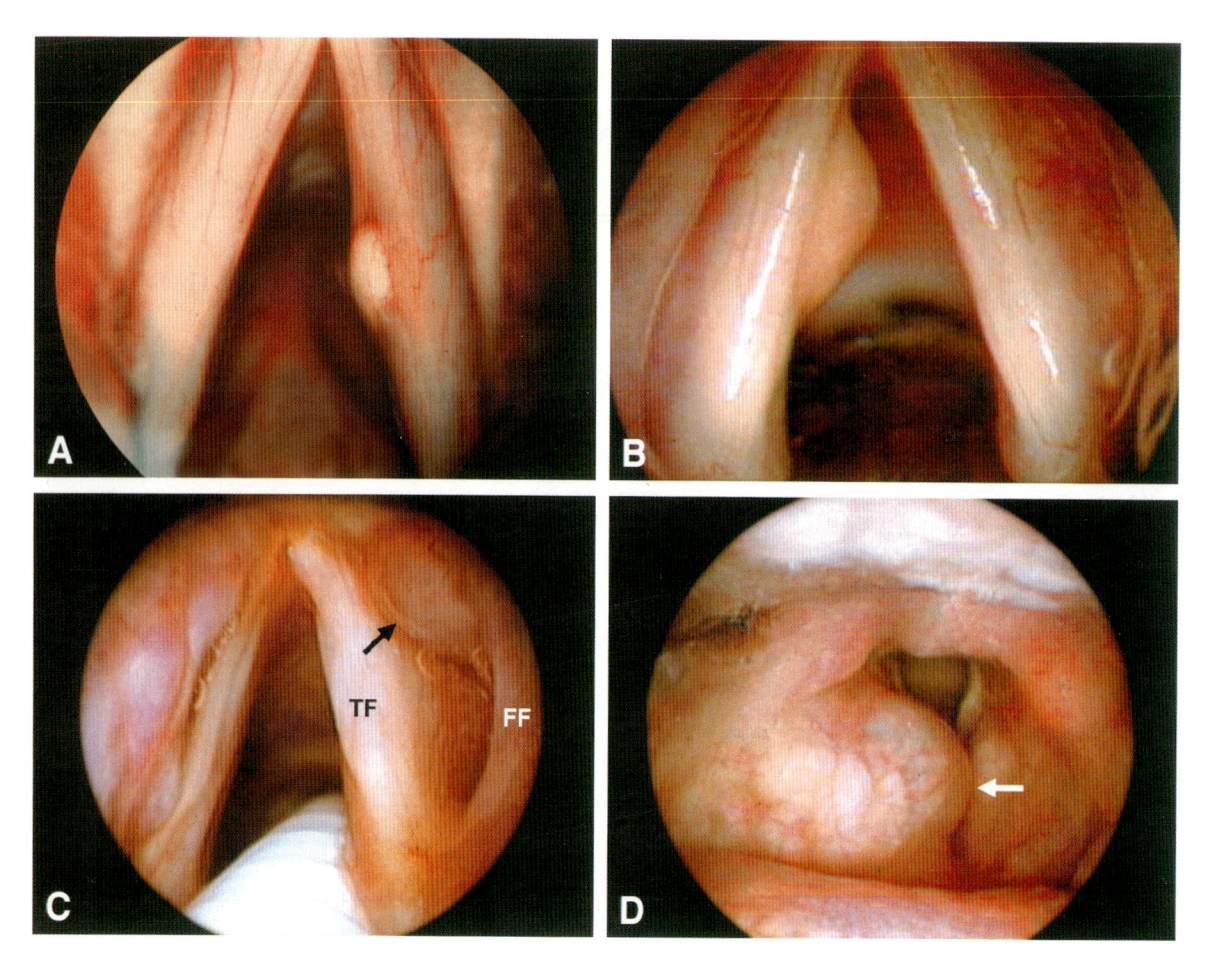

Laryngeal Cysts

Figure 9-18A. Epidermoid true vocal fold cyst. This intraoperative telescopic laryngoscopic view displays a right true vocal fold epidermoid cyst. These cysts characteristically are round white masses of desquamated keratin and cholesterol debris and lie along the medial or superior aspect of the middle third of the true vocal fold. Stroboscopic videolaryngoscopy reveals a lack of a mucosal vibratory pattern unlike polyps, which will vibrate (see Figure 10-10). Treatment requires surgical cyst removal with mucosal preservation.

Figure 9-18B. Mucous retention cyst of the true vocal fold. Mucous retention cysts present similarly to epidermoid cysts. As this intraoperative telescopic view displays, these cysts are yellow along the inferior aspect of the middle third of the true vocal fold. They contain mucous debris from mucous gland obstruction on the inferior true vocal fold surface. Like epidermoid cysts, these cysts lack mucosal vibration on stroboscopy, and they require surgical excision.

Figure 9-18C. Anterior saccular cyst. A saccular cyst (also called laryngeal or saccular mucocele) is a mucus-containing dilated saccule that does not communicate with the laryngeal lumen. Anterior saccular cysts, as demonstrated in this intraoperative view (*arrow*), protrude medially into the larynx between the true (TF) and false (FF) folds.

Figure 9-18D. Internal laryngocele. Like a saccular cyst, a laryngocele is a dilated mucus-containing saccule. Unlike a saccular cyst, however, a laryngocele communicates with the larynx lumen. This 90-degree transoral telescopic view in the office shows a typical right internal laryngocele (*arrow*) extending posterosuperiorly into the area of the false and aryepiglottic folds.

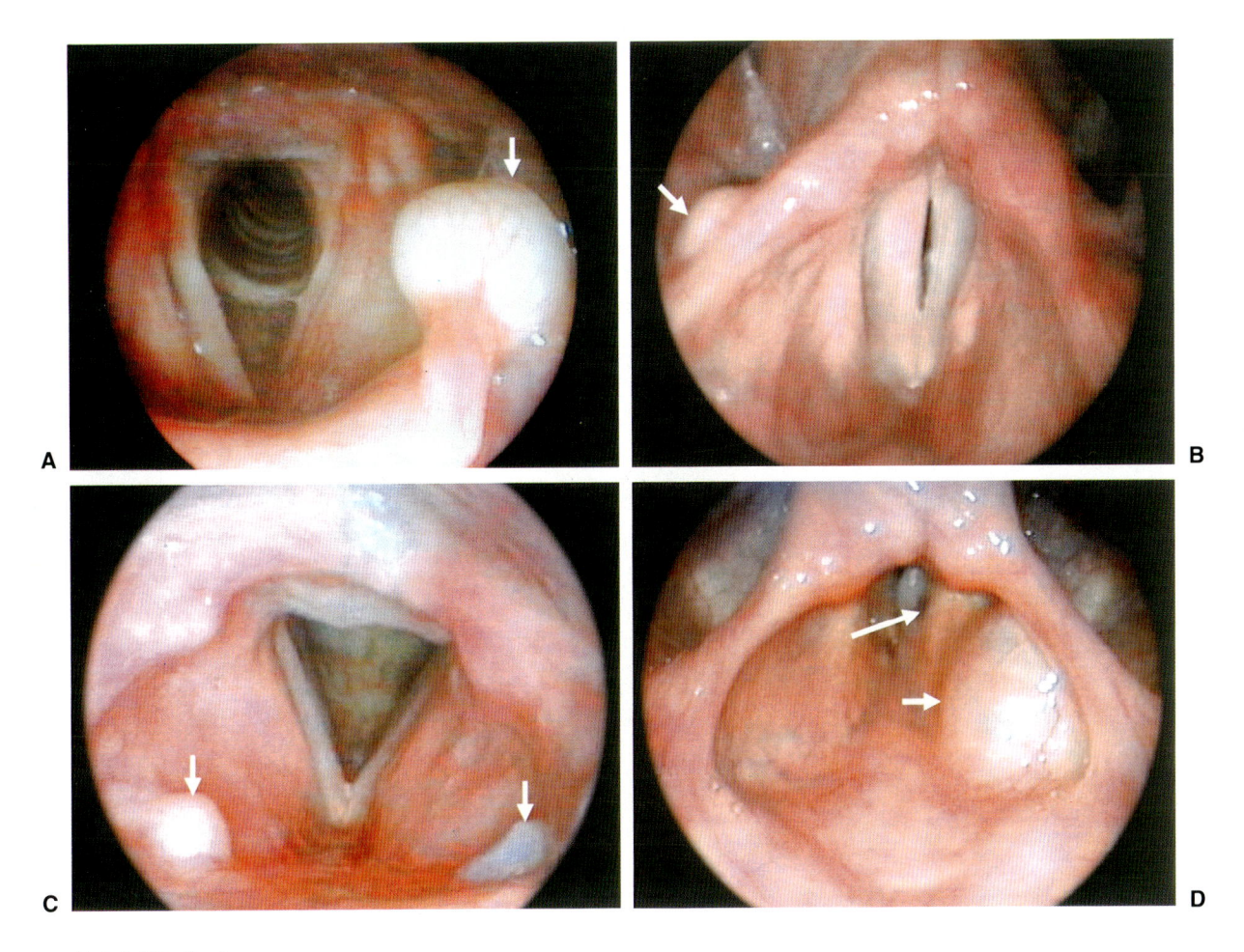

Epiglottic Cysts

Figure 9-19A. Aryepiglottic fold cyst. Epiglottic cysts are caused by mucus retention in the dilated collecting ducts of submucosal glands and are named according to site. These are the most common laryngeal cysts. This 70-degree transoral telescopic view in the office highlights a left aryepiglottic fold cyst (*arrow*).

Figure 9-19B. Aryepiglottic fold cyst. This 70-degree telescopic view shows a right aryepiglottic fold cyst.

Figure 9-19C. Epiglottic cysts. These cysts (*arrows*) were found incidentally on 90-degree transoral telescopic laryngoscopy and were of no pathologic or clinical significance. (Courtesy of K. J. Lee, M.D., New Haven, CT.)

Figure 19D. Epiglottic cyst. This large epiglottic cyst (*short arrow*) resembled a laryngocele but did not protrude from the ventricle (*long arrow*).

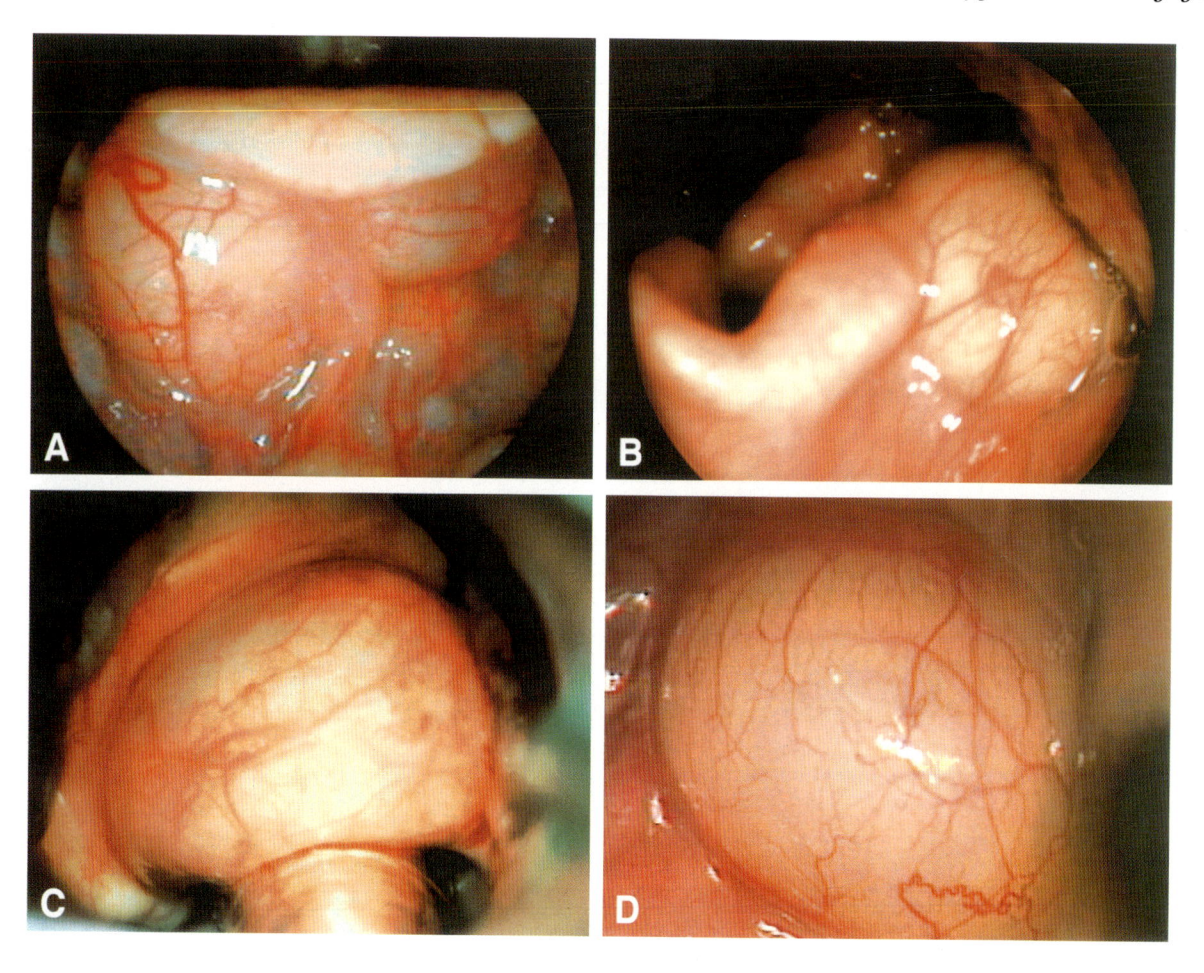

Vallecular Cysts

Figure 9-20A. Vallecular cysts. This 41-year-old woman suffered from a chronic sore throat, globus sensation, and occasional difficulty swallowing. Her gastroenterologist treated her GERD without any relief of these symptoms. Otolaryngologic referral and examination (90-degree transoral telescopy in the office) revealed a large right vallecular cyst and a smaller left cyst. The epiglottis was seen at the top of this view and the midline glossoepiglottic fold was seen between the cysts. Upon removal the contents was noted to be a very tenacious mucus. The patient's symptoms resolved after surgery.

Figure 9-20B. Vallecular cyst. This woman presented with a pharyngeal foreign body sensation and intermittent choking spells. The office telescopic exam revealed this left vallecular cyst, which was pedunculated and fairly mobile. Occasionally the cyst would flop into the supraglottic area and cause chocking. Note the omega epiglottis.

Figure 9-20C. Epiglottic cyst. This intraoperative 0-degree telescopic videolaryngoscopic exam reveals a large laryngeal surface epiglottic cyst. The epiglottis surrounds the cyst laterally and anteriorly (*top of view*), and the endotracheal tube is seen (*bottom of view*).

Figure 9-20D. Vallecular cyst. A close-up view of the smaller cyst in Figure 9-20A reveals the smooth round cyst wall and prominently displays the surface vessels.

Endoscopy of the Larynx (Videolaryngoscopy)

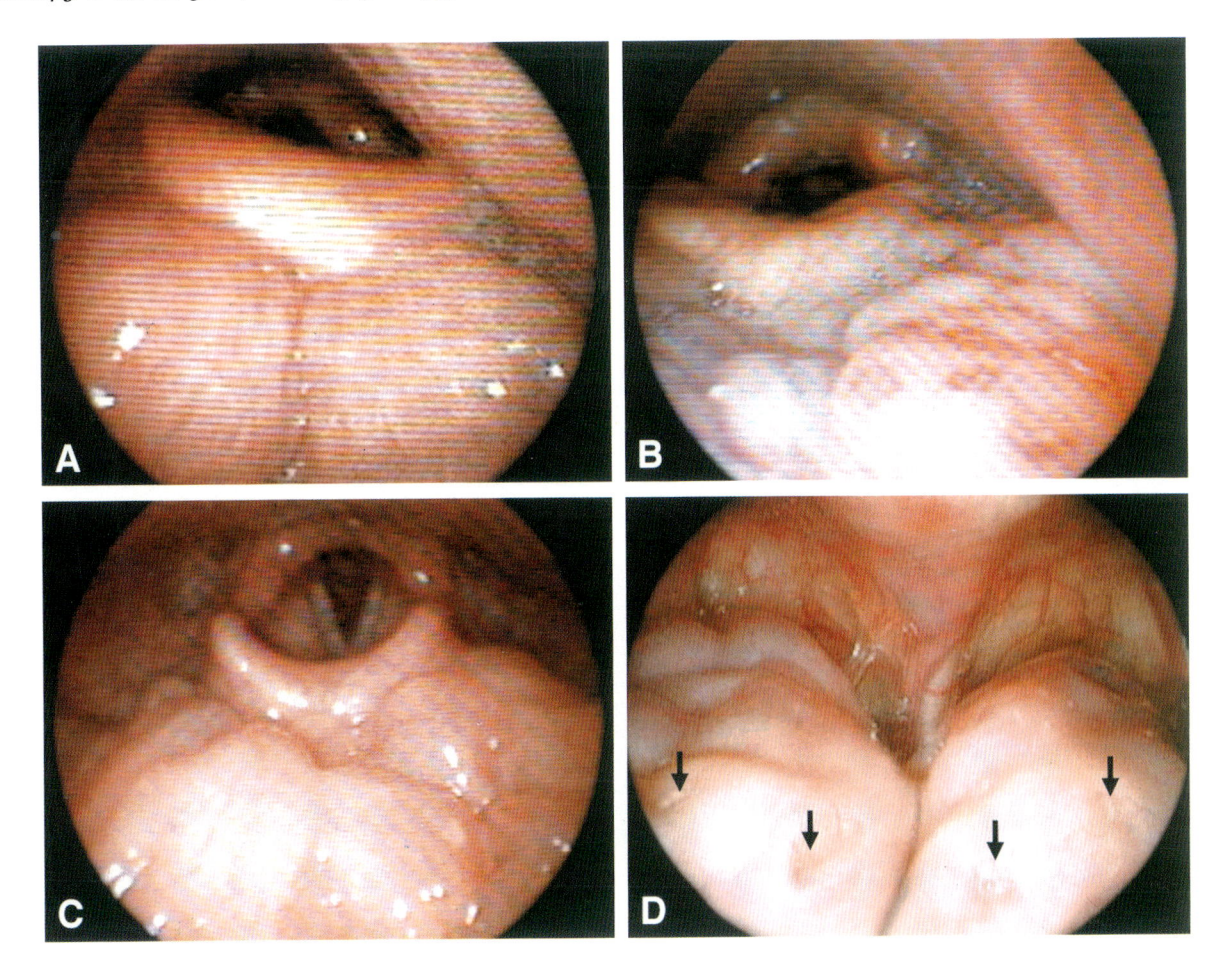

Lingual Tonsil Hypertrophy

Figure 9-21A. Lingual tonsil hypertrophy. This patient presented with a chronic globus sensation that gradually became more prominent. Fiberoptic laryngoscopy reveals bilateral markedly hypertrophied smooth distinct lingual tonsils that displaced the epiglottis posteriorly. This patient's symptoms resolved after a lingual tonsillectomy.

Figure 9-21B. Acute lingual tonsillitis. This patient complained of acute throat pain. This fiberscopic exam demonstrates hypertrophied cryptic irregular acutely infected lingual tonsils (L>R) that partially obscured the epiglottis.

Figure 9-21C. Lingual tonsil hypertrophy. The lingual tonsils make up the anteroinferior portion of Waldeyer's ring of lymphoid tissue in the pharynx. These enlarged lingual tonsils are spilling over the pharyngoepiglottic fold, which may cause a sensation of food sticking.

Figure 9-21D. Follicular lingual tonsillitis. This close-up 70-degree transoral telescopic exam of the vallecula reveals bilateral cryptic (*arrows*) lingual tonsil hypertrophy. The lingual surface of the epiglottis is at the top of the view and the midline glossoepiglottic fold extends down from the epiglottis to the base of tongue.

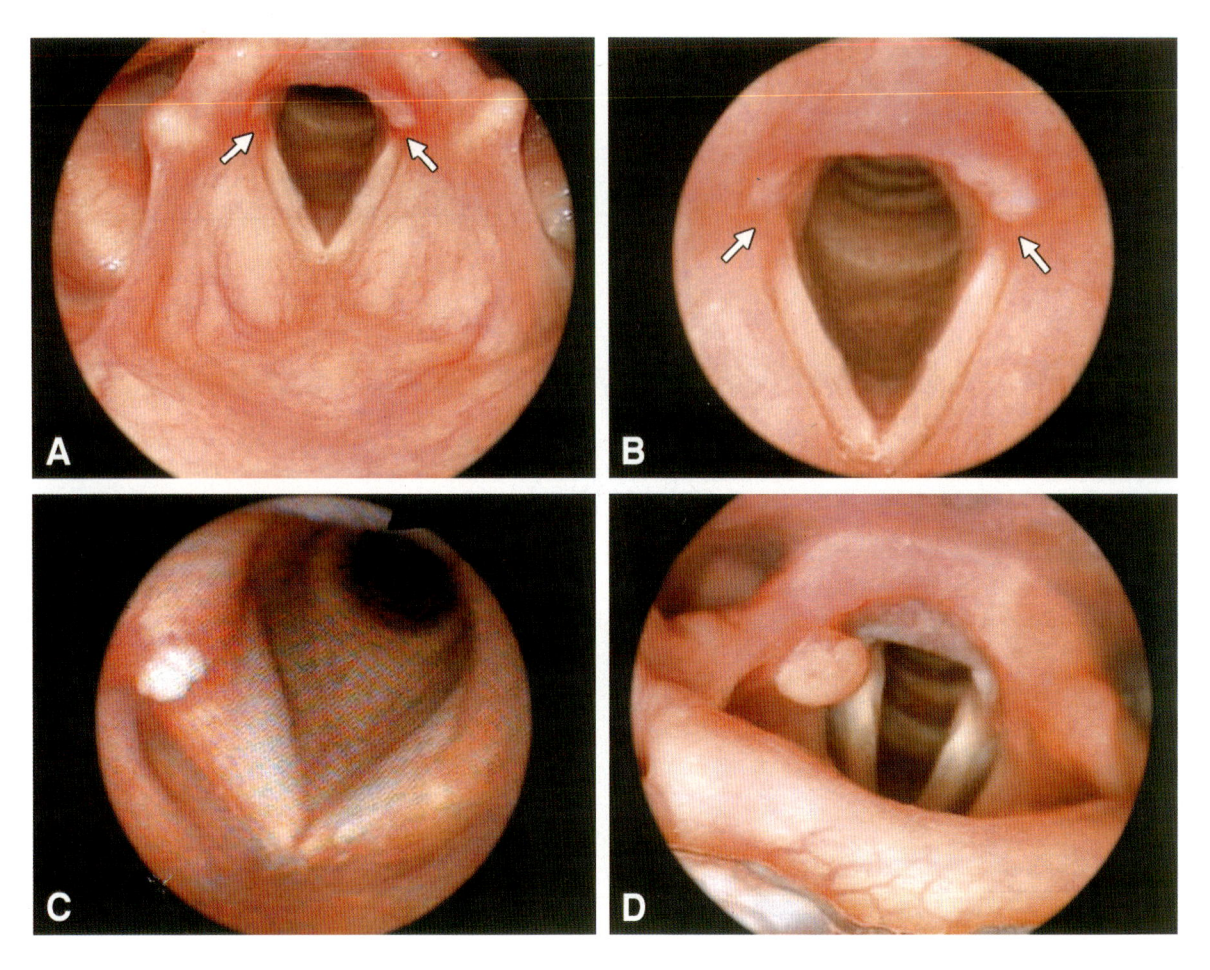

Arytenoid Contact Ulcers

Figure 9-22A. Vocal process contact ulcers. Acute and chronic voice abuse may result in contact ulcers, usually on the vocal processes of the arytenoids. This patient had bilateral vocal process contact ulcers (*arrows*) with surrounding inflammation, seen here on 90-degree transoral telescopic laryngoscopy.

Figure 9-22B. Vocal process contact ulcers. This same patient also had small bilateral true vocal fold nodules. Treatment for both contact ulcers (*arrows*) and nodules is voice rest and speech therapy. Antireflux measures may also be implemented as GERD can mimic contact ulcers and exacerbate existing ulcers. Note also that this 70-degree transoral telescopic view clearly demonstrates the cricoid cartilage and the first two tracheal rings.

Figure 9-22C. Vocal process contact ulcer. This fiberscopic view of the larynx demonstrates a right vocal process contact ulcer with an overlying fibrinous coat and surrounding inflammation. The fiberscope wide-angle lens provides a wide close-up view but also distorts the image (see Figure 10-6). The bulging inferior aspect of the true vocal folds is the conus elasticus on each side. Also visible is the right ventricle.

Figure 9-22D. Arytenoid granuloma. This 70-degree telescopic exam reveals a postintubation right arytenoid granuloma. This granuloma was located unusually high on the arytenoid, near the cuneiform cartilage. Reevaluation for surgery three months later revealed complete spontaneous healing of this granuloma.

Endoscopy of the Larynx (Videolaryngoscopy)

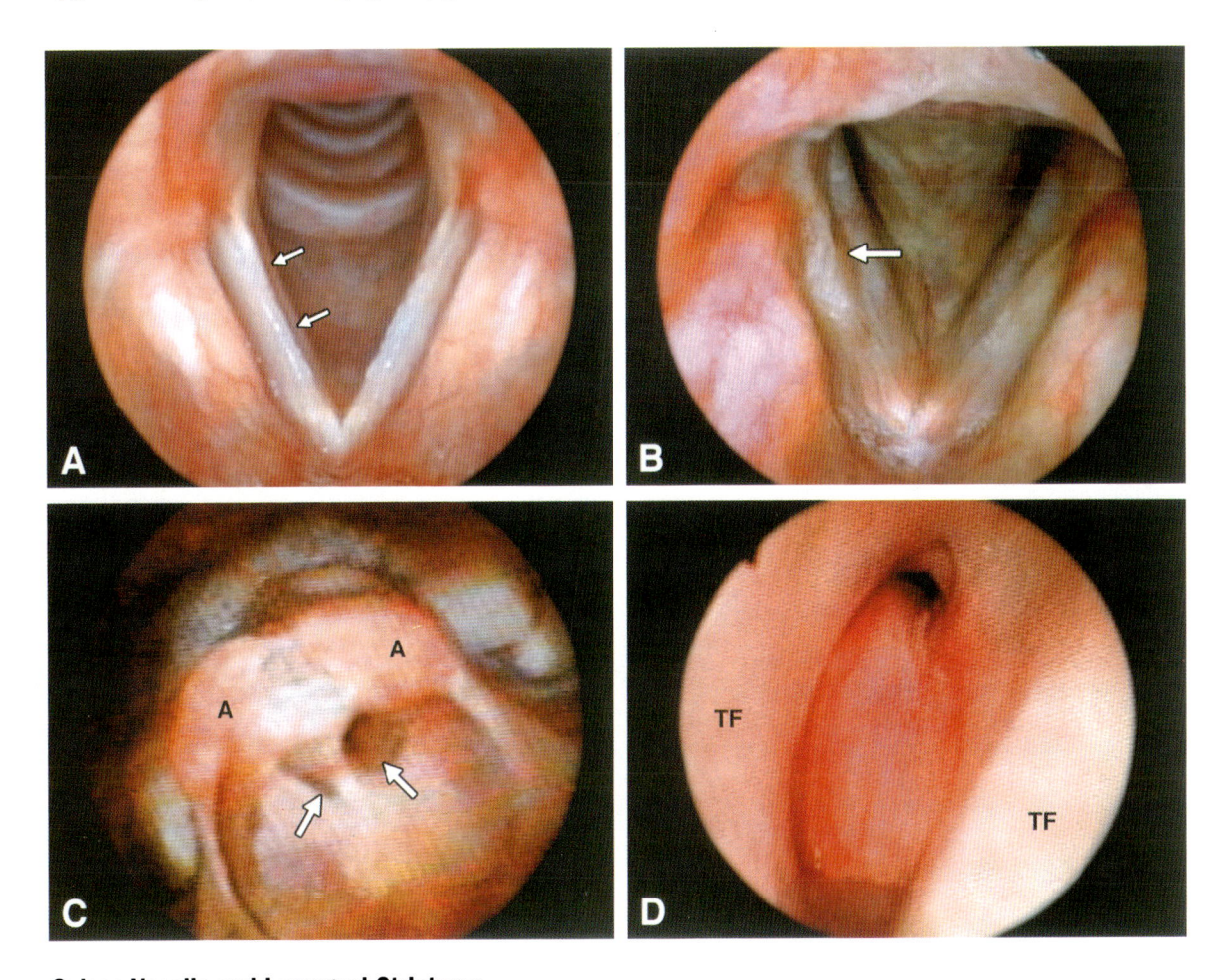

Sulcus Vocalis and Laryngeal Strictures

Figure 9-23A. Sulcus vocalis. This transoral 70-degree telescopic view of the glottis reveals a fine sulcus or furrow (*arrows*) along the medial edge of the membranous true vocal fold. This uncommon congenital condition, sulcus vocalis, results from a sulcus in the superficial lamina propria, possibly from an open epidermoid cyst. Typically the true vocal folds are bowed, resulting in a breathy husky voice. Treatment may include Teflon injection or sulcus excision.

Figure 9-23B. Sulcus vergeture. This variant of sulcus vocalis is also characterized by an atrophic depression along the free margin of the vocal fold (*arrow*).

Figure 9-23C. Supraglottic stricture. This one-year-old infant suffered laryngeal trauma in an automobile accident. She required a tracheotomy. Follow-up fiberscopic laryngoscopy demonstrated the narrow supraglottic openings leading to her glottis (*arrows*). The arytenoids were also scarred. Attempts to excise the stenosis with the CO_2 laser failed.

Figure 9-23D. Subglottic stricture. This 32-year-old man developed a subglottic stricture from a prolonged intubation complicated by chronic GERD and local infection. This transnasal fiberscopic view of the subglottis reveals the true vocal folds (TF) at the lateral portions of this view and the narrow subglottic opening at the top of this view. Thick scar tissue was seen anteriorly along the full length of the subglottis. This patient was tracheotomy-dependent until surgical correction was accomplished.

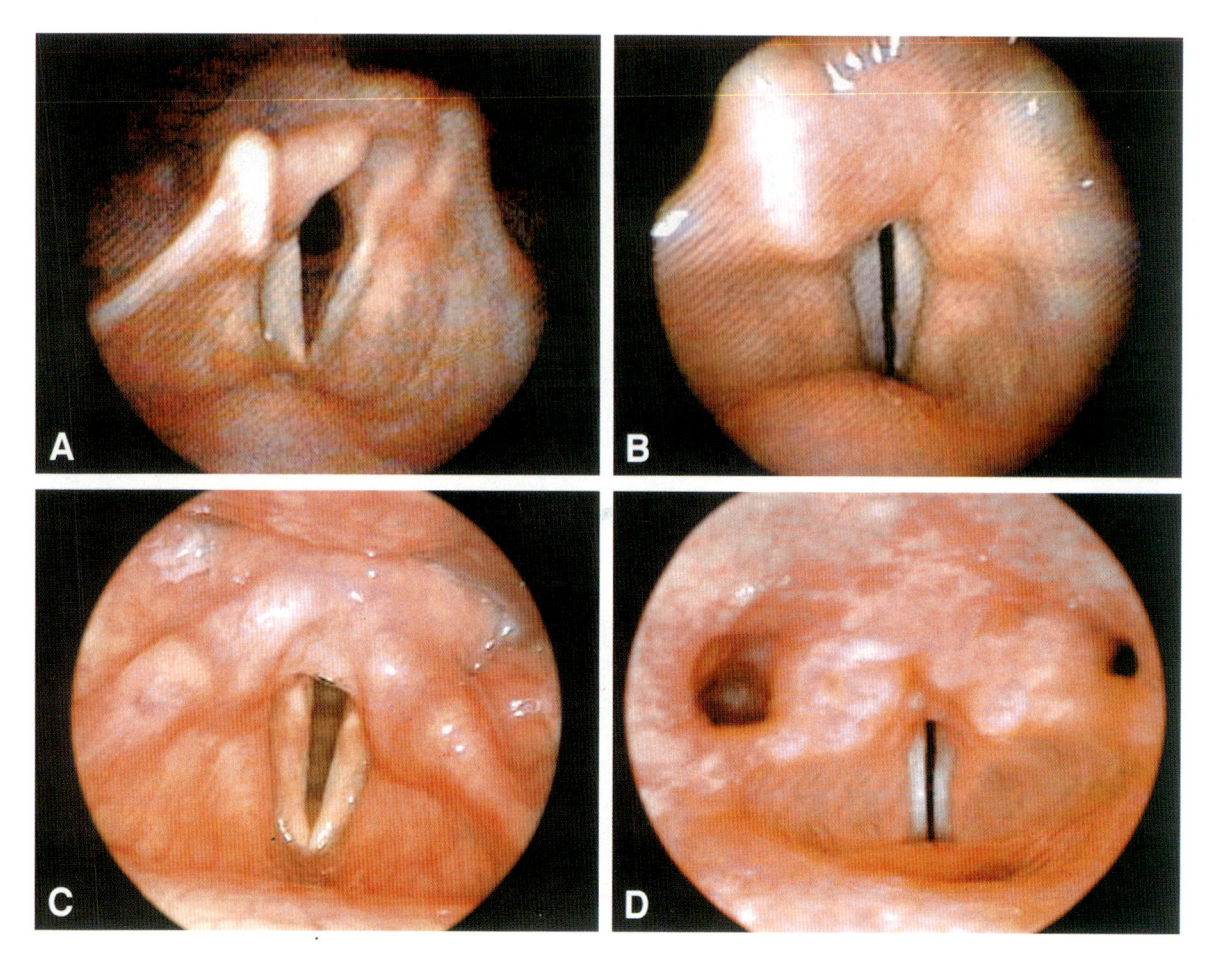

True Vocal Fold Paralysis

Figure 9-24A. Right recurrent laryngeal nerve paralysis. This patient suffered an injury to the right recurrent laryngeal nerve during a previous right thyroid lobectomy. The patient had a hoarse voice that tired easily. Fiberscopic laryngoscopy during inspiration revealed the right paralyzed true vocal fold in the paramedian position.

Figure 9-24B. Right recurrent laryngeal nerve paralysis. The same larynx on phonation demonstrated the lack of right true vocal fold movement, staying in the paramedian position. The left true vocal fold medialized fairly well, but there was still incomplete glottic closure (see also Figure 10-7G). This patient may benefit from a Teflon injection or an Isshiki Type I thyroplasty medialization.

Figure 9-24C. Bilateral recurrent laryngeal nerve paralysis. This patient had bilateral recurrent laryngeal nerve injuries from a total thyroidectomy. The bilaterally paralyzed vocal folds rested in the paramedian position, leaving her with breathy hoarseness.

Figure 9-24D. Bilateral recurrent laryngeal nerve paralysis. This 70-degree telescopic laryngoscopic exam reveals bilateral recurrent laryngeal nerve paralysis leaving the true vocal folds in the median position due to unopposed cricothyroid muscle function via the superior laryngeal nerves. This patient had adequate phonation but compromised respiration requiring tracheotomy and later a Kashima procedure.

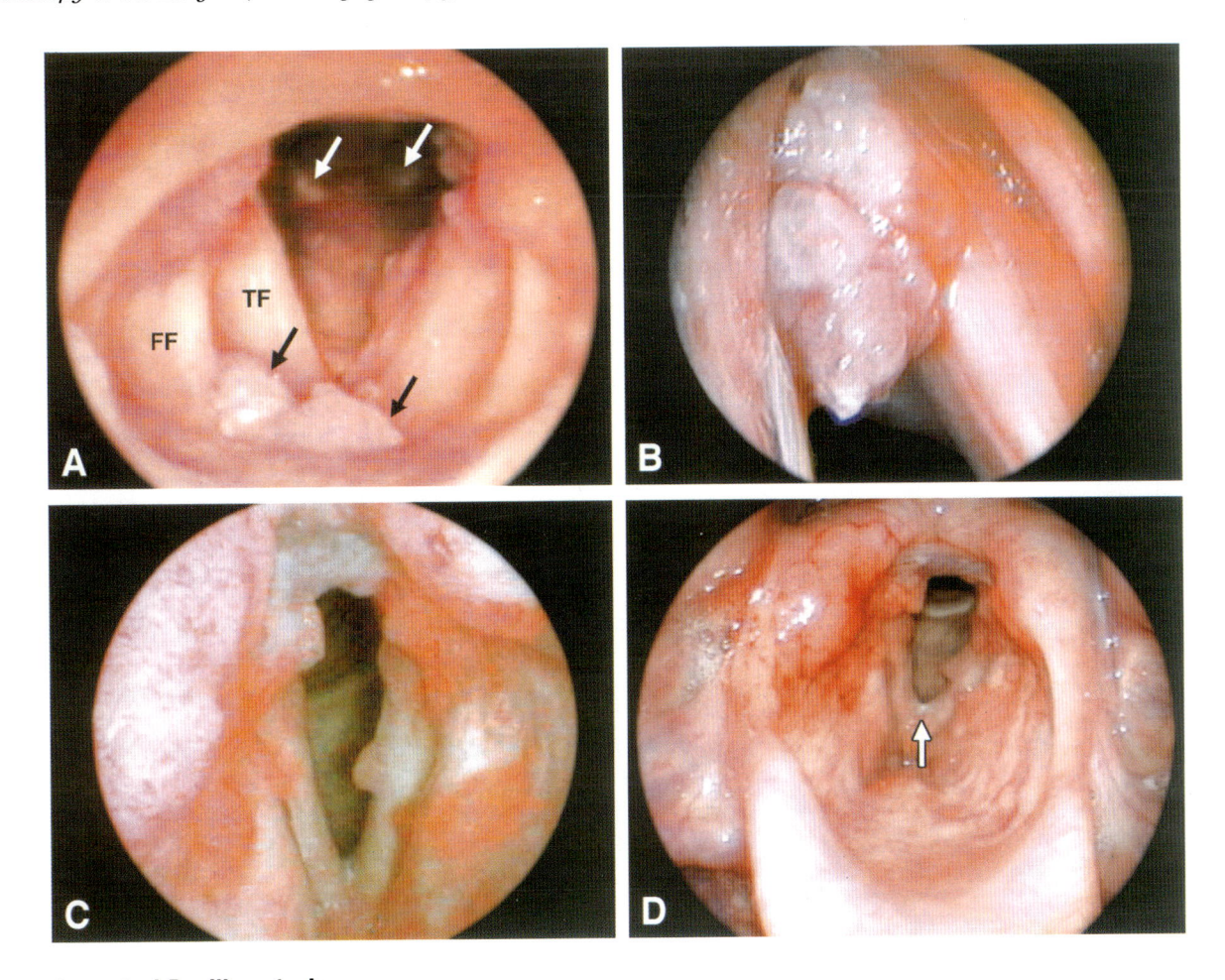

Laryngeal Papillomatosis

Figure 9-25A. Laryngeal papillomatosis. Papillomas in the larynx are typically multiple on the true and false folds and have a warty, red, friable appearance. This patient had multiple small to medium papillomas (*black arrows*) on his true (TF) and false (FF) vocal folds and even in his trachea (*white arrows*).

Figure 9-25B. True vocal fold papilloma. This patient had a large true vocal fold papilloma as seen on this intraoperative telescopic videolaryngoscopy. Adults usually present with hoarseness, but also sometimes with upper airway obstructive symptoms.

Figure 9-25C. Laryngeal papillomatosis. This 70-degree telescopic laryngoscopic exam reveals multiple small papillomas. Human papilloma virus (HPV) types 6, 11, 16, 18 are most often associated with papillomatosis; 2% of these lesions are malignant (14% if the patient also received XRT).

Figure 9-25D. Laryngeal papillomatosis. This 90-degree office telescopic laryngeal exam demonstrates multiple papillomas. Treatment consists of surgical removal or debulking with forceps or the CO_2 laser. Nevertheless, they tend to persist or recur. This patient had multiple excisions and subsequently developed an anterior commissure web (*arrow*).

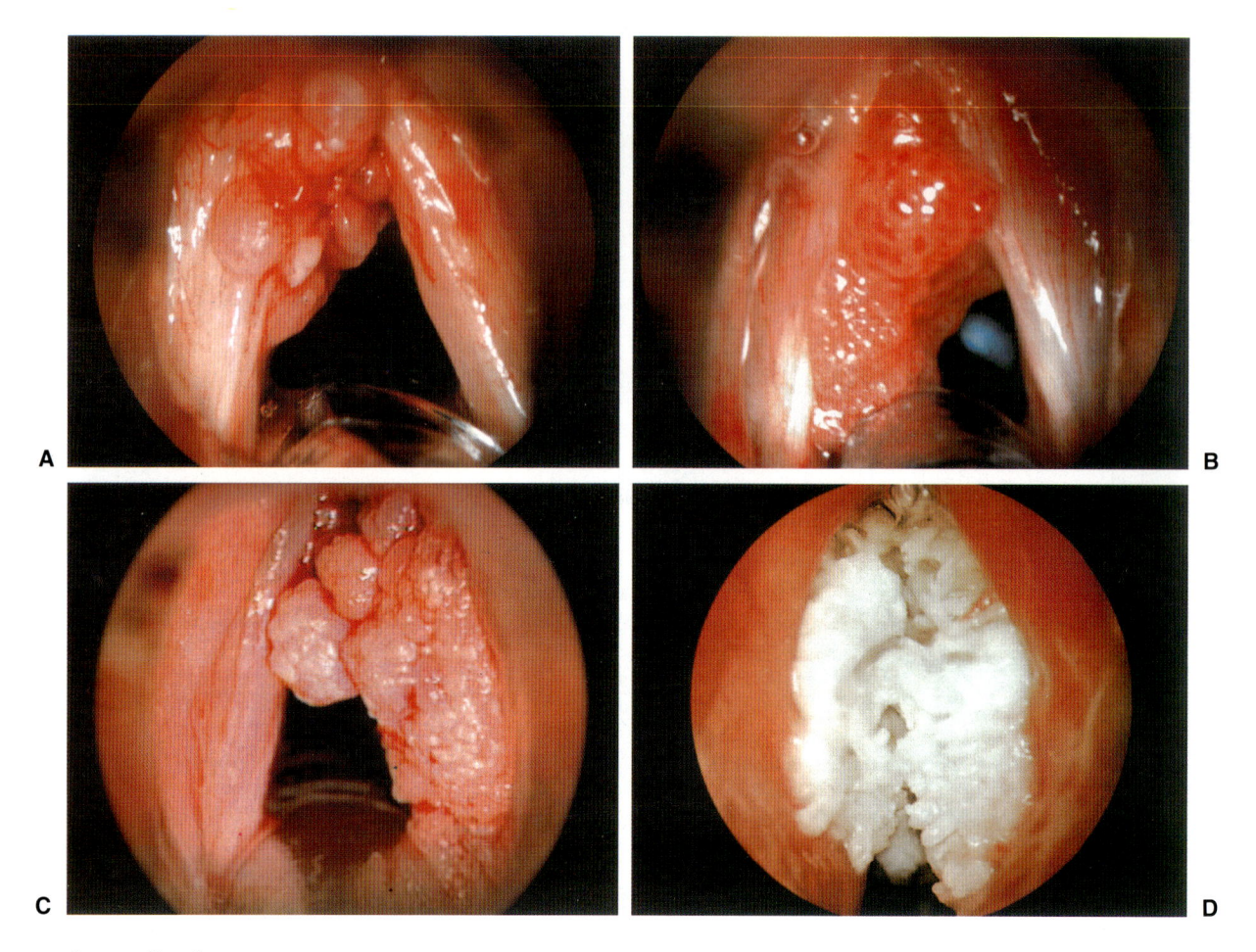

Larynx Carcinoma

Figure 9-26A. Glottic squamous cell carcinoma. This intraoperative view displays a T_2 left true vocal fold squamous cell carcinoma that extends across the anterior commissure to the anterior right true vocal fold. Surgery alone yields about an 80% cure rate, and radiation alone yields about a 60% cure rate for this lesion.

Figure 9-26B. Glottic squamous cell carcinoma. This intraoperative view shows another T_2 left true vocal fold squamous cell carcinoma that extends across the anterior commissure and subglotically. The left true vocal fold was impaired but not fixed.

Figure 9-26C. Transglottic squamous cell carcinoma. This large right T_3N_0 true vocal fold squamous cell carcinoma (SCCA) extended along the full length of the right true vocal fold and superiorly into the ventricle, thus making it a transglottic cancer (i.e., cancer extends from true fold into ventricle). The right true vocal fold was fixed. Surgery and radiation each yield about a 50% five-year survival for stage III glottic SCCA. This patient refused a total laryngectomy, so a local laser excision was performed with postoperative radiation treatment. The patient had no evidence of recurrence one year later, but he died shortly thereafter from an unrelated disease.

Figure 9-26D. Laryngeal verrucous carcinoma. The patient had been misdiagnosed with asthma due to recurrent "wheezing" until one refractory episode resulted in an otolaryngologic consultation. The patient was breathing through the posterior chink (*bottom of view*) that intermittently obstructed further with mucus. This bulky bilateral glottic verrucous carcinoma was discovered and staged as a $T_2N_0M_0$ stage II tumor. The true vocal folds were slightly mobile, limited only by the tumor bulk and not paralyzed. Ordinarily this cancer would be resected with a total laryngectomy. This tumor, however, was excised with scissors and treated with radiation. The patient had no recurrence four years postoperatively.

Endoscopy of the Larynx (Videolaryngoscopy)

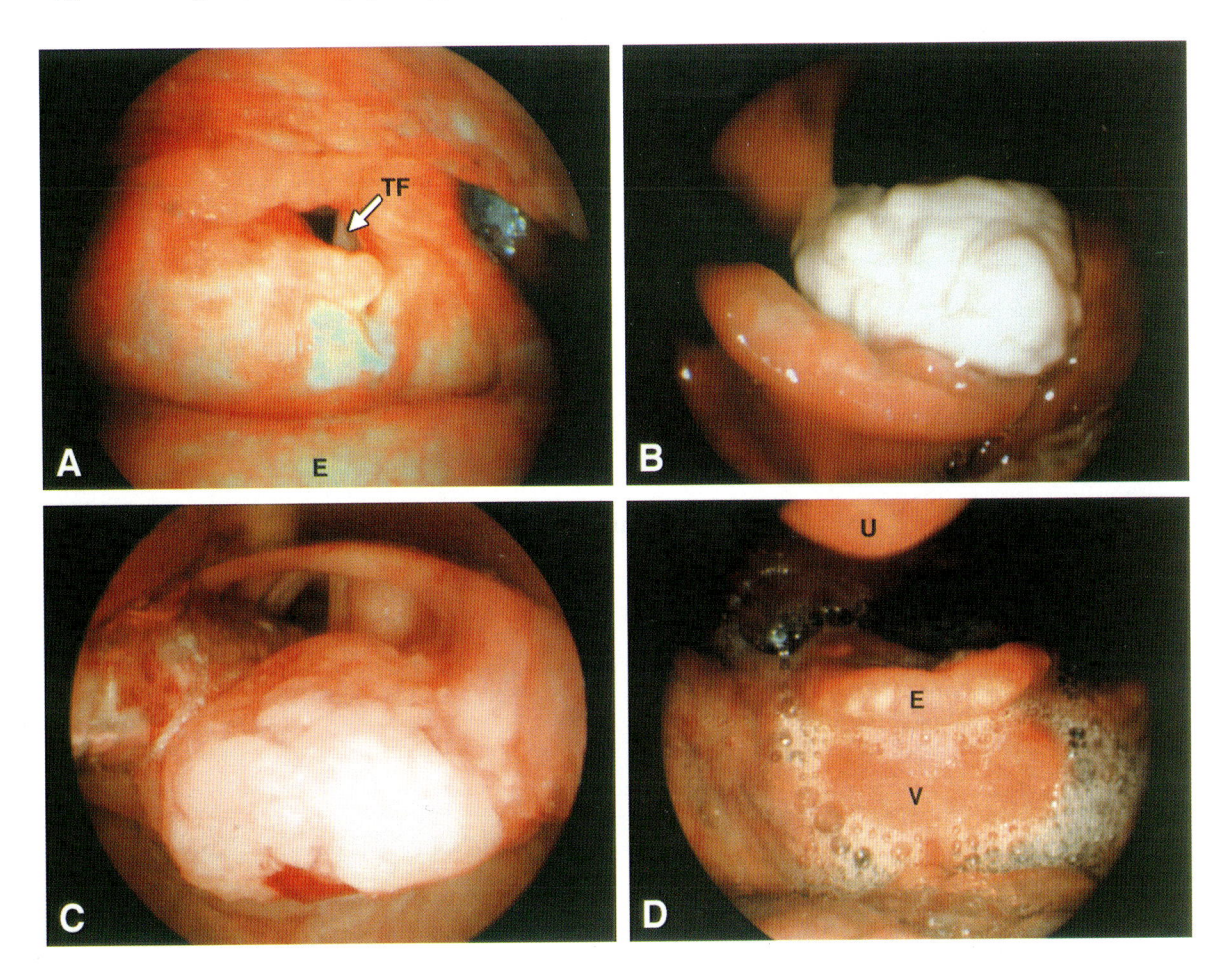

Supraglottic Squamous Cell Carcinoma

Figure 9-27A. Transglottic squamous cell carcinoma. This 70-degree transoral telescopic view of the larynx reveals a T_3 stage III right transglottic squamous cell carcinoma. The epiglottis (E) is seen at the bottom of the view, and the left true vocal fold (TF) and posterior glottis are barely visible. The patient was successfully treated with a total laryngectomy.

Figure 9-27B. Epiglottic squamous cell carcinoma. This patient presented with a globus sensation and choking spells. This 70-degree transoral telescopic exam reveals the bulky cancer emanating from the laryngeal surface of the epiglottis. The true vocal folds were mobile, and the cancer was staged as T_1N_0 stage I disease. This tumor was excised with the laser and treated with external beam radiation therapy.

Figure 9-27C. Supraglottic squamous cell carcinoma. This large bilateral supraglottic cancer was entirely above the ventricles, as was seen on another examination. This exam revealed mobile true vocal folds. The tumor did extend into the postcricoid area, making it a T_3 stage III lesion. This tumor was debulked and treated with external beam radiation therapy. The patient remains disease-free 10 years later.

Figure 9-27D. Vallecular squamous cell carcinoma. This advanced stage IV bilateral vallecular (V) squamous cell carcinoma displaced the epiglottis (E) posteriorly. The uvula (U) is visible at the top of the view. The patient was treated with a total laryngectomy and bilateral functional neck dissections.

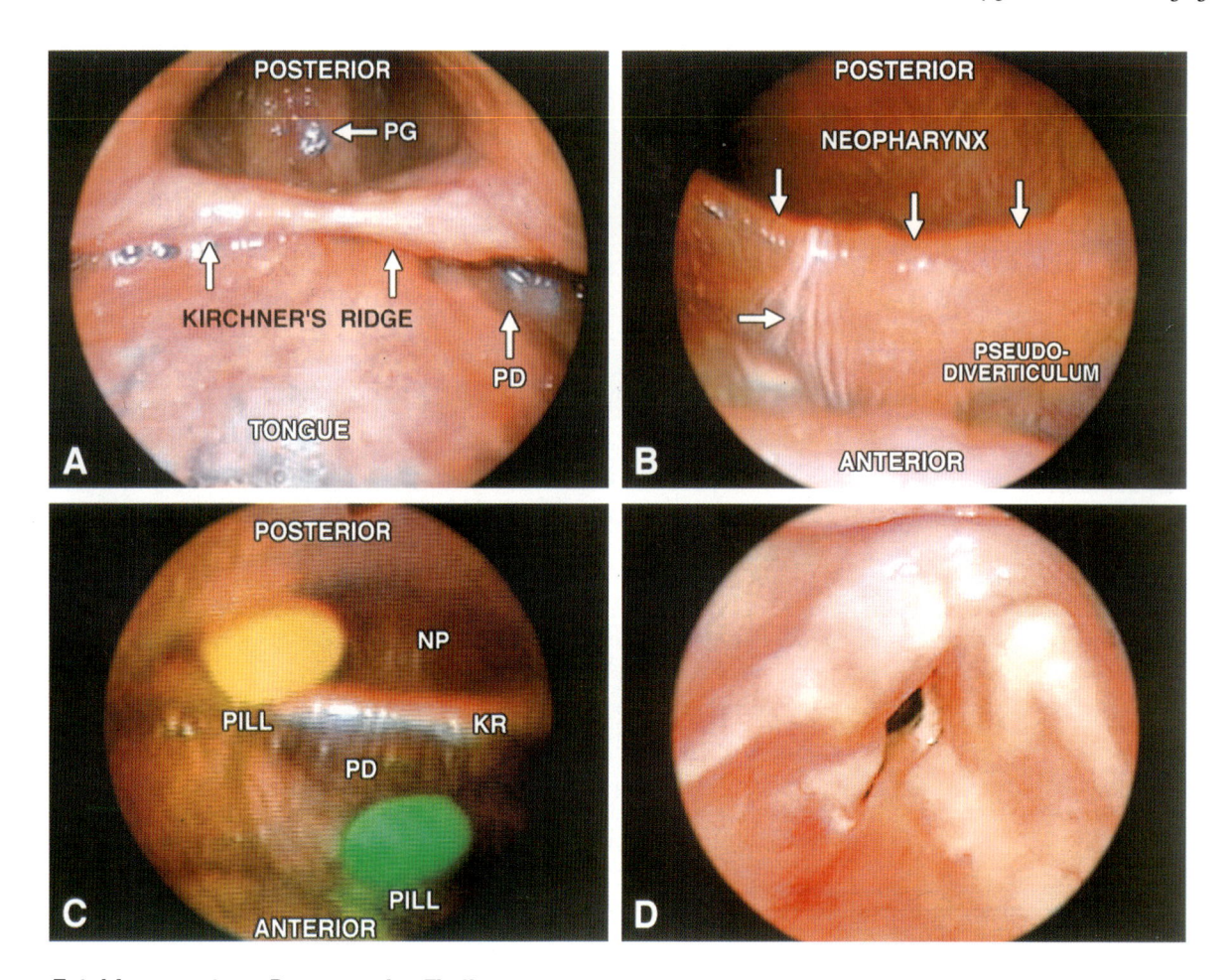

Total Laryngectomy Postoperative Findings

Figure 9-28A. Total laryngectomy postoperative findings. This 90-degree transoral telescopic view of the postlaryngectomy neopharynx reveals important postoperative findings. The tongue at the bottom of the view is anterior, and the top of the view is posterior. Upon removal of the larynx the anterior neopharynx lies just deep to the skin flap and strap muscles. When there is separation of the top portion of the anterior neopharynx closure, where it joins the base of the tongue, a salivary sinus tract forms under the skin flap or a pharyngocutaneous fistula develops. These defects heal quickly and mucosalize, leaving behind a pseudodiverticulum (PD) anterior to the neopharynx. The top of the anterior neopharynx thus forms a transverse ridge (Kirchner's ridge) either unilaterally or bilaterally. This finding was common after total laryngectomy as even asymptomatic separation of the top of the neopharynx closure was common. Also seen on this view is a pseudoglottis (PG) where the patient has a muscular narrowing that resembles a glottis in the neopharynx.

Figure 9-28B. Pseudodiverticulum and Kirchner's ridge. The 70-degree transoral telescopic exam reveals a prominent Kirchner's ridge (*vertical arrows*) and a deep pseudodiverticulum following a total laryngectomy. Mucus that accumulated in the pseudodiverticulum pouch flows into the neopharynx (seen on video) to be swallowed (*horizontal arrow*).

Figure 9-28C. Postlaryngectomy swallow. Patients may complain of a foreign body sensation, regurgitation, food sticking, and dysphagia. This transnasal fiberscopic videoendoscopic view of a swallow revealed one pill (yellow) being swallowed effectively into the neopharynx toward the esophagus, and the other pill (green) sticking in the pseudodiverticulum (PD). This view occurs quickly and can be appreciated only on reviewing the video in slow motion. Kirchner's ridge (KR) is the top of the anterior wall of the neopharynx after separation from the base of tongue.

Figure 9-28D. Partial laryngectomy postoperative findings. This man presented with breathy hoarseness after a previous partial laryngectomy. On 70-degree transoral telescopic laryngoscopy, the arytenoids moved well bilaterally but the anterior true vocal folds were scarred, leaving a large anterior gap in the glottis.

CHAPTER 10
STROBOSCOPY OF THE LARYNX (STROBOSCOPIC VIDEOLARYNGOSCOPY, STROBOVIDEOLARYNGOSCOPY)*

Stroboscopic videolaryngoscopy (strobovideolaryngoscopy) is a videolaryngoscopic examination of vocal fold vibrations with synchronized strobe lighting. It can be accomplished by using a flexible fiberscope or a rigid telescope. Many terms have been used to describe this procedure, including stroboscopic videolaryngoscopy, strobovideolaryngoscopy (RT Sataloff), videostroboscopy of the larynx, laryngeal stroboscopy, and laryngostroboscopy.

Stroboscopic examination of the larynx was first performed in 1878 by Oertel, who examined the vocal folds via indirect laryngoscopy under strobe lighting created with a disc rotating in synchrony with the patient's phonatory frequency. Now electronic stroboscopes flash rapid pulses of light along consecutive points of the vocal fold cycle in conjunction with rigid or flexible endoscopy of the larynx. An illusion is created where the vocal folds appear to move in "slow motion" by fusing multiple points along several successive vibratory cycles. This imaging technique allows careful analysis of vocal fold morphology, motion, and symmetry, along with mucosal wave progression, vibratory amplitude, and glottic closure.

Strobovideolaryngoscopy provides a more precise evaluation of the dysphonic patient. It is a sensitive technique for evaluating subtle, previously undetectable laryngeal lesions. This technique is useful in differentiating small vocal fold lesions, estimating the depth of invasion of early laryngeal cancers, and analyzing different types of vocal fold paralysis.

Equipment needed for strobovideolaryngoscopy includes (1) topical anesthesia and decongestant, (2) 3.6- or 4.4-mm laryngeal fiberscope (Olympus ENF-P3 or L3, respectively), (3) 70-degree rigid strobolaryngoscope (Karl Storz 8706CJ, Nagashima SFT-1 rigid telescope, or Kay 9105), (4) stroboscope (Kay Elemetrics Rhino-Laryngeal stroboscope model 9100, Nagashima laryngostroboscope LS-3A, or Brüel and Kjaer Rhino-Larynx stroboscope model 4914), (5) laryngophone, (6) microphone, (7) video camera, (8) video monitor, (9) video recorder, and (10) video printer. The Kay Elemetrics stroboscope is computer-integrated, allowing image digitization and manipulation as well as easy data retrieval.

Vocal fold motion and mucosal wave progression are best appreciated on motion video. Still videoprints, however, do demonstrate many of the important findings during these examinations.

*This chapter was written in collaboration with Ken Yanagisawa, M.D., and Edward M. Weaver, M.D.

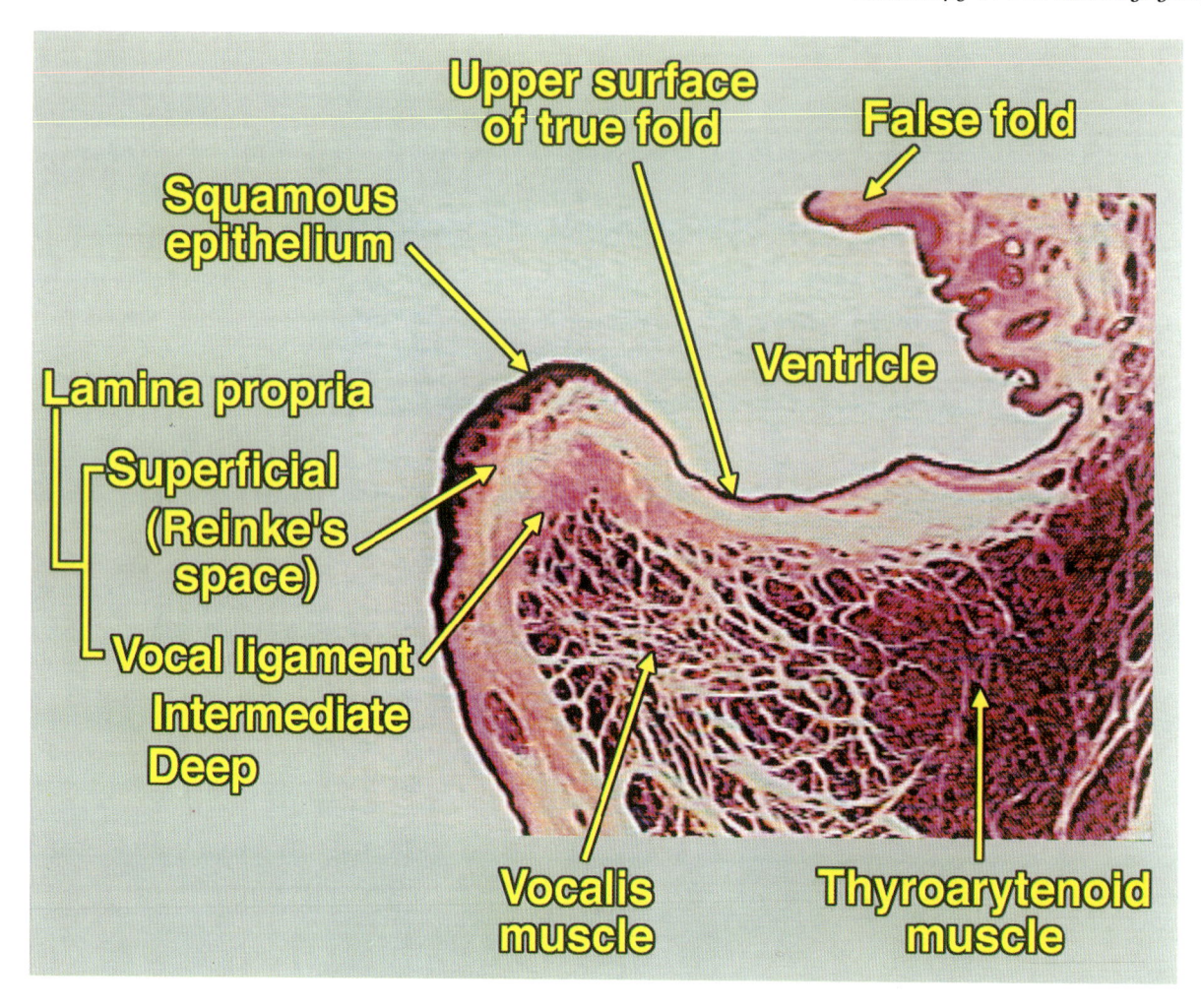

OVERVIEW OF VOCAL FOLD ANATOMY

Figure 10-1. Coronal section of vocal fold. This enlarged vocal fold coronal section demonstrates key elements of the layered structure of the true vocal fold. There are three layers: epithelium, lamina propria, and muscle. The epithelium is a nonkeratinizing stratified squamous epithelium. The lamina propria has three layers: superficial, intermediate, and deep. The superficial layer (Reinke's space) consists of loose connective tissue. The intermediate and deep layers consist of elastic and collagenous fibers that condense to form the vocal ligament. The vocalis muscle lies deep to the lamina propria. From a functional perspective, the epithelium and superficial lamina propria form the cover of the vocal fold; the intermediate and deep lamina propria form the transition zone; and the muscle forms the body. Phonation is created by vibrations of the vocal fold covers. As air flows past the properly positioned vocal folds, symmetric mucosal waves travel vertically on the loose vocal fold covers. The quality of phonation is affected by vocal fold position, length, mass, and tension as well as many other variables. Also demonstrated on this coronal section is the ventricle, the inferior edge of the false vocal fold, and the thyroarytenoid muscle. (Courtesy of John A. Kirchner, M.D., Yale University, New Haven, CT.)

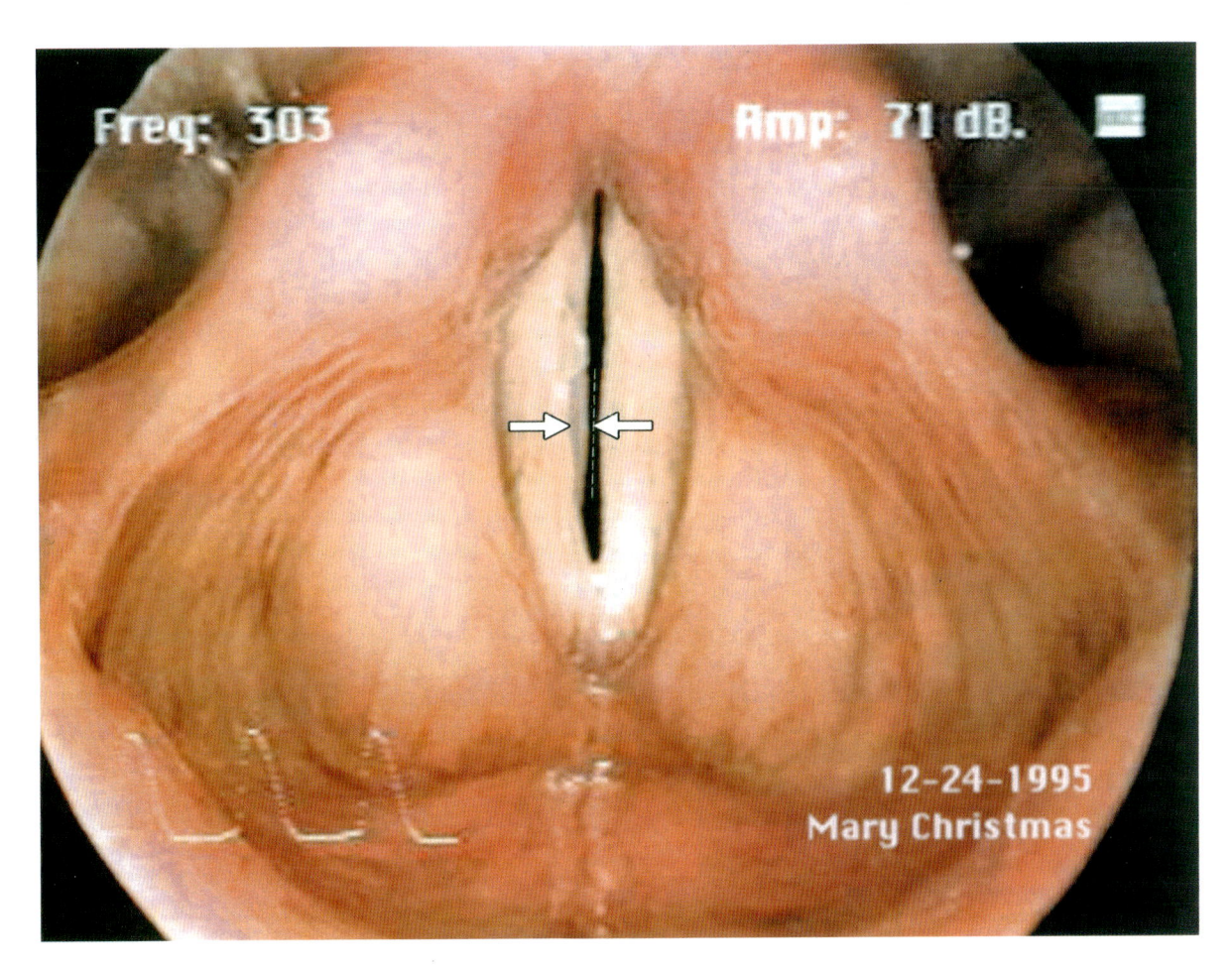

Figure 10-2. A 70-degree telescopic strobovideolaryngoscopic view of the true vocal folds. During high-frequency phonation the vocal folds elongate and the mucosal wave amplitude decreases. Low-pitch phonation corresponds to shortening of the vocal fold and increased mucosal wave amplitude. The amplitude is the distance from the midline of the glottis to the edge of the vocal fold during the open phase of its vibration. The amplitude of this high-frequency mucosal wave is marked (*arrows*), based on the stroboscopic exam. A trough of the mucosal wave is visible along the medial aspect of the right true vocal fold. The frequency is recorded in the upper left corner, the loudness in the upper right corner, the phonation wave form in the lower left corner, and the name and date in the lower right corner.

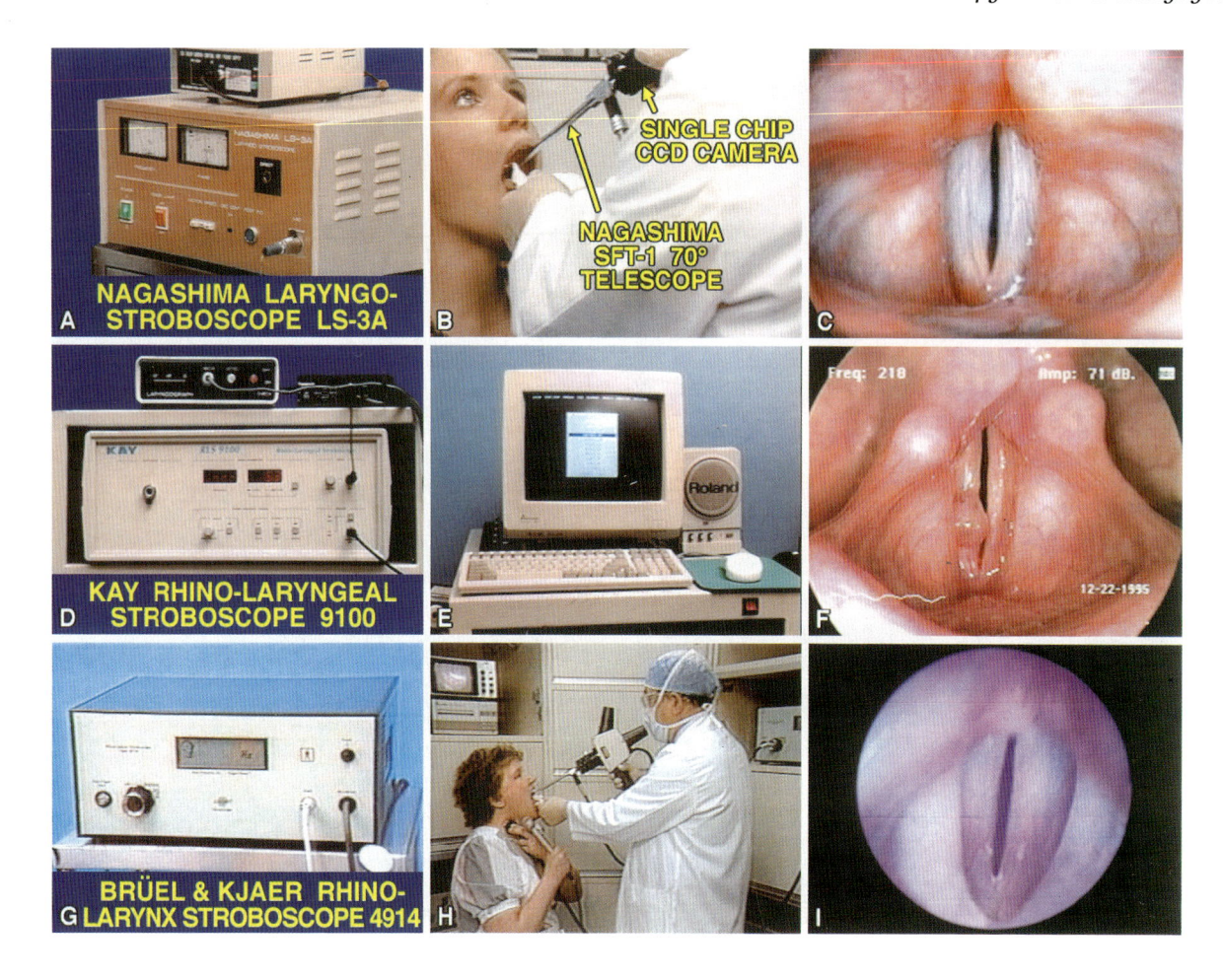

TECHNIQUES OF STROBOVIDEOLARYNGOSCOPY

Technique

Figure 10-3. With the patient topically anesthetized with 4% lidocaine spray and (when necessary) 3% ephedrine spray, the fiberscope or 70-degree telescope connected to a single- or three-chip CCD video camera are passed until the appropriate laryngeal image is noted. A laryngophone is placed against the patient's neck to measure the fundamental frequency of the voice, and a separate unidirectional microphone is held in front of the mouth (Nagashima) or attached to the video camera (Kay Elemetrics) for high-quality voice recordings. Once the image is centered and focused, videotape recording is begun. The patient is asked to phonate at normal (modal), high, and low pitch at normal loudness, followed by louder phonation. *Top row:* The Nagashima Laryngostroboscope LS-3A system. Figure 10-3A shows the stroboscope unit itself. The 70-degree rigid telescope is positioned just above the larynx in Figure 10-3B. A fiberscope can be used instead but produces a lower-quality image (see Figures 10-4–10-6). A typical videoprint of an image produced by this system is shown in Figure 10-3C. *Middle row:* The Kay Elemetric Rhino-Laryngeal Stroboscope 9100 system. Figure 10-3D shows the stroboscope unit. This stroboscope system is computer-integrated (Figure 10-3E), which allows image digitization and manipulation and provides automatic labeling and easy retrieval. A typical videoprint obtained with this system is shown in Figure 10-3F. Note the labels. This patient had a right true vocal fold sessile polyp. *Bottom row:* The Brüel and Kjaer Rhino-Larynx Stroboscope 4914 system. Figure 10-3G shows the stroboscope unit. The 70-degree rigid telescope is positioned above the larynx. The patient holds the laryngophone over her larynx with her left hand and the microphone with her right hand. The image is displayed on the video monitor behind the patient (Figure 10-3H). Figure 10-3I shows a typical videoprint.

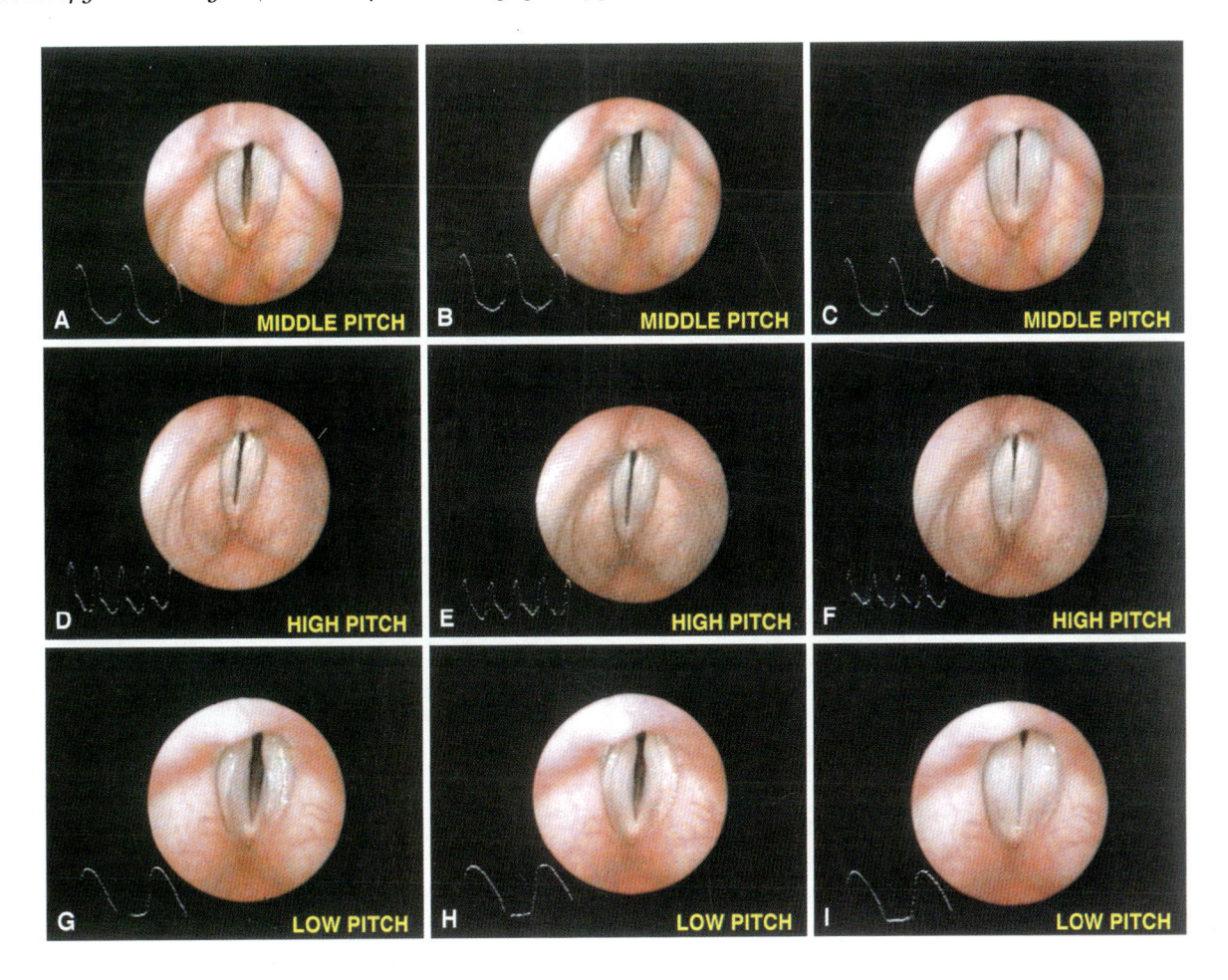

Comparison of Fiberscopic Versus Telescopic Strobovideolaryngoscopy

Figure 10-4. Fiberscopic strobovideolaryngoscopy. The fiberscopic strobovideolaryngoscopic views were obtained during middle, high, and low pitch phonation. Open and closed phase images are displayed. The middle pitch depicts nodal (normal) voice. The high pitch phonation occurs with an elongated, thinned true vocal fold and smaller amplitude than low pitch (Figure 10-4D versus 10-4G). The larger, slower low-pitch mucosal wave is much easier to see on strobovideolaryngoscopy than the high pitch wave. The low-pitch sequences in Figures 10-3G–10-3I reveal the traveling mucosal wave, especially on the right true vocal fold. A wave crest is seen on the superior surface in Figure 10-3G (*white streak*) and is then seen on the superior lateral surface in Figure 10-3H; then it disappeared on Figure 10-3I as a new crest is seen on the medial edge where the glottis is now in the closed phase. These high-quality fiberscopic views are small and have a grainy texture compared to the rigid telescopic views (Figure 10-5). Despite inferior image quality, the fiberscopic exam offers some advantages: (1) technical ease of exam, (2) ability to view true vocal folds even in the setting of an anomalous epiglottis or obstructing lesion, (3) patient maintains normal speaking position, and (4) flexibility in fiberscope tip position.

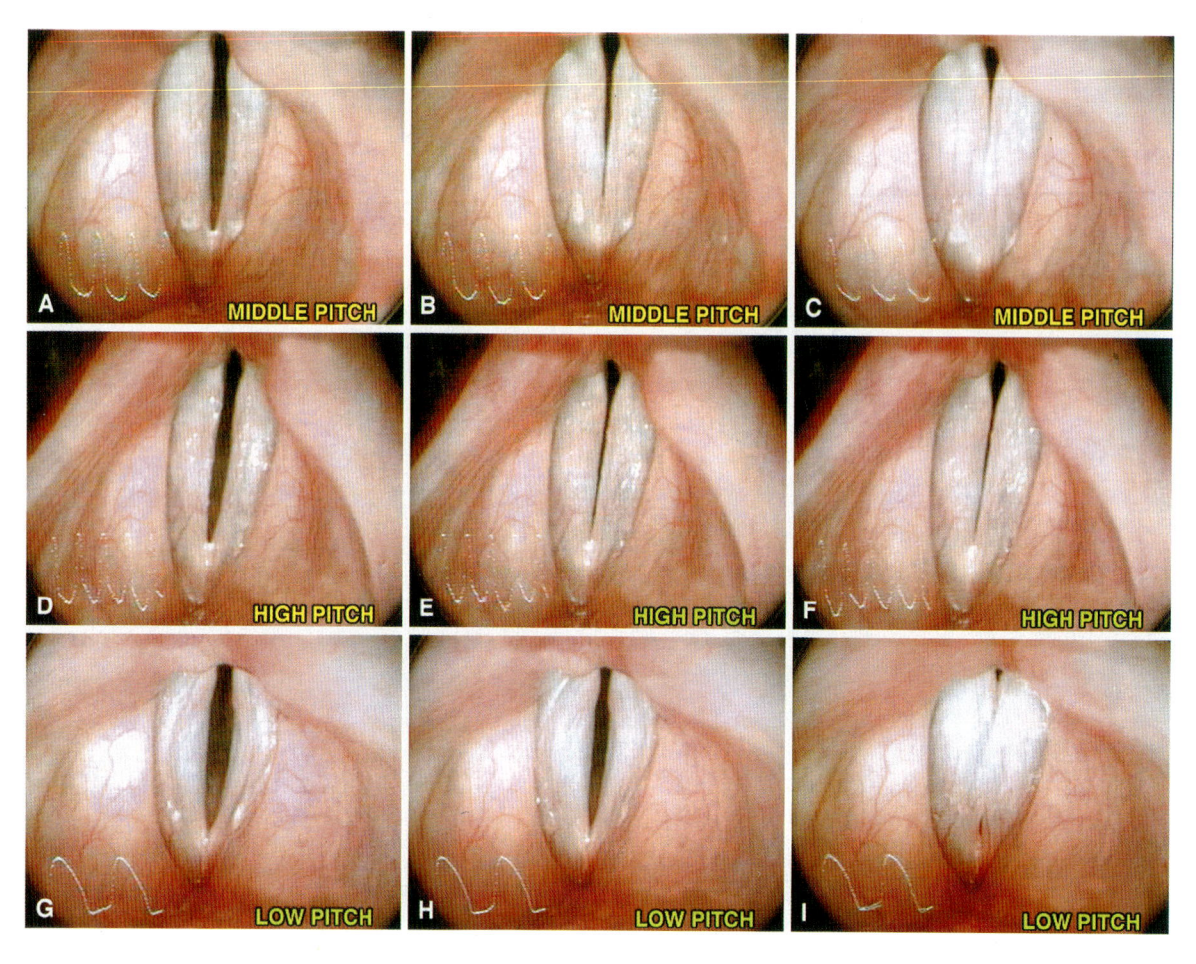

Figure 10-5. Seventy-degree telescopic strobovideolaryngoscopy. These telescopic strobovideolaryngoscopic views obtained during middle, high, and low pitch phonation are analogous to those in Figure 10-4. Again subtle vertically traveling mucosal waves can be seen on the low-pitch sequence (Figures 10-5G–10-5I). The telescopic images are brighter, larger, and clearer than the fiberscopic images. Disadvantages to this technique include the following: (1) Hyperactive gag reflex, anomalous epiglottis, or obstructing lesions make this exam very difficult, and (2) the patient is in an unnatural position for phonation. Overall, telescopic strobovideolaryngoscopy yields superior stroboscopic examinations.

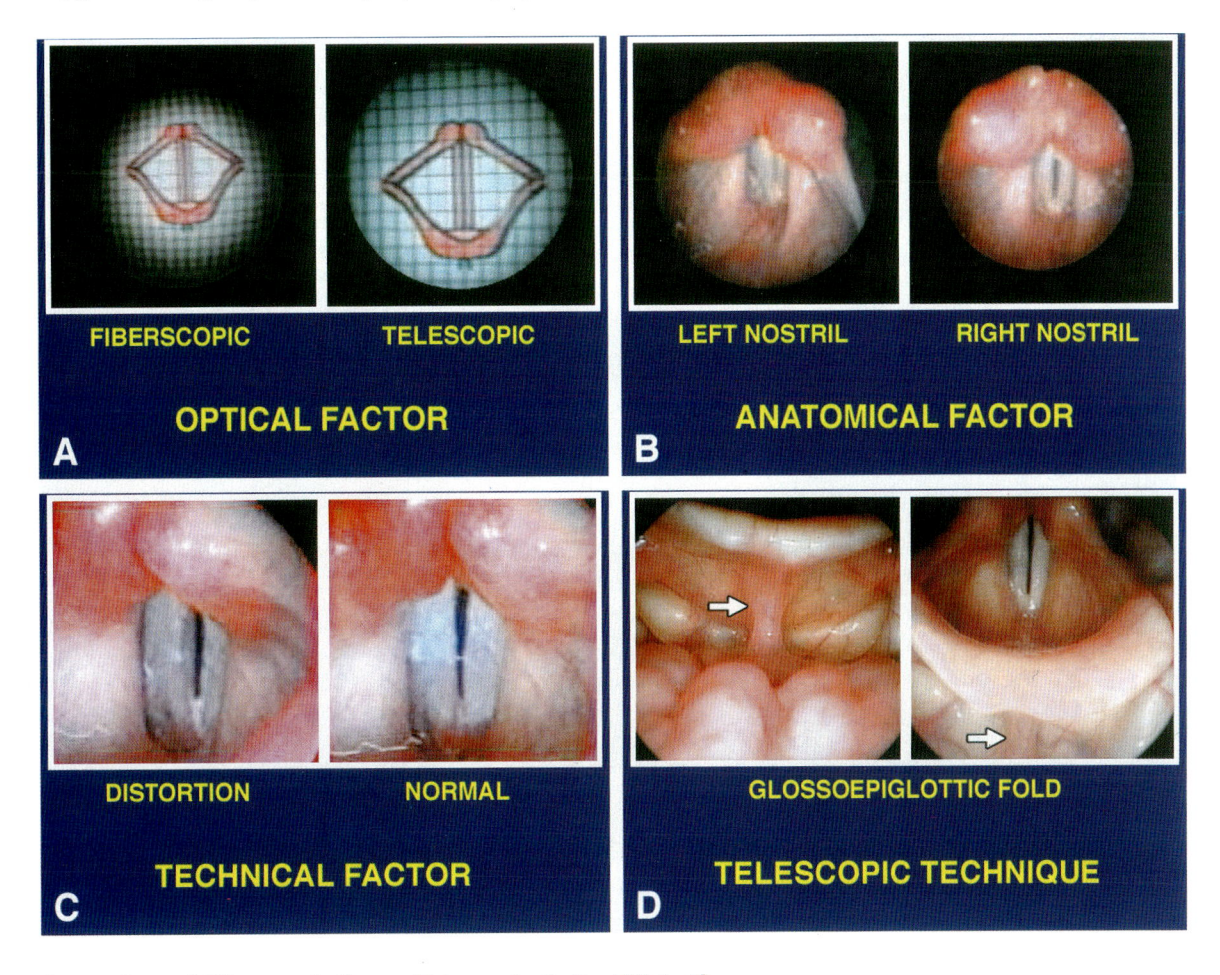

Comparison of Fiberscopic Versus Telescopic Optical Distortion

Figure 10-6A. Optical factor. The fiberscope wide-angle lens causes distortion at the periphery of its view. This distortion is clearly demonstrated as the grid curves at the periphery in the fiberscopic view. The telescope has little distortion.

Figure 10-6B. Anatomic factor. The transnasal fiberscope can be positioned to one side due to abnormal nasal passage anatomy such as a marked septal ridge or deviation. The view through the left nostril suggests an asymmetry of the true vocal folds. When viewed through the other nostril, however, the true vocal folds are symmetric. The left transnasal view angles the fiberscope to one side because of a nasal septal deviation. In correcting for this deflected position, the true vocal folds appear asymmetric. This issue is very important in the assessment of vocal fold symmetry with strobovideolaryngoscopy.

Figure 10-6C. Technical factor. Similar to the fiberscope distortion due to the nasal anatomic factor (Figure 10-6B), the positioning of the rigid telescope, such as tilting of the telescope tip sideways, can result in a distorted view of the vocal folds. The telescopic view on the left shows asymmetry of the vocal folds resulting from passage of the rigid telescope lateral to the midline. When the telescope is repositioned in the midline (*right*), the vocal folds are symmetric.

Figure 10-6D. Glossoepiglottic fold. The midline glossoepiglottic fold serves as a midline marker for positioning the fiberscope or telescope (*arrows*). By following this fold over the epiglottis, the vocal folds can be visualized without technical distortion.

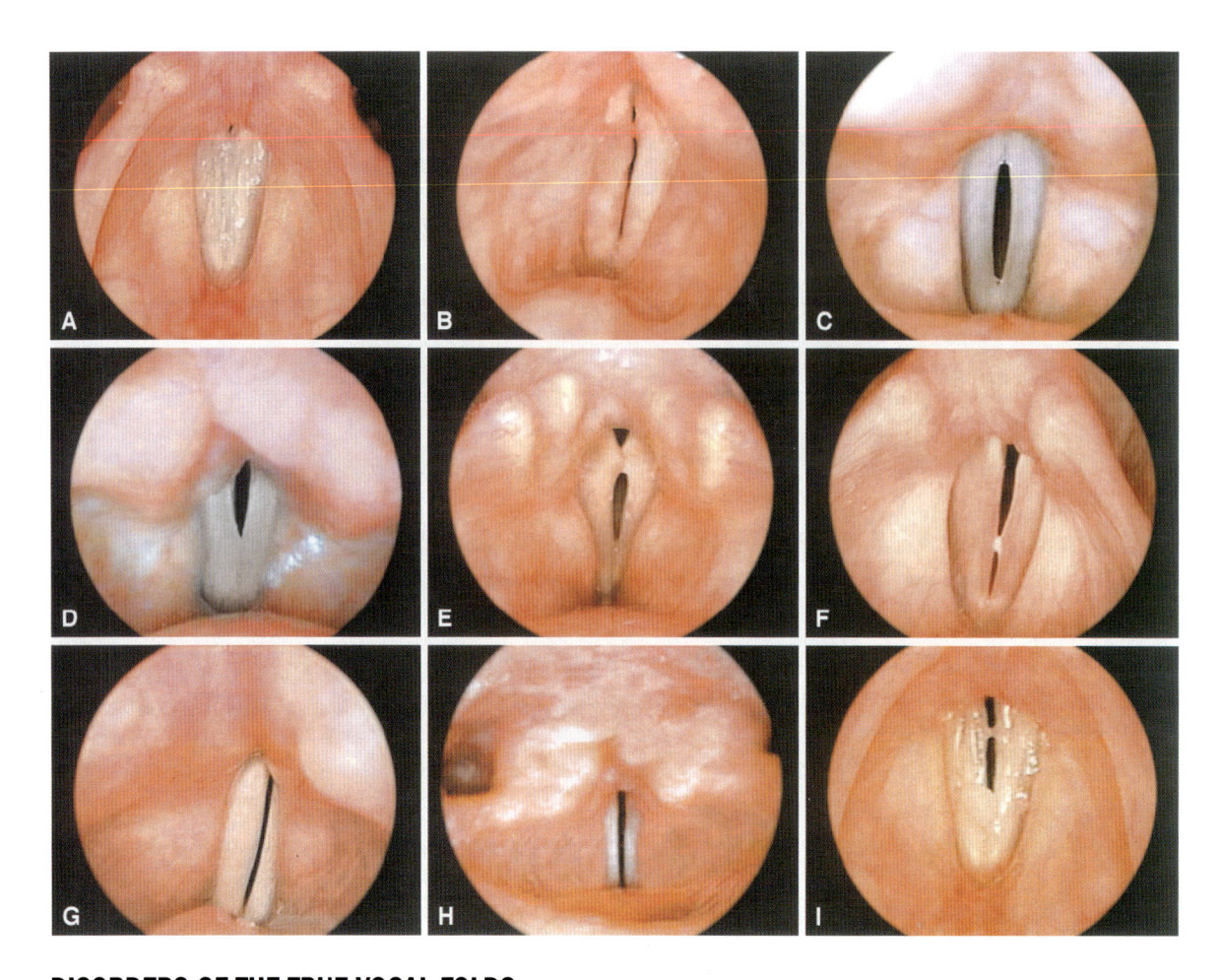

DISORDERS OF THE TRUE VOCAL FOLDS

Glottic Closure Patterns Observed with Strobovideolaryngoscopy

These patterns are observed at the time of maximal glottic closure during normal pitch and loudness.

Figure 10-7A.   Complete closure. Complete closure is the normal pattern where the medial edges of the true vocal folds meet along their entire length. Overclosure can be mistaken for normal complete glottic closure. Overclosure can occur with Reinke's edema or extensive sessile polyps, for example.

Figure 10-7B.   Irregular closure. This pattern is characterized by irregular glottic edges along most of its length. Cancer, leukoplakia, laryngitis sicca, vocal fold surgery changes, and mucus can all cause this pattern.

Figure 10-7C.   Spindle-shaped closure. This closure pattern is also called "bowing." It is seen with vocal fold paralysis, sulcus vocalis, atrophy, the aged vocal folds, or postoperative changes.

Figure 10-7D.   Posterior gap. This pattern is seen in Reinke's edema, sessile vocal fold polyposis, or vocal fold surgical changes.

Figure 10-7E.   Anterior and posterior gaps. This pattern could also be called a posterior hourglass closure. This abnormal closure pattern was due to prominent arytenoid vocal processes that left closure gaps anterior and posterior to their closure point.

Figure 10-7F.   Hourglass closure. This closure pattern is shaped like an hourglass and is often caused by vocal fold nodules, a small polyp, or any other small, smooth, protuberant lesion in the middle third of the vocal folds.

Figure 10-7G.   Incomplete closure. The glottic edges are smooth but the vocal fold edges do not meet in this closure pattern. The patient had a unilateral left vocal fold paralysis.

Figure 10-7H.   Incomplete closure. This midline incomplete closure was the result of bilateral recurrent laryngeal nerve vocal fold paralysis that left the vocal folds in a paramedian position.

Figure 10-7I.   Pseudo-hourglass closure. This odd glottic closure pattern appears to include a posterior hourglass pattern. In fact both the anterior polypoid mass and the posterior "nodules" were mucus. Upon clearing the throat these lesions disappeared. It is important, therefore, to be sure the patient coughs and clears any residual mucus before performing strobovideolaryngoscopy.

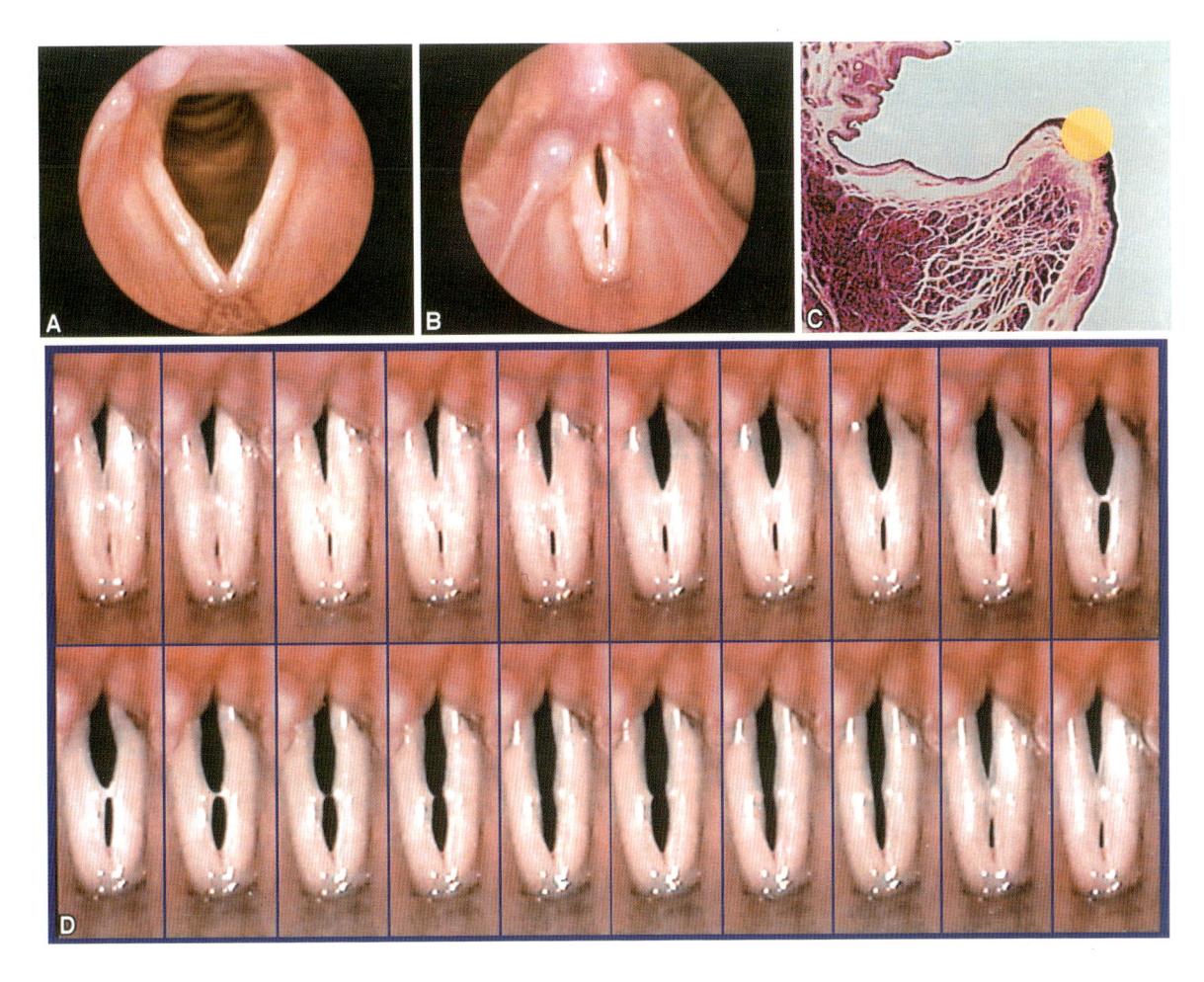

Vocal Fold Nodules

Figure 10-8A. Vocal fold nodules on abduction. Nodules usually occur bilaterally as a result of chronic vocal abuse. They typically occur along the medial vocal fold edges at the junction of the anterior and middle one thirds of the vocal folds (see Figure 9-13).

Figure 10-8B. Vocal fold nodules on adduction. During adduction an hourglass glottis is formed with incomplete closure anterior and posterior to the nodules.

Figure 10-8C. Microphotographic representation of a vocal fold nodule (schematic). The nodule forms in the superficial layer of the lamina propria. They are usually fibrous and firm but may be edematous.

Figure 10-8D. Stroboscopic composite of one glottic cycle. The vocal nodules are symmetric, causing incomplete ("hourglass") glottic closure, reduced amplitude, and absent mucosal wave along the nodules. Mucosal wave changes are best appreciated on motion video.

Vocal Fold Polyp

Figure 10-9A. Vocal fold polyp on abduction. Vocal fold polyps usually occur unilaterally and are caused by acute voice abuse. They can, however, occur bilaterally (usually asymmetrically) and with a variety of causes (see Figures 9-14–9-16).

Figure 10-9B. Vocal fold polyp on adduction. Glottic closure is incomplete due to the bulk of the soft tissue mass. The true vocal folds are asymmetric.

Figure 10-9C. Microphotographic representation of a vocal fold polyp (schematic). The polyp forms in the superficial layer of the lamina propria and may become large and bulky.

Figure 10-9D. Stroboscopic composite of several glottic cycles. The vibratory movements of the vocal folds are asymmetric with incomplete glottic closure and reduced vocal fold amplitude. A pliable or edematous polyp will maintain a mucosal wave, whereas a fibrous or hemorrhagic polyp will lack a mucosal wave. Vibratory movements and mucosal wave changes are best appreciated on motion video.

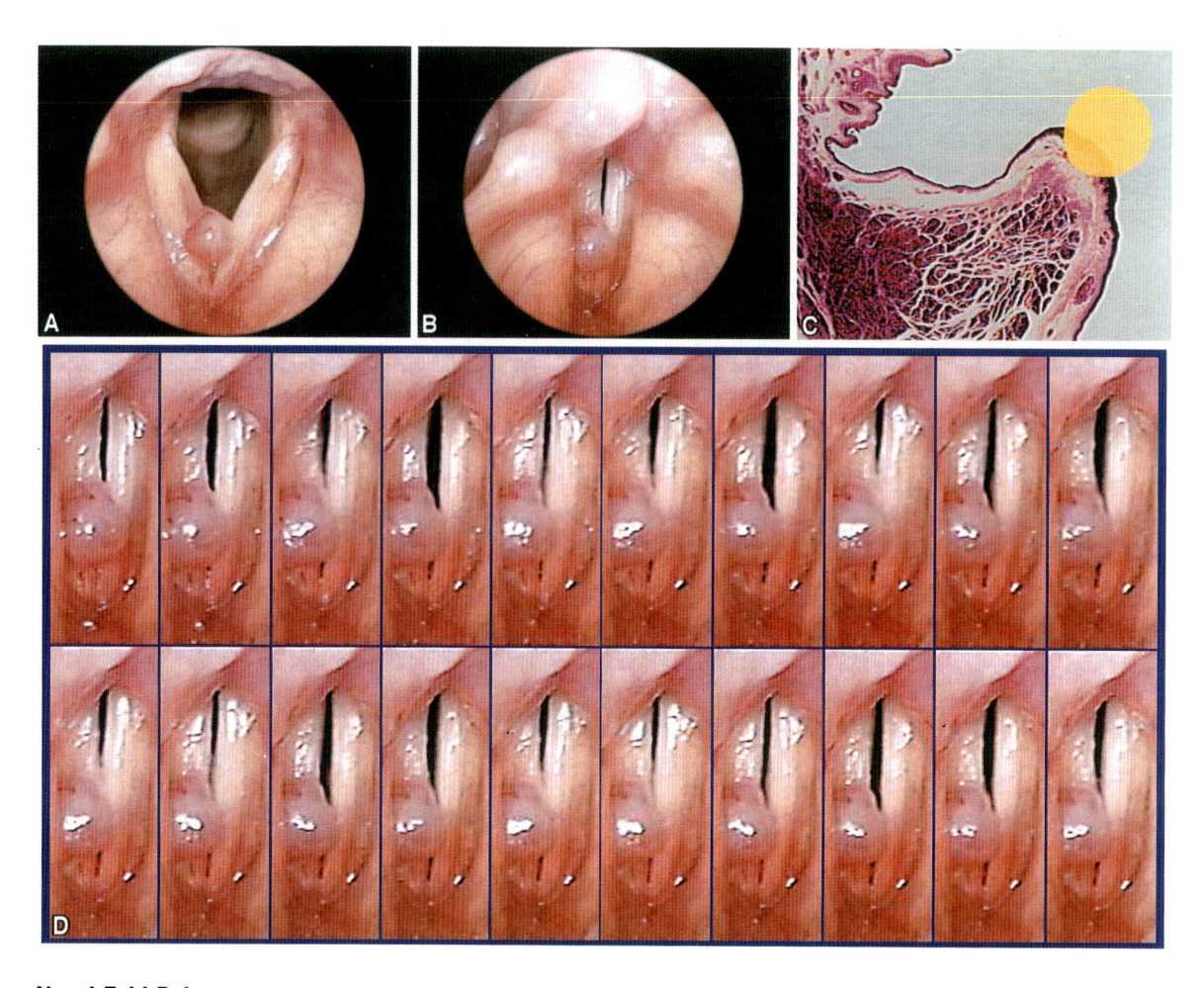

Vocal Fold Cyst

Figure 10-10A. Vocal fold cyst on abduction. Vocal fold cysts are almost always unilateral as is this right true vocal fold cyst. Most such cysts are epidermoid or mucous retention cysts that lie in the middle one-third of the true vocal folds (see Figure 9-18).

Figure 10-10B. Vocal fold cyst on adduction. Glottic closure is incomplete during phonation, and a protuberant cyst often hinders contralateral vocal fold vibration. The true vocal fold asymmetry and impingement on the contralateral true vocal folds are seen in this view.

Figure 10-10C. Microphotographic representation of a true vocal fold cyst (schematic). The round cyst lies in the superficial layer of the lamina propria with a cyst wall encasing it.

Figure 10-10D. Stroboscopic composite of glottic cycles. Cysts tend to be stiffer than polyps and nodules. They cause an incomplete anterior gap, posterior gap, or hourglass glottic closure; vibration asymmetry; very small vibration amplitude on the affected side; and no mucosal wave over the cysts. The limitation of vibration of cysts is much greater than that of nodules or polyps, therefore allowing strobovideolaryngoscopy to differentiate cysts from nodules or polyps. Vibration and mucosal wave changes are best appreciated on motion video.

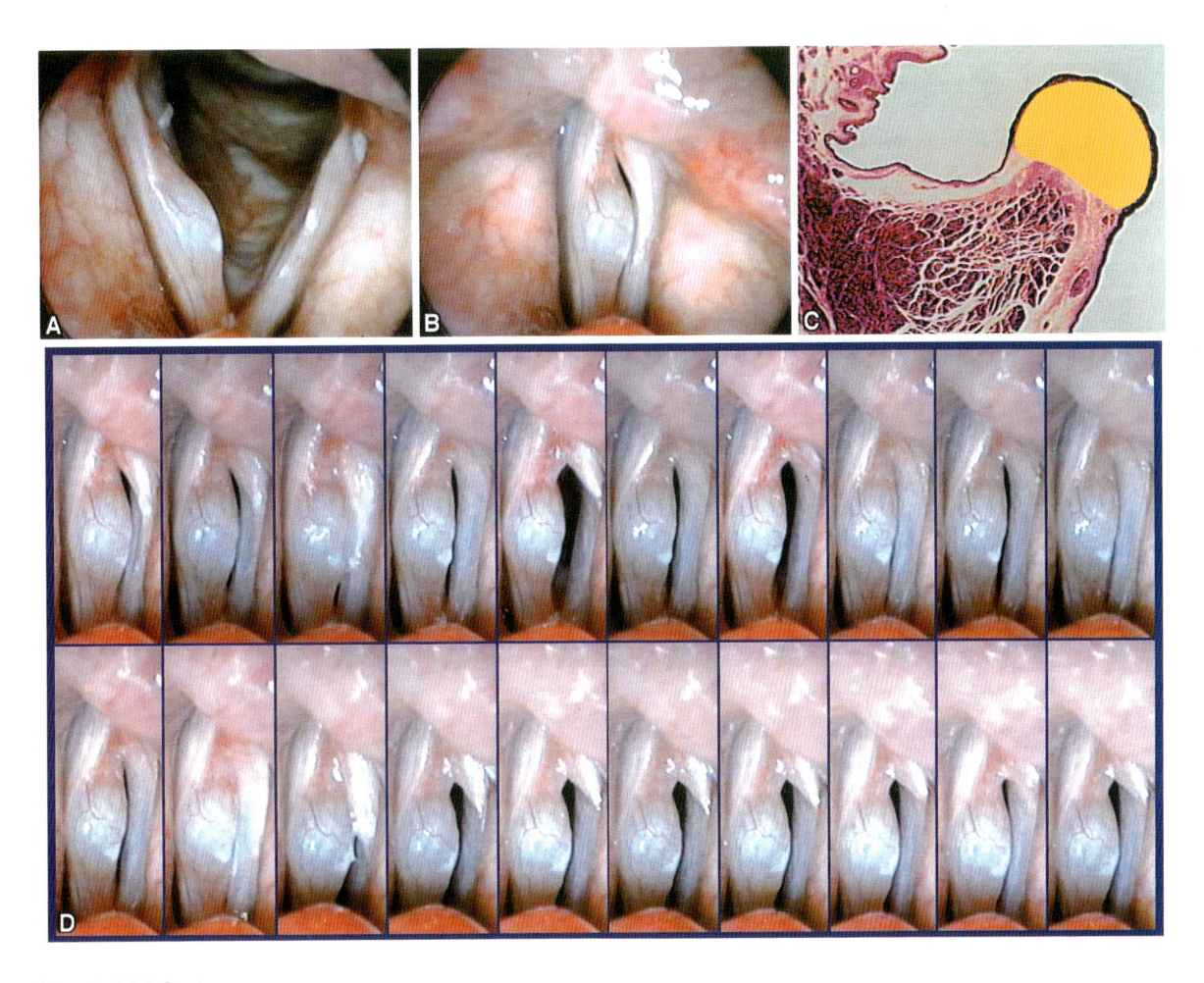

Vocal Fold Leukoplakia

Figure 10-11A. Vocal fold leukoplakia on abduction. Leukoplakia is more commonly unilateral but may occur bilaterally and anywhere on the true vocal folds. It may be large or small, exophytic or plaque-like. One must take care to remove adherent mucus in order to examine the lesion adequately.

Figure 10-11B. Vocal fold leukoplakia on adduction. Depending on the location and extent of the lesion the glottic closure may be affected. The contralateral true vocal fold mucosa appears thickened adjacent to the original right true vocal fold lesion.

Figure 10-11C. Microphotographic representation of true vocal fold leukoplakia (schematic). Leukoplakia originates from the epithelium and may extend into the superficial layer of the lamina propria. It invades more deeply only when malignant.

Figure 10-11D. Stroboscopic composite of glottic cycles. The irregular right true vocal fold has no mucosal wave over the lesion. Vibratory movements are usually asymmetric and limited, especially when the lesion is malignant. Thus, strobovideolaryngoscopy is a sensitive technique for early vocal fold cancer detection. Mucosal wave and vibratory movement abnormalities are best appreciated on motion video.

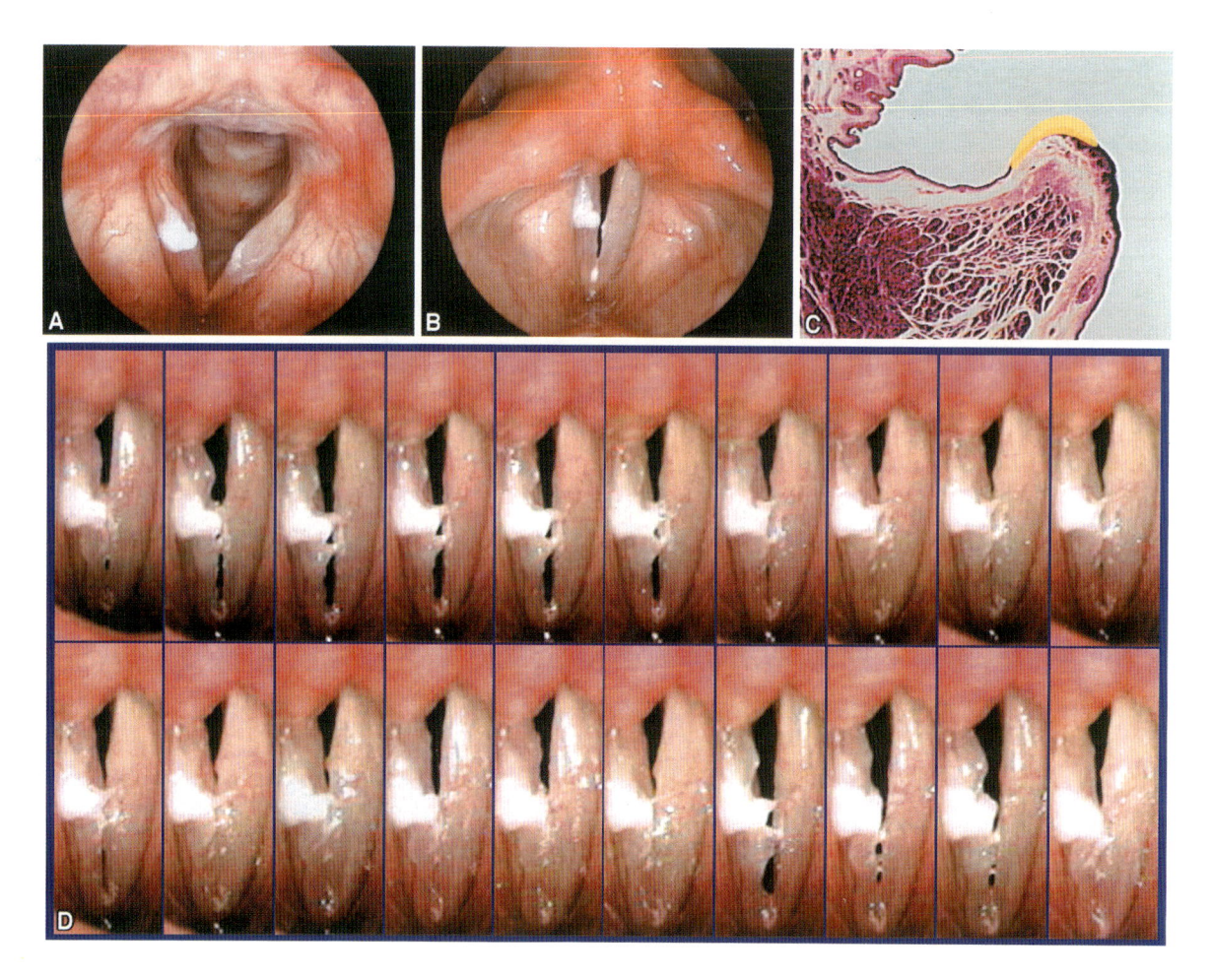

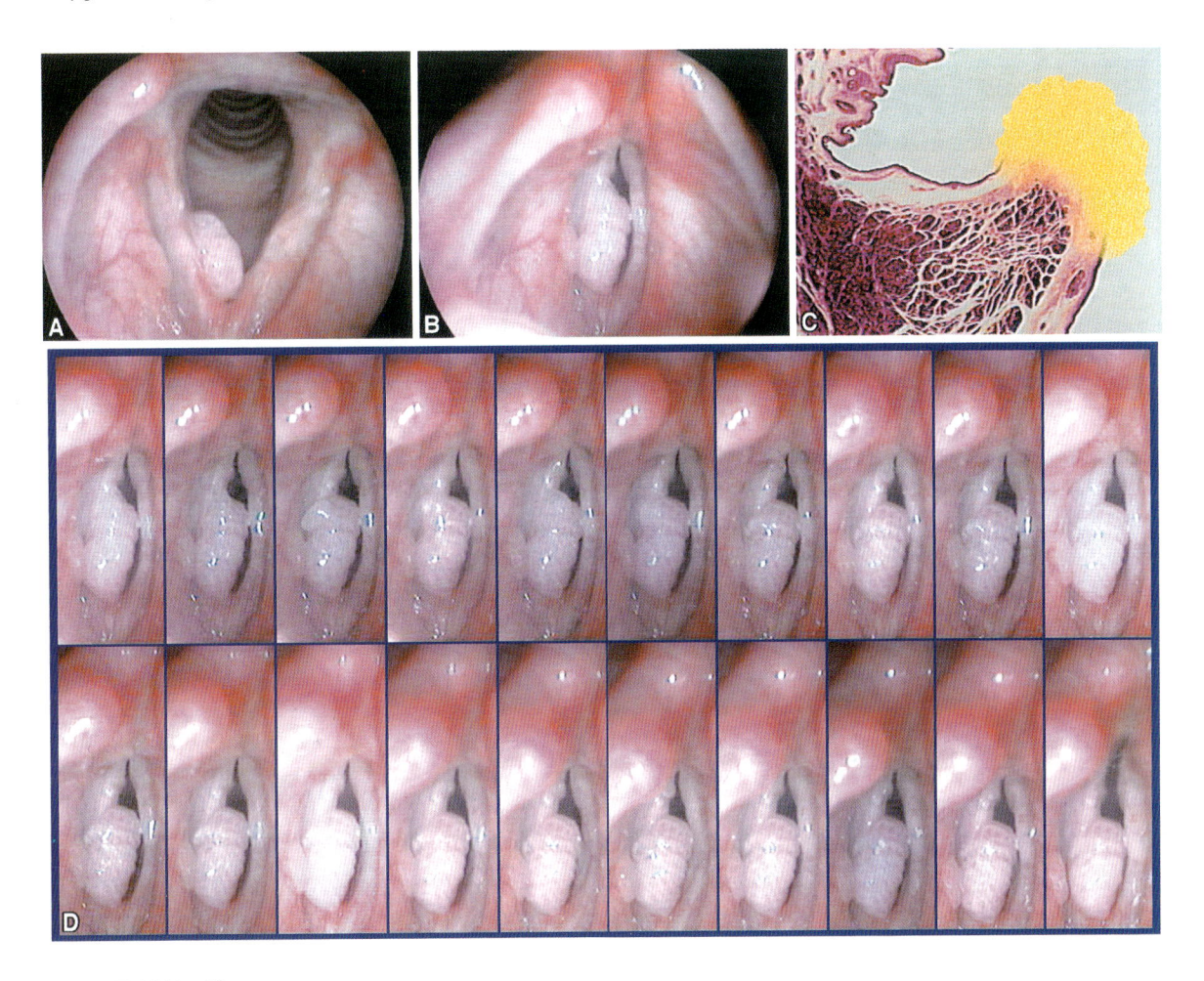

Vocal Fold Papilloma

Figure 10-12A. Vocal fold papilloma on abduction. Laryngeal papillomas usually occur multiply and occur anywhere in the larynx. They have an irregular, warty, exophytic surface (see Figure 9-25).

Figure 10-12B. Vocal fold papilloma on adduction. True vocal fold papillomas usually compromise glottic closure by mass effect and impingement on the contralateral true vocal fold function.

Figure 10-12C. Microphotographic representation of a true vocal fold papilloma (schematic). Papillomas are benign neoplasms that originate in the epithelium but can invade the lamina propria and even into muscle. These lesions are caused by the human papilloma virus.

Figure 10-12D. Stroboscopic composite of glottic cycles. The lesion inhibits true vocal fold vibration and has no mucosal wave. A larger lesion prevents adequate glottic closure and impinges on the contralateral true vocal fold function. Motion disturbances are easily appreciated on motion video.

Chapter 11
Simultaneous Velolaryngeal Videoendoscopy

Simultaneous velolaryngeal videoendoscopy is the simultaneous examinations of the velum palatini (soft palate) via rigid transnasal videonasopharyngoscopy and the larynx via transnasal fiberscopic videolaryngoscopy. Both examinations are video- and audio-recorded in order to study the coordinated movements and positioning of the larynx and soft palate during respiration, phonation, swallowing, coughing, straining, singing, and during other routine laryngeal functions.

The equipment used for this dual exam includes (1) flexible fiberscope (Olympus ENF-P3), (2) Hopkins 4.0-mm 18-cm-long 70-degree rigid nasal telescope (Karl Storz 7200C), (3) xenon light source, (4) two video cameras, (5) two video monitors, (6) two video recorders, (7) microphone, (8) video printer, and (9) nasal topical anesthetic and decongestant.

These examinations are best appreciated on motion video with real-time audio. Still videoprints, however, do demonstrate many of the important findings during these examinations.

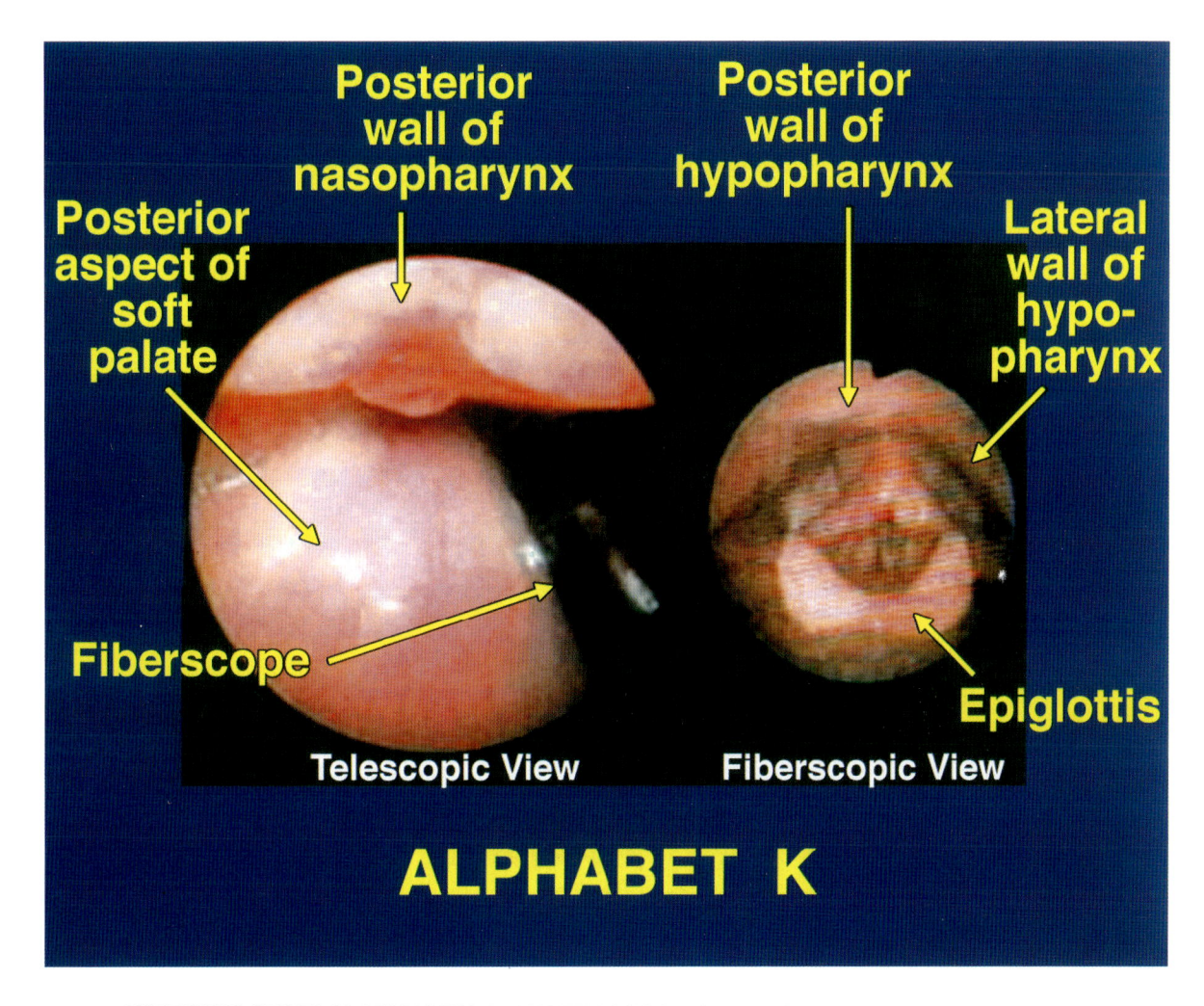

OVERVIEW OF VELOLARYNGEAL VIDEOENDOSCOPIC ANATOMY

Figure 11-1. Simultaneous velolaryngeal videoendoscopy with a closed velopharyngeal port. The 70-degree rigid transnasal nasopharyngoscopic view is seen on the left with the patient articulating the plosive /k/ which closes the velopharyngeal port by raising the soft palate. The posterior nasopharyngeal wall is visible at the top of the view, and the flexible fiberscope is seen traversing across the soft palate and diving down into the pharynx. The flexible fiberscopic view of the larynx is seen on the right simultaneously.

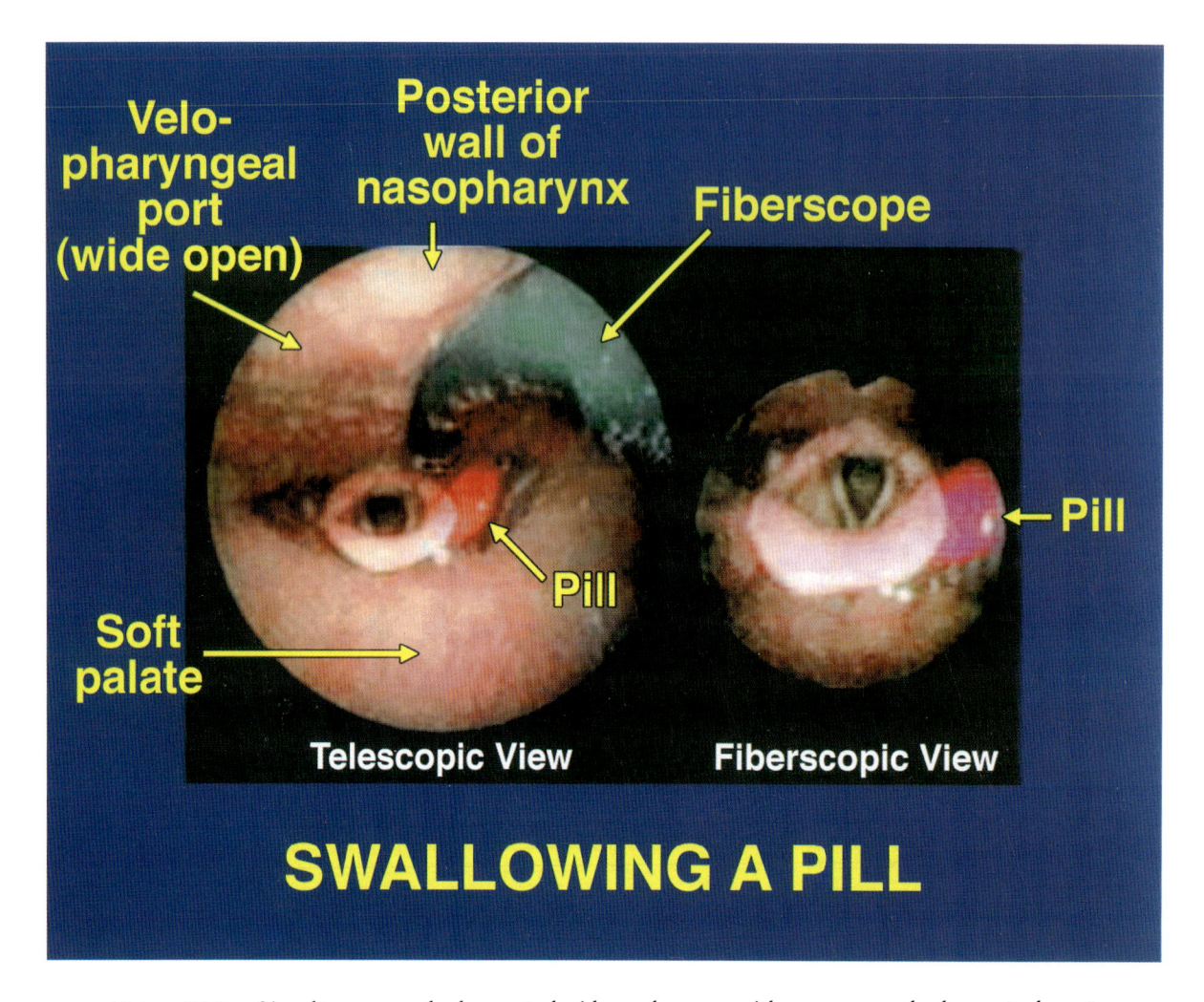

Figure 11-2. Simultaneous velopharyngeal videoendoscopy with an open velopharyngeal port. The nasopharyngoscopic view reveals an open velopharyngeal port making the larynx visible from the nasopharynx as the soft palate drops and relaxes anteriorly (*bottom of view*). The flexible fiberscope arises from the left choana passing down to the larynx. The right picture shows the laryngoscopic view. Interestingly, the patient opens the glottis widely in between swallows despite the red pill temporarily sticking in the left vallecula.

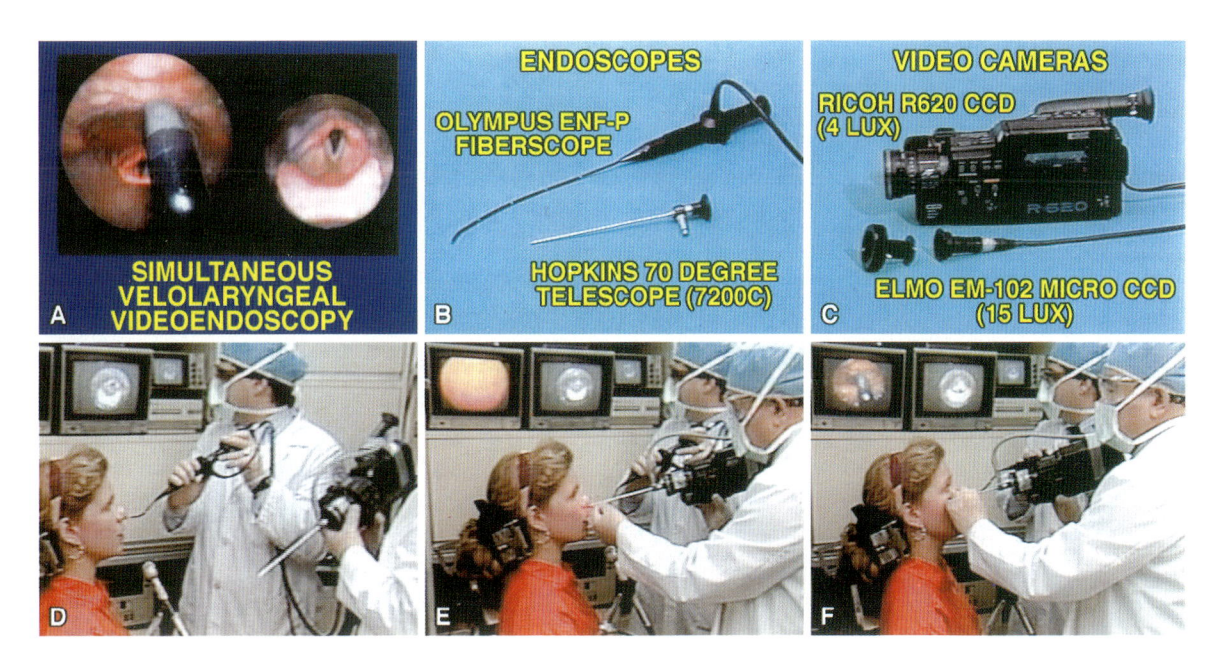

TECHNIQUES OF SIMULTANEOUS VELOLARYNGEAL VIDEOENDOSCOPY

Figure 11-3A. Simultaneous velolaryngeal videoendoscopy. The simultaneous video image of the nasopharynx (*left*) and the larynx (*right*) in combination with simultaneous audio allows examination of the coordinated movements of the soft palate during normal laryngeal functions. This example demonstrates that the velopharyngeal port opens widely during nasal respiration.

Figure 11-3B. Endoscopes. The flexible fiberscope is used to view the larynx. The Hopkins 4.0-mm 70-degree rigid nasal telescope is used to view the soft palate.

Figure 11-3C. Cameras. An Elmo EM-102 Micro CCD (15 lux) camera was attached to the fiberscope to document the laryngeal exam. A Ricoh home video camera (4 lux) was attached to the rigid telescope to document the simultaneous soft palate exam. Each camera is connected to a video recorder and a monitor. Each video recorder also audio-records the exam.

Figure 11-3D. Fiberscopic laryngoscopy. First the patient's nasal passages are sprayed with topical nasal anesthetic and decongestant. The right nasal cavity is further treated with a cotton pledget soaked with anesthetic and decongestant for the rigid telescopic exam. The flexible fiberscope is passed through the left nasal cavity along the middle meatus (this position ultimately yields the most stable images) to examine the nasopharynx and soft plate before continuing down the pharynx. Once in proper position for the laryngeal exam, it is fixed to the subject's nose and handed to an assistant. The image is seen on the right monitor behind the subject.

Figure 11-3E. Seventy-degree transnasal rigid nasopharyngoscopy. Next the rigid 70-degree telescope is passed through the right nasal cavity to the nasopharynx. The 70-degree telescope provides the best images of the velopharyngeal port and soft palate (see Figure 7-4). The image is on the left monitor behind the subject.

Figure 11-3F. Simultaneous velolaryngeal videoendoscopy. The images from each endoscope are viewed side by side during the exam and are video- and audio-recorded for review.

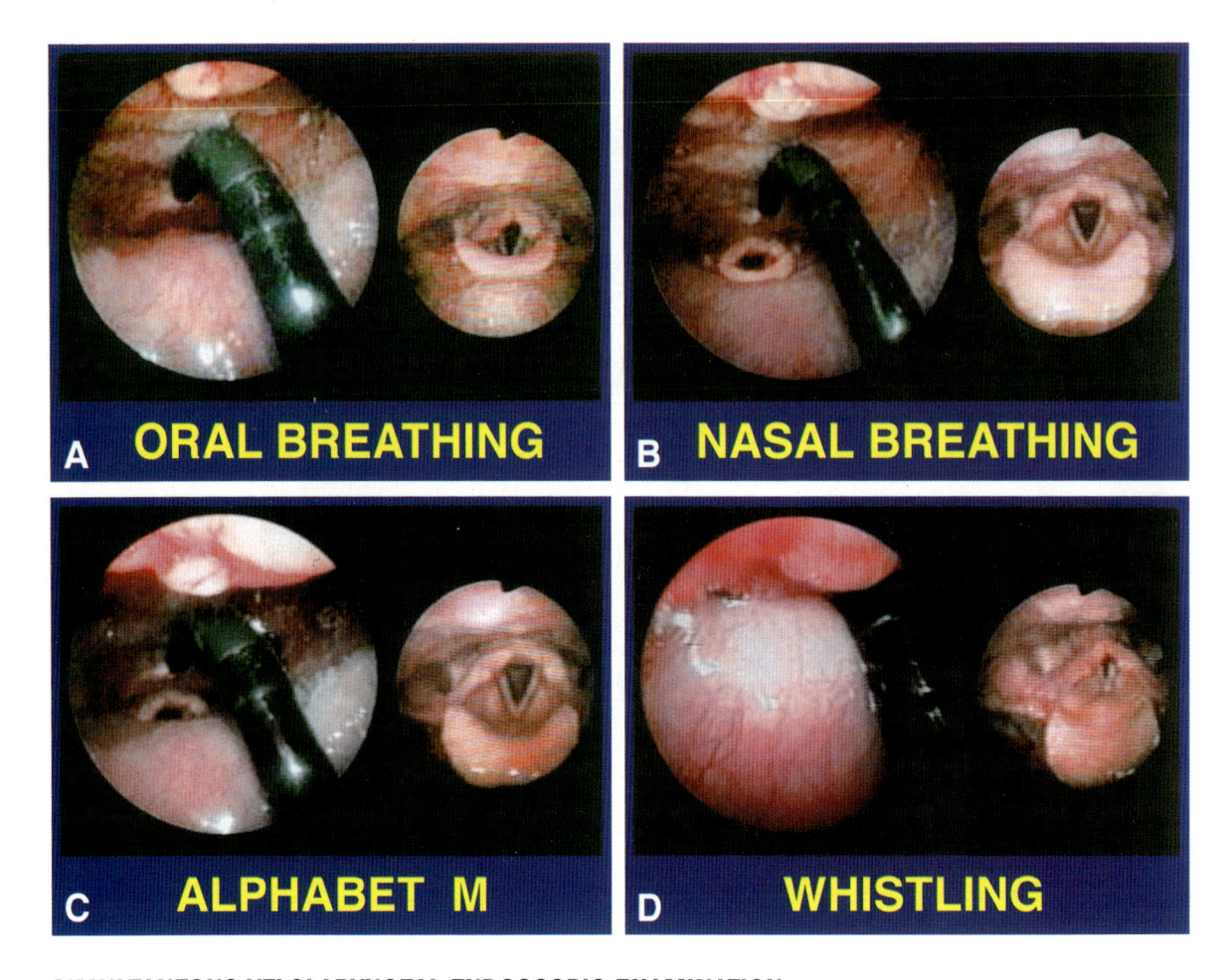

SIMULTANEOUS VELOLARYNGEAL ENDOSCOPIC EXAMINATION

Breathing

Figure 11-4A. Oral breathing. During oral respiration the soft palate rises to close the velopharyngeal port (*left*). The glottis is open widely to accommodate air flow.

Figure 11-4B. Nasal breathing. During nasal breathing the soft palate drops and relaxes forward to open the velopharyngeal port. The air can then flow through the nose. Again the glottis is wide open.

Phonating and Whistling

Figure 11-4C. Saying the alphabet. Articulation of certain speech sounds requires specific soft palate positioning. When saying /k/ the soft palate rises to close the velopharyngeal port (Figure 11-1). When articulating the nasal consonants /m/ or /n/ the port opens widely as seen here. *Note:* The patient can say "M" and open the velopharyngeal port to facilitate passage of the flexible fiberscope through the nasopharynx.

Figure 11-4D. Whistling. Whistling is accompanied by velopharyngeal closure so as not to lose force and waste air out the nose.

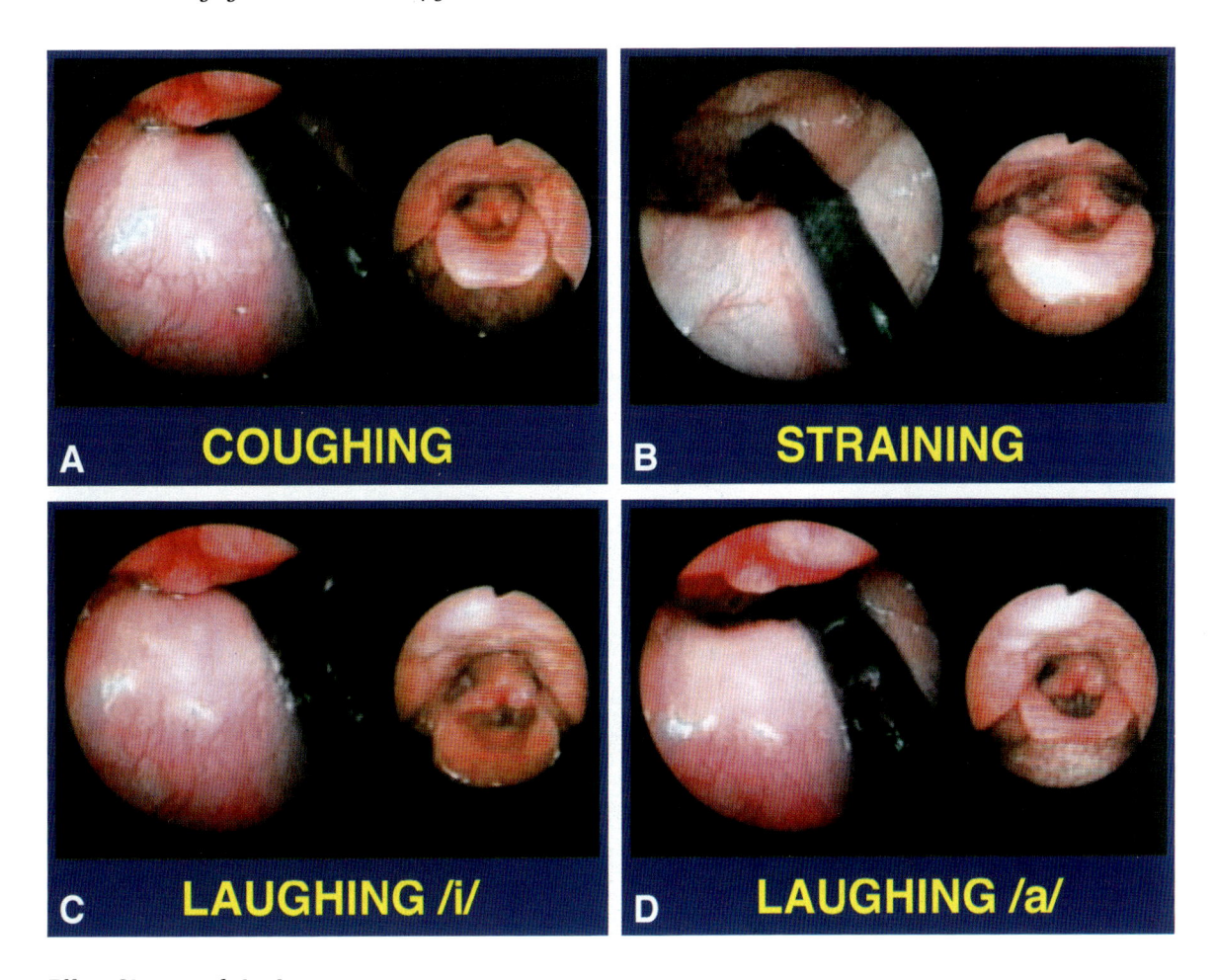

Simultaneous Velolaryngeal Videoendoscopy 163

A COUGHING **B STRAINING**

C LAUGHING /i/ **D LAUGHING /a/**

Effort Closure of the Larynx

Figure 11-5A. Coughing. In preparation for the expulsive phase the velopharyngeal port and ventricular (false) folds are closed in order to build subglottic pressure (see also Figure 9-5A). When the air escapes during the expulsive phase, the laryngeal inlet and glottis open widely, and the velopharyngeal port begins to open.

Figure 11-5B. Straining. The soft palate is partially raised but the velopharyngeal port is wide open during straining. The aryepiglottic sphincter and ventricular folds are tightly closed.

Figure 11-5C. Laughing. Laughing is accompanied by soft palate and laryngeal convulsions. The soft palate position, however, is vowel-dependent. When laughing on /i/ (e.g., "hee, hee, hee") the soft palate rises high, closing the port.

Figure 11-5D. Laughing. When laughing on /a/ (e.g., "ha, ha, ha") the soft palate drops leaving an open velopharyngeal port. This view catches a convulsion seen in the soft palate (nearly closed) and the larynx (glottis tightly closed).

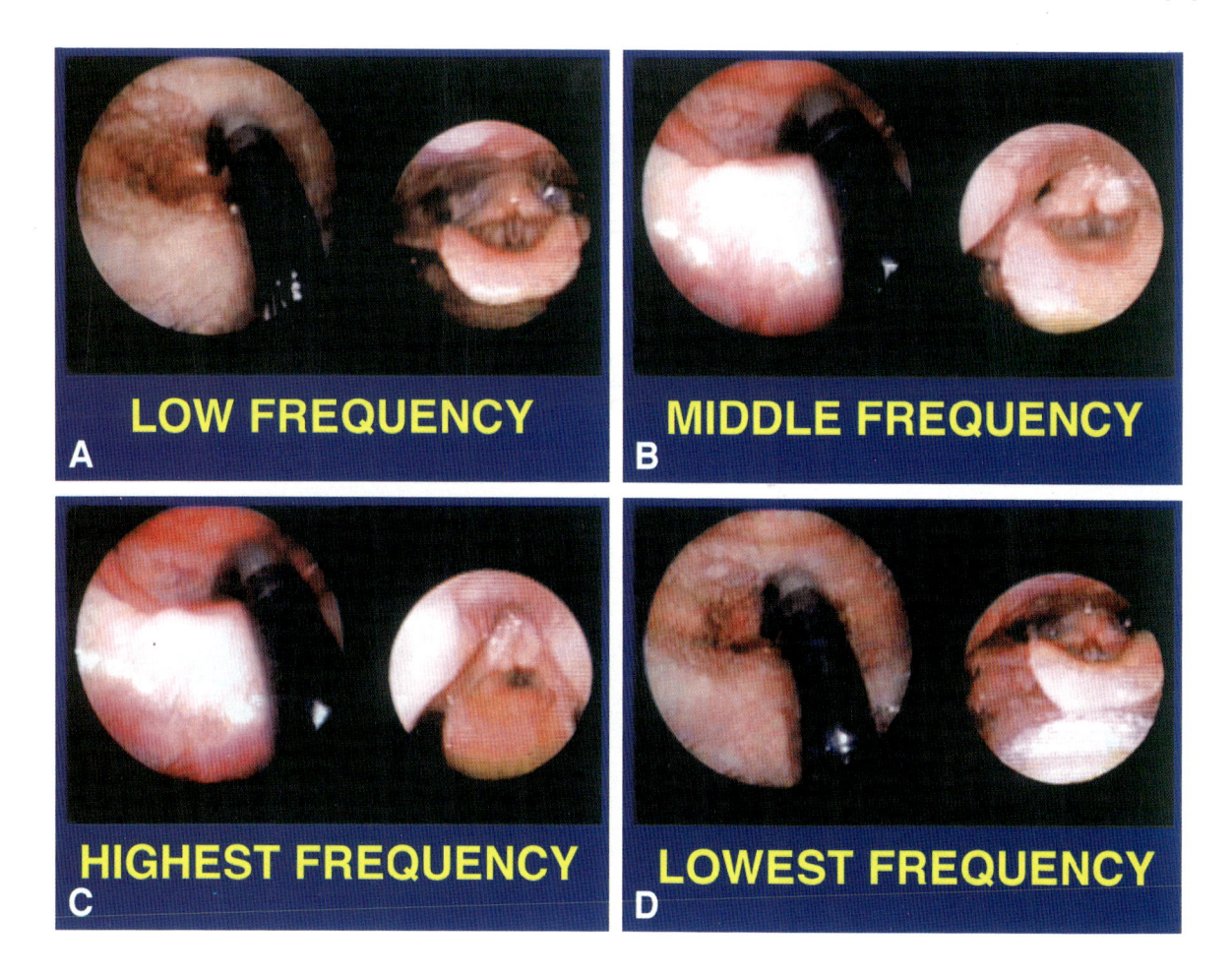

A **LOW FREQUENCY**

B **MIDDLE FREQUENCY**

C **HIGHEST FREQUENCY**

D **LOWEST FREQUENCY**

Siren

Figure 11-6A. Low-frequency range. Slow-motion simultaneous velolaryngeal endoscopy clearly demonstrates the changes in the larynx, hypopharynx, and velopharyngeal port during a continuous pitch change from low frequency to high frequency and back to low frequency again (siren). Figure 11-6 represents four points in this video sequence. Starting in the low-frequency range the velopharyngeal port is open, and the hypopharynx is open. The larynx remains descended.

Figure 11-6B. Middle-frequency range. As the pitch gradually increases into the middle-frequency range the velopharyngeal port closes, and the hypopharynx begins to narrow. Note the lateral pharyngeal walls begin to contract. The larynx also begins to rise.

Figure 11-6C. High-frequency range. At the peak frequency the port remains closed, the hypopharynx is at its narrowest, the supraglottic larynx is contracted and narrow, and the larynx is elevated.

Figure 11-6D. Lowest-frequency range. As the pitch lowers again, everything returns to baseline (port open, hypopharynx open, supraglottic larynx open, and larynx descended).

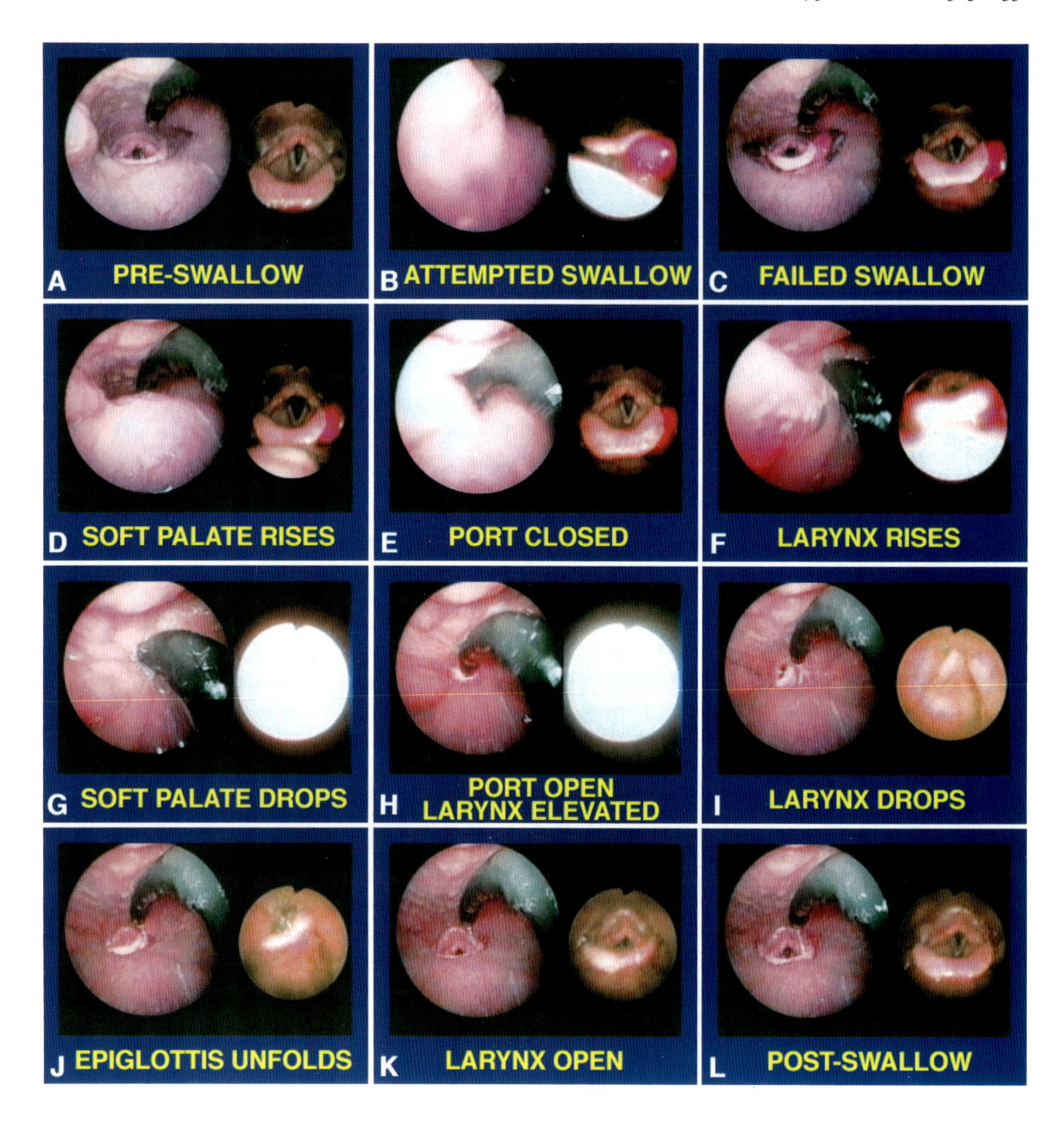

A PRE-SWALLOW	**B** ATTEMPTED SWALLOW	**C** FAILED SWALLOW
D SOFT PALATE RISES	**E** PORT CLOSED	**F** LARYNX RISES
G SOFT PALATE DROPS	**H** PORT OPEN LARYNX ELEVATED	**I** LARYNX DROPS
J EPIGLOTTIS UNFOLDS	**K** LARYNX OPEN	**L** POST-SWALLOW

Swallowing

Figure 11-7A. Pre-swallow. The velopharyngeal port and larynx are both open before the swallow. The following sequence comprises views taken from a super-slow-motion run of video.

Figure 11-7B. Attempted swallow. The soft palate rises to close the velopharyngeal port, and the pill slides along the left vallecula toward the piriform sinus.

Figure 11-7C. Failed swallow. The pill sticks in the left vallecula, seen through both endoscopes. In between swallows, the subject breathes and opens the glottis despite the presence of the pill still in the vallecula.

Figure 11-7D. Soft palate rises. A second swallow begins with the soft palate rising and the velopharyngeal port beginning to close. The larynx is still open at this point.

Figure 11-7E. Velopharyngeal port closed. Now the port is closed but the larynx remains open.

Figure 11-7F. Larynx rises. The port is closed and the larynx begins to rise, with the epiglottis starting to fold down over the larynx. As the larynx rises, it touches the fiberscope lens, thereby obscuring the view of the larynx.

Figure 11-7G. Soft palate begins to relax. The velopharyngeal port begins to open again as the soft palate starts to drop and relax. The larynx is still elevated and covered with the epiglottis.

Figure 11-7H. Velopharyngeal port open and larynx elevated. The soft palate drops down and the port is wide open. The fiberscope is visible with the elevated closed larynx pressed against the lens. The fiberscopic view is still obscured by the elevated larynx, and the pill is out of sight.

Figure 11-7I. The port is wide open. The nasopharyngoscopic view reveals the larynx beginning to drop and the epiglottis beginning to unfold. The fiberscopic view shows that the larynx has dropped slightly because it is no longer pressed against the lens and obscuring the view. The epiglottis is seen mostly folded posteriorly over the larynx. The pill is gone.

Figure 11-7J. Epiglottis unfolds. The larynx continues to drop and the epiglottis continues to unfold.

Figure 11-7K. Larynx open. The larynx has fallen and the epiglottis is nearly completely unfolded. The glottis begins to open.

Figure 11-7L. Post-swallow. The epiglottis has completely unfolded. The larynx is in its original position. The soft palate remains relaxed and forward. The pill is gone. The patient is ready for another swallow.

Chapter 12
Rigid and Contact Endoscopy in Microlaryngeal Surgery*

Rigid and contact endoscopy in microlaryngeal surgery are techniques developed by Mario Andrea and Oscar Dias for the anatomic and the *in vivo* histologic examinations of the larynx and its superficial mucosa. Rigid endoscopy in microlaryngeal surgery (REMS) is similar to the previously described telescopic videolaryngoscopy performed in the operating room (Figure 9-4). Zero-, 30-, 70-, and 120-degree telescopes are used to examine fully the larynx through the suspended direct laryngoscope. REMS is followed by contact endoscopy in microlaryngeal surgery (CEMS) whereby a contact endoscope with 60× and 150× magnification capability is used to examine the superficial mucosa histology through the direct laryngoscope before performing the microsurgical procedure. Both REMS and CEMS are recorded on video for later review and comparison to the histology sections.

REMS with video recording is an excellent method of examining and documenting laryngeal anatomy and pathology, while CEMS allows one to assess the mucosal histology and histopathology *in situ*. CEMS may allow one to confirm the preoperative diagnosis of mucosal lesions (e.g., papilloma) by their characteristic histologic appearance, or it may allow one to assess surgical margins after a laryngeal cancer resection.

Equipment required for REMS includes (1) direct laryngoscope, (2) rigid Hopkins 5.0-mm 24-cm-long 0-, 30-, 70-, and 120-degree endoscopes (Karl Storz 8712AA, BA, CA, and DA, respectively), (3) xenon light source, (4) operating microscope, and (5) laryngoscope suspension system. CEMS requires, in addition (1) a contact laryngoscope [a rigid 4.0-mm 24-cm-long 30-degree Hamou microcolpohysteroscope (Karl Storz 26156B) was used originally; subsequently the contact laryngoscope (Karl Storz 8715A) (5.0- and 8.0-mm 24-cm-long 0-degree) was designed by Mario Andrea and Oscar Dias, specifically for the assessment of the vocal fold epithelium, offering significant advantages for the clinical use of contact endoscopy in the larynx], (2) saline serum, (3) Spongostan, and (4) 1% methylene blue. Videoendoscopy equipment includes (1) a video camera, (2) a video monitor, (3) a video recorder, and (4) a video printer.

*This chapter was written in collaboration with Mario Andrea, M.D., Ph.D. and Oscar Dias, M.D., Ph.D.

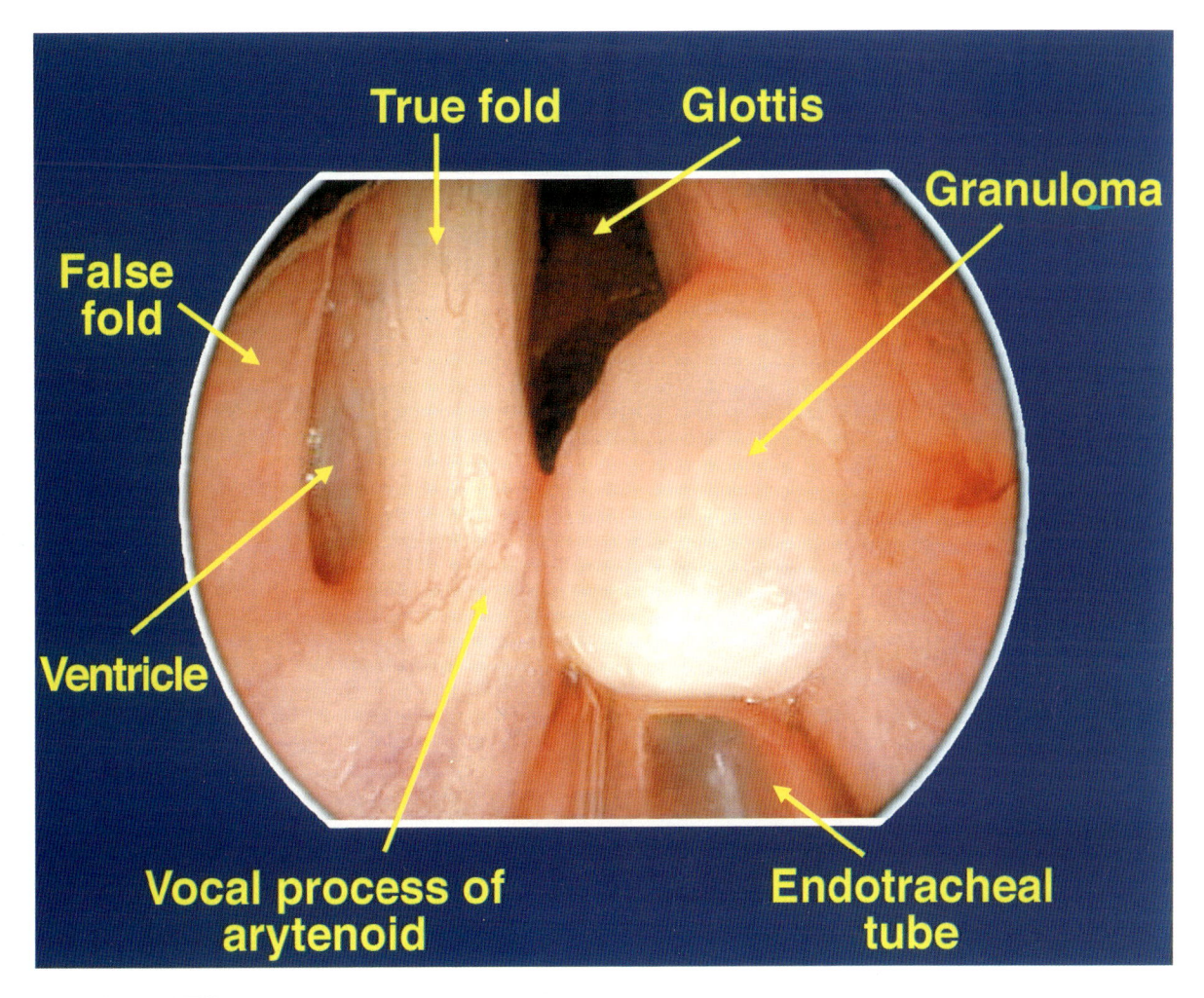

OVERVIEW

REMS

Figure 12-1. Zero-degree REMS. This close-up view of the larynx provides a detailed exam of important laryngeal structures. This is an operative procedure; thus, like the operating room techniques of videolaryngoscopy (Figure 9-4), the larynx is oriented with the anterior structures at the top of the view and with the posterior structures at the bottom. This view clearly displays the true vocal folds, ventricle, glottis, and part of the arytenoids. A large posterior granuloma and the endotracheal tube are also displayed.

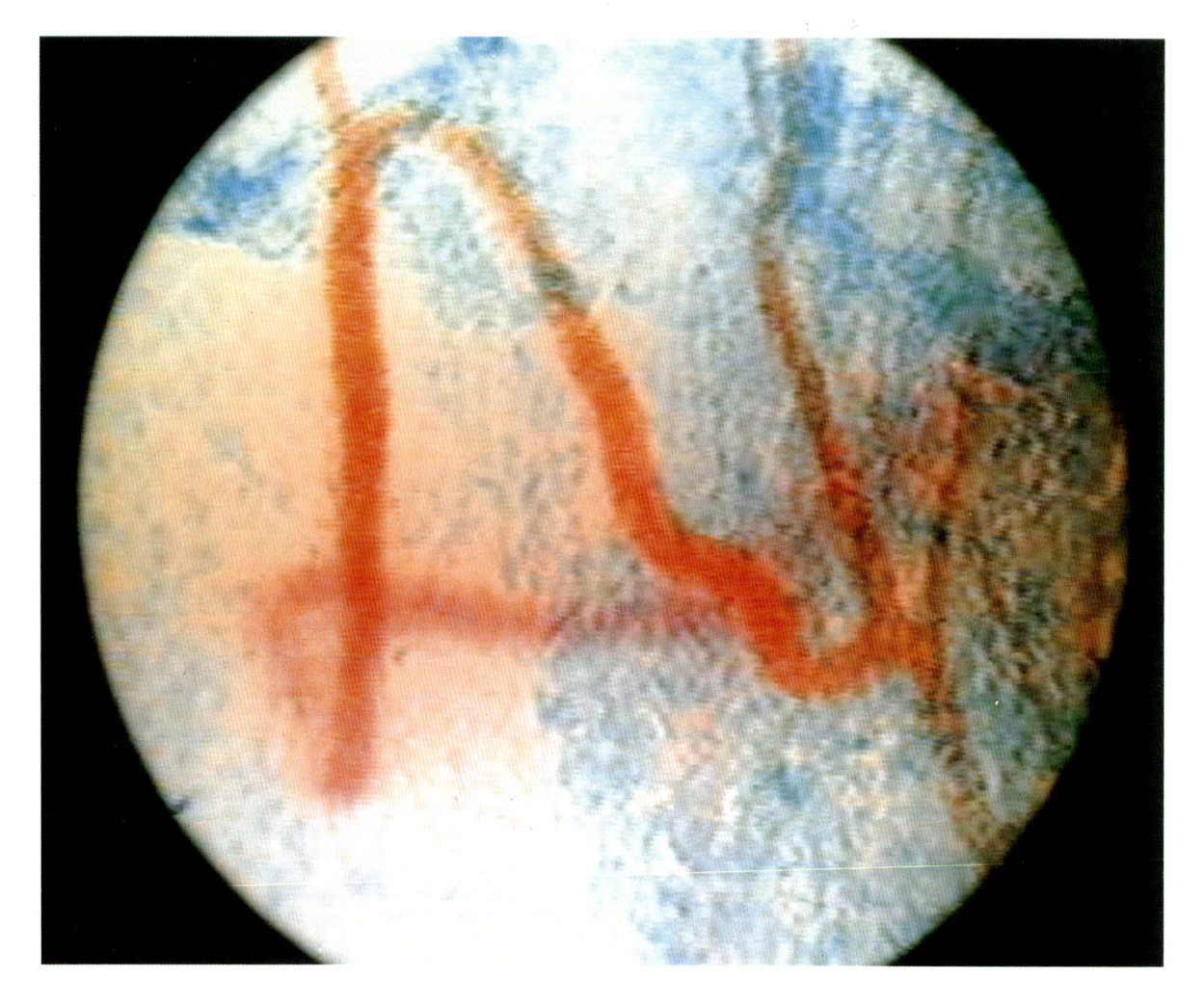

CEMS

Figure 12-2. 60× CEMS. Contact endoscopy (60×) reveals normal mucosal microvasculature of the true vocal fold. Methylene blue staining *in vivo* enhances the cellular structures, especially when viewed with the 150× contact endoscope. Here the background staining is noted.

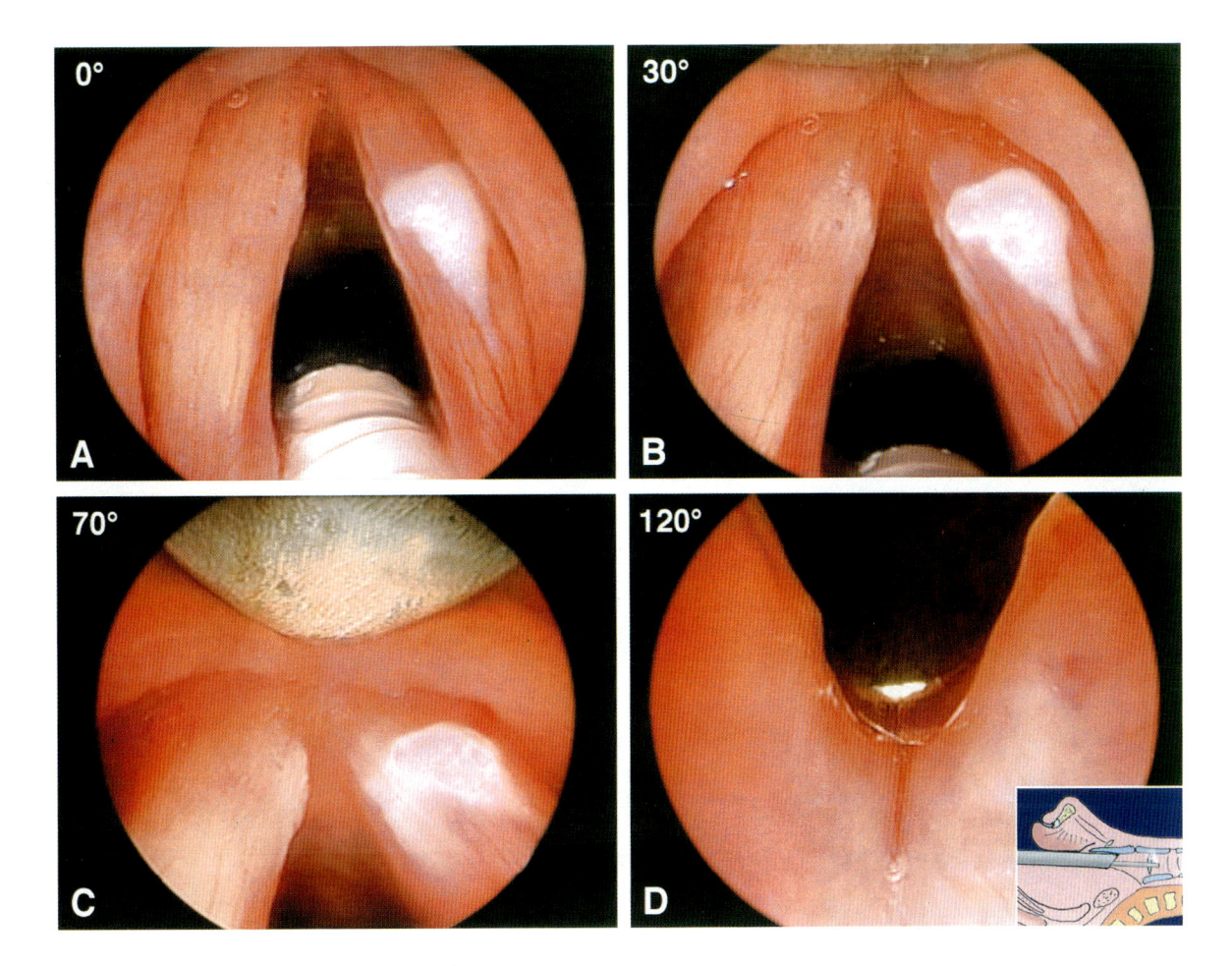

TECHNIQUES OF REMS AND CEMS

REMS

Figure 12-3A. Zero-degree REMS. Just like telescopic videolaryngoscopy in the operating room (Figure 9-4), REMS and CEMS require suspension laryngoscopy in the intubated anesthetized patient. The rigid 5.0-mm endoscopes then are passed through the direct laryngoscope for a detailed laryngeal examination prior to a microsurgical procedure. This 0-degree REMS reveals a clear close-up view of the superior surface of the true vocal folds and ventricles. The right true vocal fold leukoplakia is seen.

Figure 12-3B. Thirty-degree REMS. The 30-degree rigid endoscope produces a good view of the anterior commissure (*top middle of view*) and the anterior subglottis (*middle of view*). The medial true vocal fold surfaces and the ventricles begin to come into fuller view with the 30-degree endoscope compared to the 0-degree endoscope. A small area of the left anterior medial true vocal fold leukoplakia becomes visible on this view. The distal blade of the direct laryngoscope can barely be seen at the very top of this view.

Figure 12-3C. Seventy-degree REMS. The 70-degree rigid endoscope provides a direct view of the anterior commissure and medial surfaces of the true vocal folds. The laryngoscope is seen at the top of this view, and the left medial true vocal fold lesion is now more visible. The ventricles can be well visualized when this endoscope is directed laterally.

Figure 12-3D. One-hundred-twenty-degree REMS. For this view the rigid endoscope tip is positioned just beyond the true vocal folds as the scope looks back up the larynx (*inset*). This view demonstrates the inferior surface of the true vocal folds and anterior commissure. The laryngoscope is seen just above the glottis.

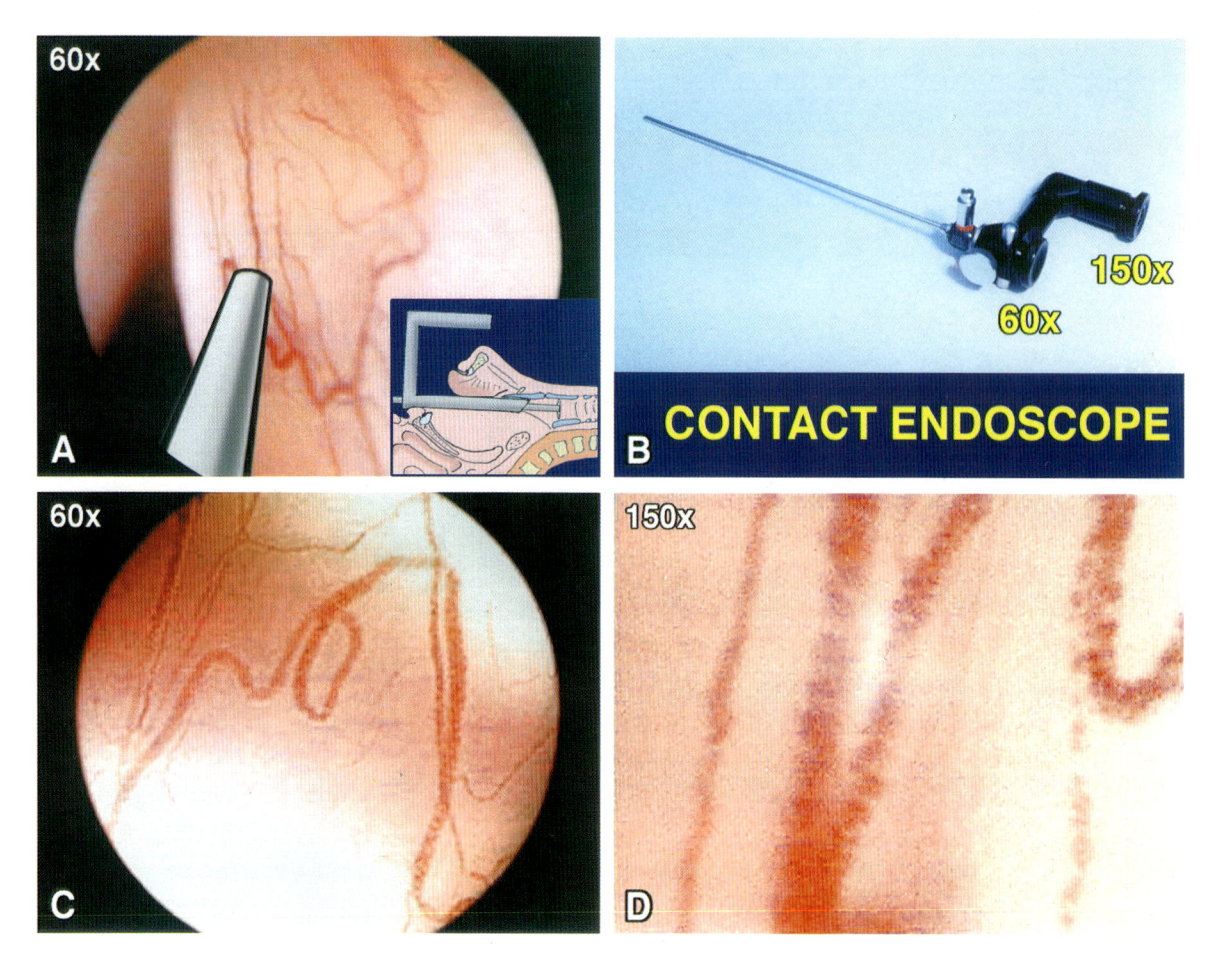

CEMS

Figure 12-4A. Contact endoscope. The contact endoscope is positioned near the mucosa of interest just before cleaning the mucosal surface with Spongostan soaked in saline serum. The area is then carefully suctioned and 1% methylene blue is applied. The endoscope is gently advanced to the mucosa where the stained superficial epithelium becomes visible at magnifications of 60× or 150×. Video recording allows direct comparison of the contact endoscopic view to the histologic sections.

Figure 12-4B. Contact endoscope. Andrea first used the Hamou microcolpohysteroscope (60× and 150×) shown here for developing contact laryngoscopy. Now a new contact laryngoscope (Karl Storz 8715A) offers significant advantages for the use of contact endoscopes in the larynx (better imaging and easier manipulation).

Figure 12-4C. 60× CEMS. This 60× contact endoscopic view of normal true vocal fold mucosa without methylene blue staining gives a detailed picture of the normal microvasculature.

Figure 12-4D. 150× CEMS. This 150× contact endoscopic view of the same microvasculature reveals individual red blood cells. When the mucosa is stained with methylene blue, individual epithelial cells are visible (Figure 12-5).

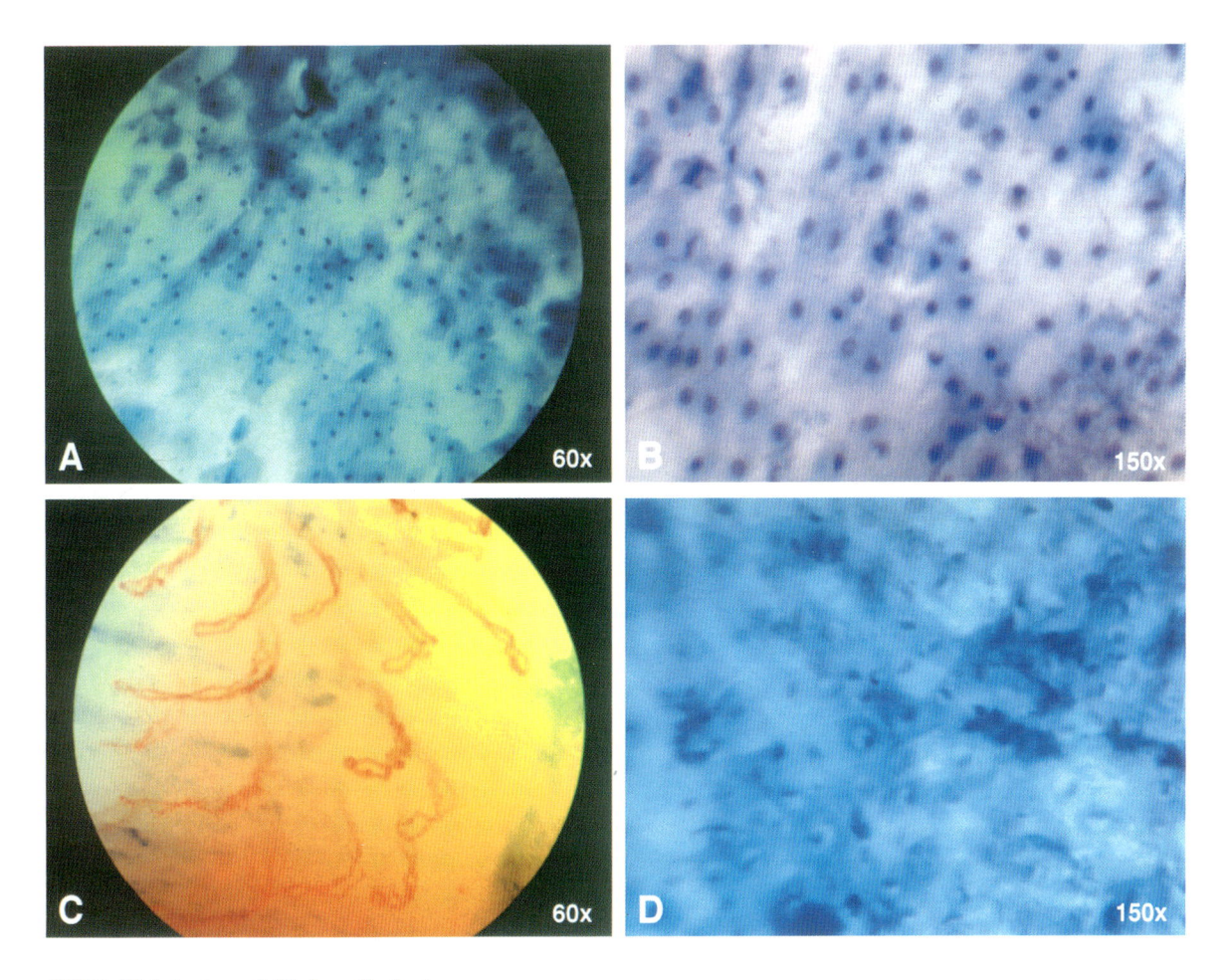

CEMS Histology and Histopathology

Figure 12-5A. Normal true vocal fold histology at 60× magnification. This 60× CEMS view after methylene blue staining demonstrates a homogeneous pattern of the epithelial cellular population and normal nuclear (dark blue) and cytoplasmic (light blue) morphology including regular shape, dimension, and nuclear/cytoplasm ratio. (Photography by Mario Andrea, M.D., Ph.D. and Oscar Dias, M.D., Ph.D.)

Figure 12-5B. Normal true vocal fold histology at 150× magnification. The 150× CEMS allows a more detailed exam of the nuclear morphology. (Photography by Mario Andrea, M.D., Ph.D. and Oscar Dias, M.D., Ph.D.)

Figure 12-5C. 60× CEMS of laryngeal papilloma. This 60× CEMS view reveals the classic papillary arrangement of papillomatosis. Each papilla has a central axis vessel. (Photography by Mario Andrea, M.D., Ph.D. and Oscar Dias, M.D., Ph.D.)

Figure 12-5D. 150× CEMS of laryngeal papilloma. This higher-magnification view of a laryngeal papilloma reveals balloon cells (crescentic peripherally displaced nucleus and a vacuolated cytoplasm) and inflammatory cells (large regular nuclei). Occasionally, neutrophil infiltrates can be seen in the epithelium. (Photography by Mario Andrea, M.D., Ph.D. and Oscar Dias, M.D., Ph.D.)

Chapter 13
Endoscopy of the Middle Ear (Middle Ear Videoendoscopy)*

Middle ear endoscopy is the examination of the middle ear cavity using a rigid telescope or flexible fiberscope. When the exam is documented with a video camera, the procedure is called *middle ear videoendoscopy.*

Middle ear endoscopy can be accomplished by transcanal telescopic examinaton through either a myringotomy in the intact tympanic membrane or an existing tympanic membrane perforation. This technique was pioneered by Nomura in 1982 and advocated more recently by Poe as an office procedure to precede (and sometimes replace) middle ear exploration. Transmastoid telescopy at the time of otosurgery allows a more thorough intraoperative exam that may aid in determining the extent of pathology and discerning anatomical anomalies.

Equipment required for middle ear endoscopy includes (1) 1.9-mm 12-cm-long 5- and 25-degree ototelescopes (Richard Wolf endoscopes used by Poe) or 1.9-mm 0- and 30-degree ototelescopes (Karl Storz 28-301A&D, respectively) for transtympanic membrane endoscopy, (2) Hopkins 2.7-mm 11-cm-long 0- and 30-degree and 4.0-mm 6-cm-long 0- and 30-degree ototelescopes (Karl Storz 1230A&B and 1215A&B, respectively) for otosurgical endoscopy, (3) 1.0-mm 5-cm-long flexible fiberscope (Machida MES-10 used by Poe) for eustachian tube and middle ear endoscopy in some cases, (4) xenon light source, and (5) myringotomy set. A specially designed protective shield or sidearm telescope may be used. Middle ear videoendoscopy also requires (1) video camera, (2) video monitor, (3) video recorder, and (4) video printer.

Middle ear endoscopy is a useful adjunct to the ear exam in both the office and the operating room. A patient with a possible perilymph fistula, for example, may be spared a middle ear exploration if it can be ruled out by middle ear endoscopy in the office. Transmastoid telescopy during otosurgery may augment the microscopic exam by revealing the anatomy and pathology of the posterior portion of the attic and facial recess. The posterior superior extent of a middle ear cholesteatoma, an anomaly of the facial nerve, or congenital anomalies of the ossicular chain, for example, may be demonstrated.

* This chapter was written in collaboration with Dennis Poe, M.D.

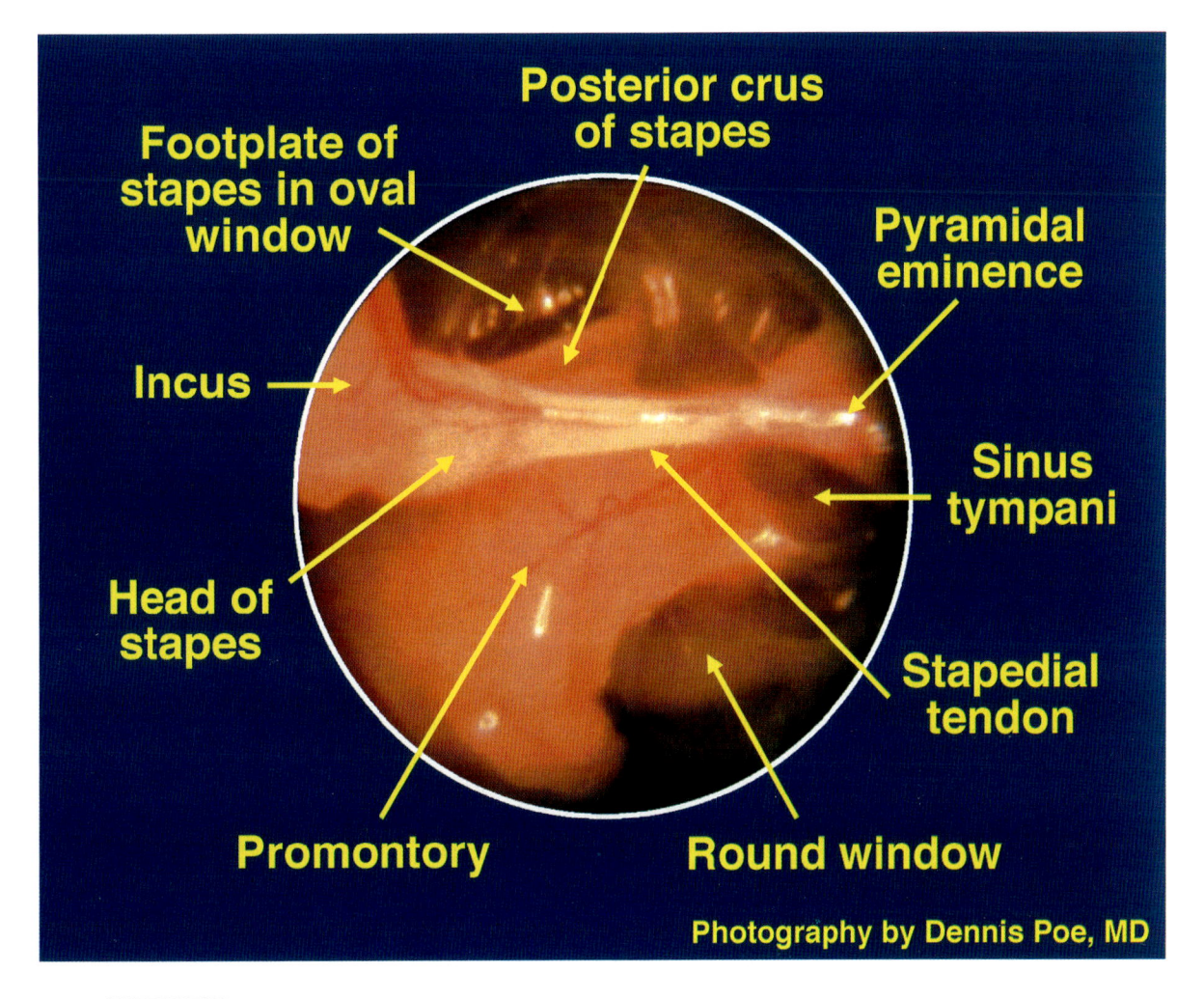

Endoscopy of the Middle Ear (Middle Ear Videoendoscopy) 175

OVERVIEW

Figure 13-1. Five-degree transtympanic telescopic view of the middle ear. This broad 1.9-mm 5-degree Wolf transtympanic ototelescopic view of the posterior left middle ear shows normal middle ear structures. The top of the view is superior, the bottom is inferior, and the right is posterior.

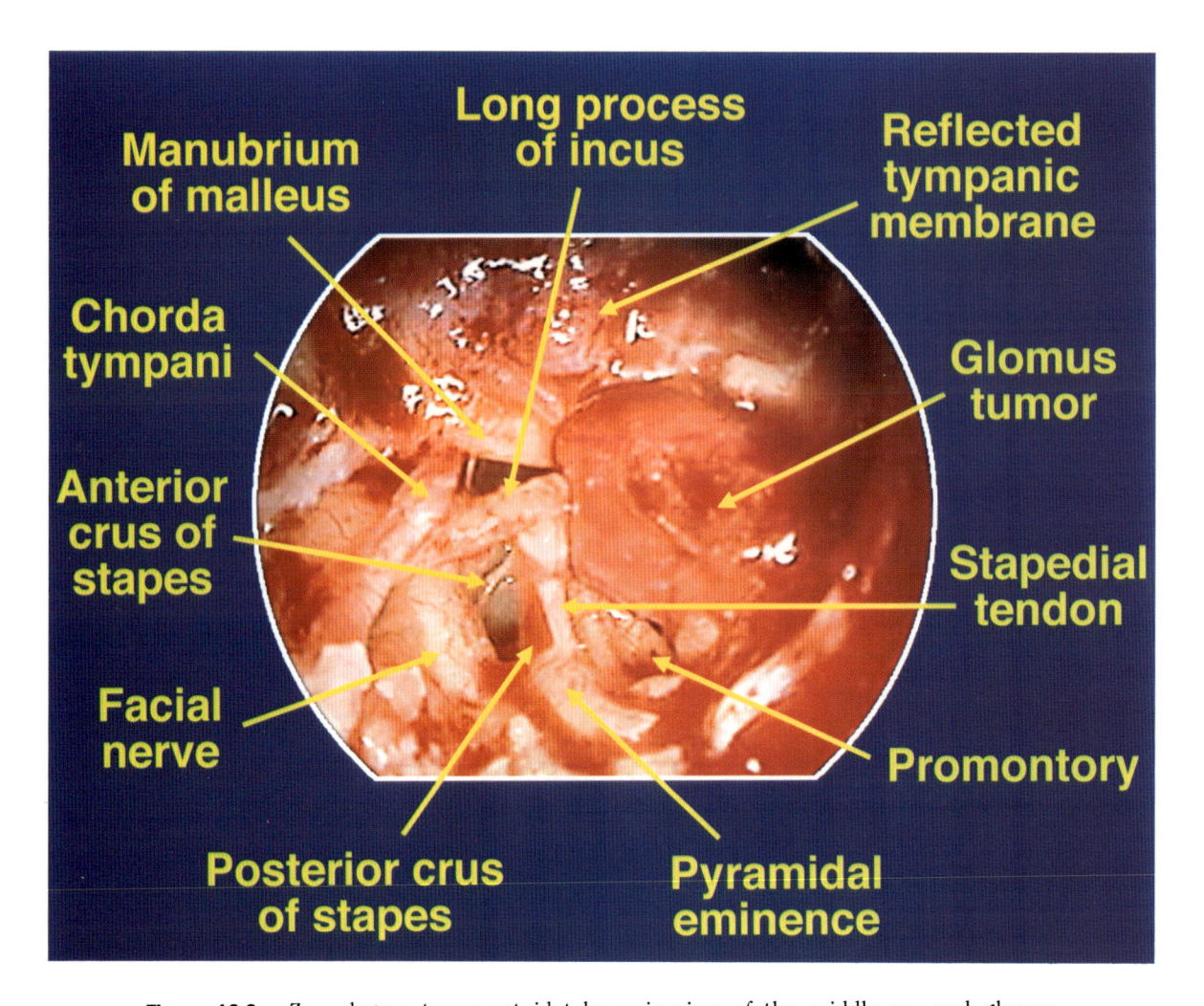

Figure 13-2. Zero-degree transmastoid telescopic view of the middle ear and glomus tumor. This intraoperative panoramic 4.0-mm 0-degree transmastoid telescopic view of the right middle ear is oriented such that the top of the view is anterior, the bottom is posterior, the left is superior, and the right is inferior. Normal middle ear structures are labeled. The tympanic membrane is reflected anteriorly. The large glomus tumor impinges on the incudostapedial joint, thus causing this patient's 40-dB conductive hearing loss preoperatively.

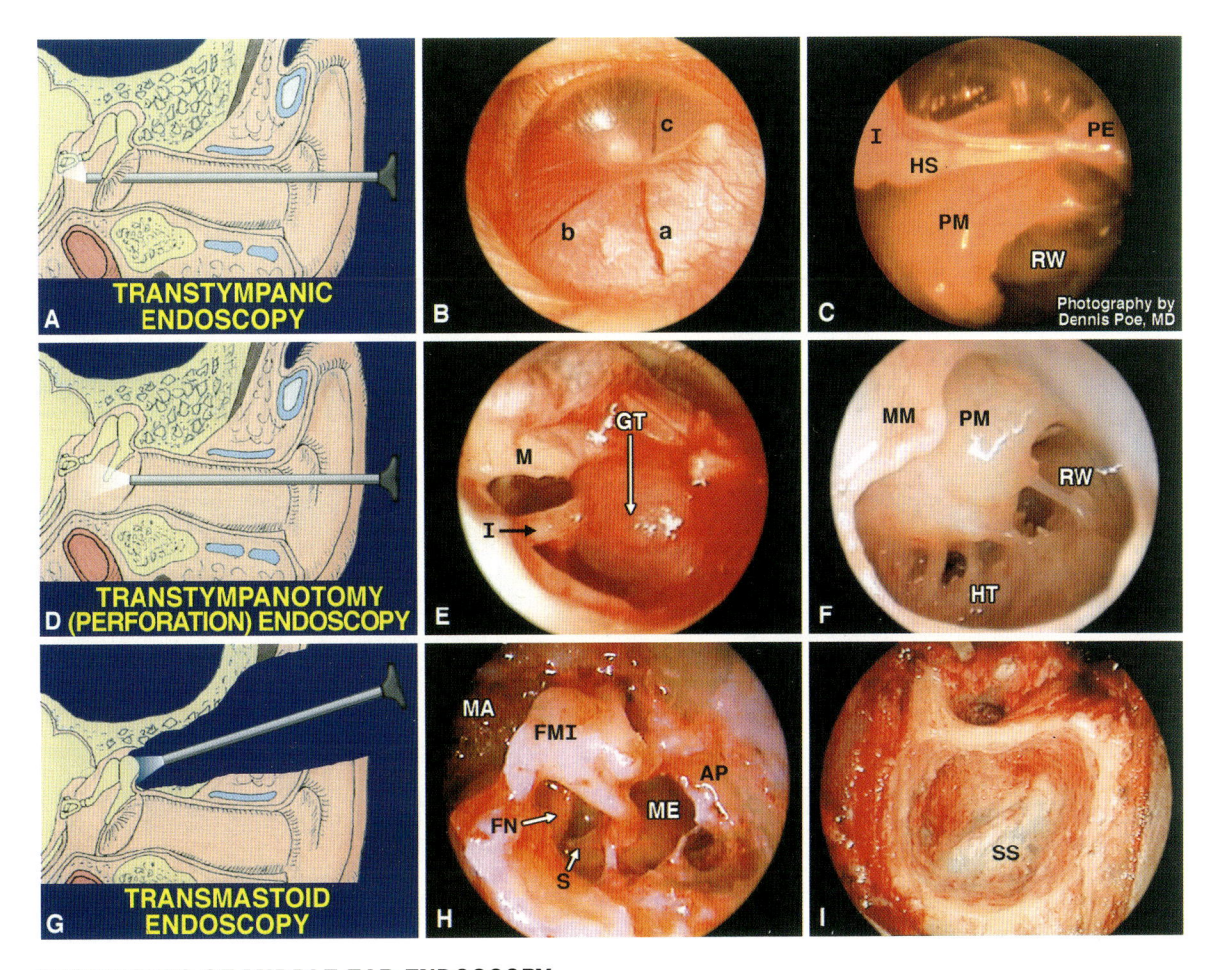

TECHNIQUES OF MIDDLE EAR ENDOSCOPY

Figure 13-3. *Top row:* Transtympanic middle ear endoscopy. A 2- to 3-mm radial myringotomy is made overlying the suspected middle ear pathology. Figure 13-3B demonstrates three left radial myringotomies. The patient is supine so the top of the view is anterior and the bottom is posterior. The posterior superior myringotomy (a) allows one to view the ossicles, the oval and round windows, the sinus tympani, and the pyramidal eminence. A rigid 1.9-mm 5- or 25-degree ototelescope is passed through the myringotomies. Figure 13-3C (see also Figure 13-1) shows the normal posterior left middle ear including the incus (I), the stapedial muscle and tendon attached from the head of stapes (HS) to the pyramidal eminence (PE), the promontory (PM), and the round window (RW). In Figure 13-3C the top of the view is superior and the right is posterior. The inferior myringotomy (b) allows one to see the hypotympanum, and the anterior myringotomy (c) allows one to view the eustachian tube orifice. Five- and 25-degree telescopes allow the examiner to see most aspects of the middle ear. The 1.0-mm flexible fiberscope may be used; however, it yields smaller images of lesser resolution. *Middle row:* Transtympanotomy or transperforation endoscopy. A larger (2.7- or 4.0-mm) rigid ototelescope can be passed into the middle ear through a tympanotomy intraoperatively or through a large tympanic membrane perforation in the office. The larger telescopes yield larger, clearer images. Figure 13-3E (see also Figures 4-20C, 4-20D, and 13-2) shows a transtympanotomic view of the right middle ear (top of the view is anterior, the right is inferior) displaying the malleus (M), the incus (I), and a large glomus tumor (GT) impinging on the incudostapedial joint. Figure 13-3F shows a transperforation view of the left middle ear displaying the malleus (MM), promontory (PM), round window niche (RW), and hypotympanum (HT). *Bottom row:* Transmastoid endoscopy. Intraoperative transmastoid middle ear endoscopy provides another means of carefully examining the middle ear during tympanomastoidectomy surgery. Figure 13-3H displays the right middle ear of a patient with external auditory canal atresia as seen through the 4.0-mm 0-degree transmastoid ototelescope (see also Figures 4-21A and 4-21D). The malleus and incus are fused (FMI) and the atretic plate is visible (AP). Also visible are the facial nerve (FN) and stapes (S). Figure 13-3I shows a 4.0-mm 0-degree telescopic wide-angle view of a right-sided simple mastoidectomy. The external canal is at the top of the view, and the sigmoid sinus (SS) is at the bottom.

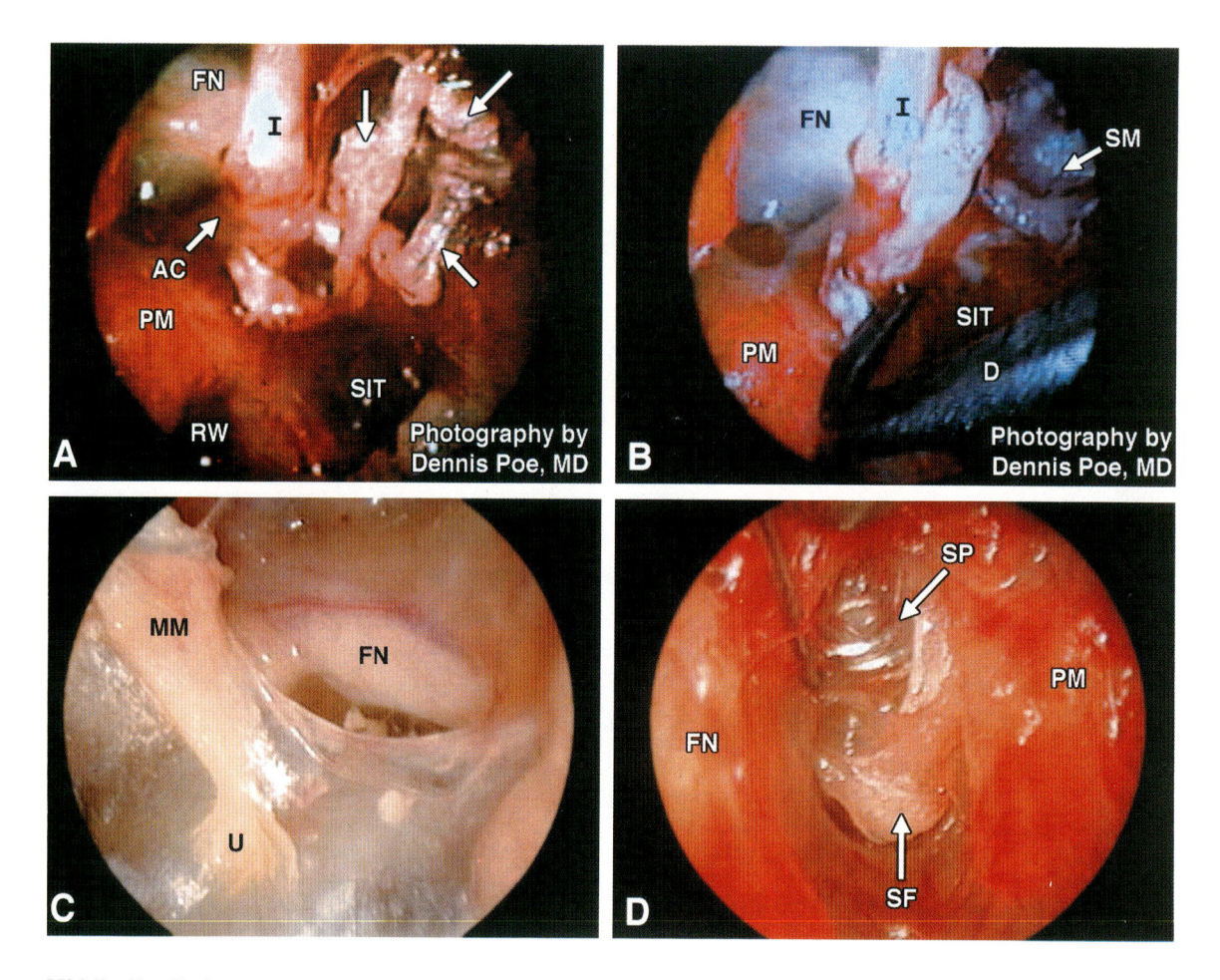

Middle Ear Endoscopy

Figure 13-4A. Cholesteatoma. This 2.7-mm 0-degree transtympanotomic left middle ear endoscopic view reveals a sinus tympani cholesteatoma (*arrows*) that caused this patient's conductive hearing loss. Also clearly seen on this view were the incus (I), promontory (PM), horizontal portion of the facial nerve (FN), round window (RW), stapes superstructure including the anterior crus (AC), and sinus tympani (SIT).

Figure 13-4B. Cholesteatoma. This 2.7-mm 30-degree transtympanotomic left middle ear endoscopic view reveals squamous matrix (cholesteatoma) (SM) in the sinus tympani (SIT). The angled telescopes enable the surgeon to see even small areas of pathology that are otherwise difficult to view. The incus (I), promontory (PM), facial nerve (FN), stapes superstructure, and curved dissector (D) were also seen in this view.

Figure 13-4C. Dehiscent facial nerve. This 4.0-mm 0-degree transperforation view of the left middle ear demonstrates a dehiscent horizontal facial nerve (FN). The posterior superior perforation also reveals the cochleariform process, visible behind the malleus manubrium (MM). The umbo (U) and part of the intact tympanic membrane are seen.

Figure 13-4D. Stapedial prosthesis. This patient underwent a stapedectomy in the past for otosclerosis. Later the patient had persistent conductive hearing loss in this right ear. This 2.7-mm 0-degree transtympanotomic telescopic view recorded at the time of middle ear exploration reveals a wire and coil stapes prosthesis (SP) attached to the stapes footplate (SF) that was fixed due to otosclerosis. The facial nerve (FN) and promontory (PM) were also seen in this view. At surgery the footplate was removed, the oval window was covered with fascia, and the prosthesis was lengthened slightly to transmit sound to the oval window.

BIBLIOGRAPHY

HISTORY—OTOLOGY

Brubaker JD, Holinger PH. The larynx, bronchi, and esophagus in Kodachrome. *J Biol Photogr Assoc* 10:83, 1941.

Buckingham RA. Photography of the ear. In: English GM, ed. *Otolaryngology,* vol 1. Hagerstown, MD: Harper & Row, 1981, Chapter 58.

Hantman I. A simple technique for photography of the drum head. *Arch Otolaryngol* 34:7–11, 1941.

Hantman I. Secretory otitis media: illustrated with photographs of the tympanic membrane in natural color. *Arch Otolaryngol* 38:561–573, 1943.

Holinger P, Brubaker JD, Brubaker JE. Open tube, proximal illumination mirror and direct laryngeal photography. *Can J Otolaryngol* 4:781–785, 1975.

Pensak ML, Yanagisawa E. Tympanic membrane photography: historical perspective. *Am J Otol* 5:324–332, 1984.

Politzer A. *Die Beleuchtungsbilder des Trommelfells im Gesunden und Kranken Zustande.* Vienna: Wilhelm Braumuller, 1865 (*The Membrane Tympani in Health and Disease,* translated by Matheson and Newton. New York: William Wood and Co., 1869).

Rudinger N. In: Stahl, E., ed. *Atlas des menschlichen Gehororganes herausgegben von Dr. Rudinger nach Natur Photographirt von J. Albert.* Munchen: Verlag der J. J. Lentnerschen Buchtandlung, 1866.

Schultz van Treek. Ein neues Instrument zur Untersuchung und Photographie des Trommelfells. *Z Hals Nas Heilk (Berlin)* 44:326–331, 1938.

Stein ST. Apparat zur photographischen Aunahme des Trommelfells. *Arch Ohren Nasen Kehlkopfheilkd* 7:56–58, 1873.

Yanagisawa E, Smith HW, Rosnagle R, Pratt LW. *Photography of the Tympanic Membrane and Middle Ear.* Scientific Exhibit, American Academy of Otolaryngology, 1979.

HISTORY—RHINOLOGY

Bozzini P. Lichtleiter, eine Erfindung zur Anschauung innerer Thelle und Krankeiten. *J Prac Arzneykunde Wundarzneykunst. (Berlin)* 1806:24.

Czermak JN. *Der Kehlkopfspiegel.* Leipzig: W. Engelmann, 1863.

Czermak JN. Zur Verwerthung des Liston-Garcia'schen Prinzips. *Wien Med Wochenschr* 11:81, 1861.

Draf W. *Endoskopie der Nasennebenhohlen.* Berlin: Springer, 1978.

Flatau TS. Laryngoskopie und hintere Rhinoskopie bei geschlossenem Mund. *Passow Beitr* 3:461, 1910.

Friedrich JP, Terrier G. Indications et resultats de l'evidement ethmoidale sous guidage endoscopique. Schweizerische Ges fur HNO. 73. Fruhjahrsversammlung St. Moritz, Juni, 1986.

Hays H. Eine neue Untersuchungsmethode fur die hintere Nase, die Tuben und den Larynx mit einem elektrischen Pharyngosckop. *Z Laryngol (Leipzig)* 2:496, 1910.

Heermann H. Uber endonasale Chirurgie unter Verwendung des binocularen Mikroskopes. *Arch Ohr Nas Kehlkopfheilk* 171:295, 1958.

Hellmich S, Herberholdt C. Technische Verbesserungen der Kieferhohlendoskopie. *Arch Klin Exp Ohr Nas Kehlkopfheilk* 199(2):678, 1971.

Hirschmann A. Uber Endoskopie der Nase und deren Nebenhohlen. *Arch Laryngol Rhinol (Berlin)* 14:194, 1903.

Kennedy DW. Functional endoscopic sinus surgery—technique. *Arch Otolaryngol* 111:643–649, 1985.

Messerklinger W. Die normalen Sekretwege in der Nase des Menschen. *Arch Klin Exp Ohr Nas Kehlkopfheilk* 195:138, 1969.

Messerklinger W. Endoscopy of the nose. Baltimore: Urban & Schwarzenberg, 1978.

Nitze M. Eine neue Beobachtungs- und Untersuchungsmethode für Harnrohre, Harnblase und Rectum. *Wien Med Wochenschr* 649, 1879.

Stammberger H. An endoscopic study of tubal function and the diseased ethmoid sinus. *Arch Otolaryngol* 243:254–259, 1986.

Valentin A. Die cystoskopische Untersuchung des Nasenrachens oder Salpingoskopie. *Arch Laryngol Rhinol (Berlin)* 13:410, 1903.

Wertheim G. Uber ein Verfahren zum Zwecke der Besichtigung des vorderen und mittleren Drittels der Nasenhohle. *Wien Med Wochenschr* 19:293, 1869.

Wigand ME, Steiner W, Jaumann MP. Endonasal sinus surgery with endoscopical control: from radical operation to rehabilitation of the mucosa. *Endoscopy* 10:2255, 1978.

Yamashita K. Endonasal flexible fiberscopic endoscopy. *Rhinology* 21:233, 1983.

Zaufal E. Zur endoskopischen Untersuchung der Rachenmundung der Tube en face und des Tubenkanals. *Arch Ohr Nas Kehlkopfheilk* 79:109, 1909.

HISTORY—LARYNGOLOGY

Benjamin B. Technique of laryngeal photography. *Ann Otol Rhinol Laryngol* 93 (Suppl 109), 1984.

French TR. On photographing the larynx. *Trans Am Laryngol* 4:32–35, 1882.

French TR. On a perfected method of photographing the larynx. *NY Med J* 4:655–656, 1884.

Garcia M. Observation on the human voice. *Proc R Soc Lond* 7:399–420, 1855.

Holinger PH, Brubaker JD, Brubaker JE. Open tube, proximal illumination mirror and direct laryngeal photography. *Can J Otolaryngol* 4:781–785, 1975.

Kleinsasser O. Entwicklung und Methoden der Kehlkopffotografie (mit Beschreibung eines neuen einfachen Fotolaryngoskopes). *HNO* 11:171–176, 1963.

Sawashima M, Hirose H. New laryngoscopic technique by use of fiber optics. *J Acoust Soc Am* 43:168–169, 1968.

Tsuiki Y. *Laryngeal Examination.* Tokyo: Kanehara Shuppan, 1956.

Ward PH, Berci G, Calcaterra TC. Advances in endoscopic examination of the respiratory system. *Ann Otol Rhinol Laryngol* 83:754–760, 1974.

Yamashita K, Oku T, Tanaka H, et al. VTR endoscopy. *J Otolaryngol Jpn* 80:1208–1209, 1977.

Yanagisawa E, Casuccio JR, Suzuki M. Video laryngoscopy using a rigid telescope and a video home system color camera—a useful office procedure. *Ann Otol Rhinol Laryngol* 90:346–350, 1981.

OTOLOGY

Brenman AK. Two devices which facilitate photography with the Zeiss operation microscope. *Trans Am Acad Ophthalmol Otolaryngol* 65:724–734, 1961.

Buckingham RA. Disorders common to the eardrum and canal. In: *Atlas of Some Pathological Conditions of the Eye, Ear and Throat.* Chicago: Abbott Laboratories, 1955.

Buckingham RA. Endoscopic otophotography. *Laryngoscope* 73:7184, 1963.

Buckingham RA. Photography of the ear. In: English GM, ed. *Otolaryngology,* vol 1. Hagerstown, MD: Harper & Row, 1981, Chapter 58.

Chen B, Fry TL, Fischer ND, et al. Otoscopy and photography, a new method. *Ann Otol Rhinol Laryngol* 88:771–773, 1979.

Chole RA. Photography of the tympanic membrane, a new method. *Arch Otolaryngol* 106:230–231, 1980.

Eichner H. Neue Moglichkeiten der Trommelfellfotografie. *Laryngol Rhinol Otol* 56:167–172, 1977.

Hawke M. Telescopic otoscopy and photography of the tympanic membrane. *J Otolaryngol* 11:35–89, 1982.

Hegener J. Die Photographie des Trommelfells. In: Denker A, Kahler O, eds. *Handbuch der Hals, Nasen, Ohren-Heilkund.* Berlin: Julius Springer, 1926, pp 944–949.

Hough JVD. Malformations and anatomical variations seen in the middle ear during the operation for mobilization of the stapes. *Laryngoscope,* 68:1337–1379, 1958.

House WF, House HP, Urban J, et al. Operating microscope observation viewer and motion picture camera. *Trans Am Acad Ophthalmol Otolaryngol* 63:228–229, 1959.

Hughes GB, Yanagisawa E, Dickins JRE, et al. Microscopic otologic photography using a standard 35 mm camera. *Am J Otol* 2:243–247, 1981.

Konrad HR, Berci G, Ward P, et al. Pediatric otoscopy and photography of the tympanic membrane. *Arch Otolaryngol* 105:431–433, 1979.

Lundborg T, Linzander S. The otomicroscopic observation and its clinical application. *Acta Otolaryngol (Stockh) Suppl* 266:3–36, 1970.

Mambrino L, Yanagisawa E, Yanagisawa K. Endoscopic ENT photography—a comparison of pictures by standard color films and newer color video printers. *Laryngoscope* 101:1229–1232, 1991.

Mann W, Munker G. A new method of otophotography. *Arch Otorhinolaryngol* 212:137–139, 1976.

Molinie M. La Photographie Stereoscopique du Tympan. *Bull Acad Med Paris* 80:655–656, 1918.

Pensak ML, Yanagisawa E, Tympanic membrane photography: historical perspective. *Am J Otol* 5:324–332, 1984.

Politzer A. *Die Beleuchtungsbilder des Trommelfells im Gesunden und Kranken Zustande.* Vienna: Wilhelm Braumuller, 1865 (*The membrane tympani in health and disease,* translated by Matheson and Newton. New York: William Wood and Co, 1869).

Schultz van Treek. Ein Neues Instrument zur Untersuchung und Photographie des Trommelfells. *Z Hals Nas Heilk (Berlin)* 44:326–331, 1938.

Selkin SG. Flexible fiberoptics for laryngeal photography. *Laryngoscope* 93:657–658, 1983.

Smith HW, Rosnagle RS, Yanagisawa E. Tympanic membrane photography. *Arch Otolaryngol* 99:125–127, 1981.

Stein ST. Apparat zur Photographischen Aunahme des Trommelfells. *Arch Ohren Nasen Kehlkopfheilkd* 7:56–58, 1873.

Yanagisawa E. Effective photography in otolaryngology—head and neck surgery: tympanic membrane photography. *Ototlaryngol Head Neck Surg* 90:399–407, 1982.

Yanagisawa E. The use of video in ENT endoscopy—its value in teaching. *ENT J* 73:754–763, 1994.

Yanagisawa E, Carlson RD. Telescopic video-otoscopy using a compact home video color camera. *Laryngoscope* 97:1350–1355, 1987.

Yanagisawa E, Smith HW, Rosnagle RS, et al. *Photography of the tympanic membrane and middle ear.* Scientific Exhibit. American Academy of Otolaryngology, 1979.

Yanagisawa K, Shi JM, Yanagisawa E, et al. Color photography of video images of otolaryngological structures using a 35 mm SLR camera. *Laryngoscope* 97:992–993, 1987.

NASAL/NASOPHARYNX

Chiang T-C, Jung PF. The nasopharyngoscope and camera examination of the primary carcinoma of nasopharynx. *Cancer* 40:2353–2364, 1977.

Clement PAR. Endoscopy in otorhinolaryngology. In: *Recent Advances in E.N.T.—Endoscopy.* Ceuterick, Belgium: Scientific Society for Medical Information, 1985, pp 11–24.

Dehaen F, Clement PAR. Endonasal surgical treatment of bilateral choanal atresia under optic control in the infant. *J Otolaryngol* 14:95–98, 1985.

Draf W. Therapeutic endoscopy of the paranasal sinuses. *Endoscopy* 10:247–254, 1978.

Draf W. The therapeutic value of paranasal sinus endoscopy. In: *Recent Advances in E.N.T.—Endoscopy.* Ceuterick, Belgium: Scientific Society for Medical Information, 1985, pp 207–216.

Friedrich JP. Sinus surgery under endoscopic guidance. In: *Recent Advances in E.N.T.—Endoscopy.* Ceuterick, Belgium: Scientific Society for Medical Information, 1985, pp 235–244.

Gilbert STJ, Pigott RW. The feasibility of nasal pharyngoscopy using the 70 degree Storz–Hopkins nasopharyngoscope. *Br J Plast Surg* 35:14–18, 1982.

Bibliography

Gordon N. Astrachan D, Yanagisawa E. Videoendoscopic diagnosis and correction of velopharyngeal stress incompetence in a bassoonist. *Ann Otol Rhinol Laryngol* 103:595–600, 1994.

Hirschmann A. Over Endoskopie der Nase und deren Nedenhohlen. Eine neue Utersuchungsmethode. *Arch Laryngol Rhinol* 14:195, 1903.

Ilum P. Endoscopic examination of the nasopharynx. *Acta Otolaryngol (Stockh)* 88:273–278, 1979.

Jaumann MP, Steiner W. Endoscopy of the nose and nasopharynx. *Endoscopy* 10:240–247, 1978.

Jaumann MP, Steiner W, Berg M. Endoscopy of the pharyngeal eustachian tube. *Ann Otol Rhinol Laryngol* 89 (Suppl 68):54–5, 1980.

Kennedy, DW. Functional endoscopic sinus surgery—technique. *Arch Otolaryngol* 111:643–649, 1985.

Kennedy DW, Zinreich SJ, Rosenbaum AE, et al. Functional endoscopic sinus surgery. *Arch Otolaryngol* 111:576–582, 1985.

Lavorato AS, Lindholm CE. Fiber-optic visualization of motion of the eustachian tube. *Trans Am Acad Ophthalmol Otolaryngol* 84:534–541, 1977.

Messerklinger W. *Endoscopy of the nose*. Baltimore: Urban & Schwartzenberg, 1978, pp. 1–178.

Messerklinger W. Endoscopic diagnosis and surgery of recurring sinusitis. In: *Recent Advances in E.N.T.—Endoscopy*. Ceuterick, Belgium: Scientific Society for Medical Information, 1985, pp. 189–196.

Ohnishi T, Yanagisawa E. Endoscopic anatomy of the anterior ethmoidal artery. *ENT J* 73:634–636, 1994.

Ohnishi T, Yanagisawa E. Lateral lamella of the cribriform plate—an important high-risk area in endoscopic sinus surgery. *ENT J* 74:688–690, 1995.

Selkin SG. Photodocumentation of laser microsurgery: preoperative, intraoperative, and postoperative techniques for still and video photographs. *Otolaryngol Head Neck Surg* 95:259–272, 1986.

Shanmugham MS. The role of fiberoptic nasopharyngoscopy carcinoma (NPC). *J Laryngol Otol* 99:779–782, 1985.

Sher AE, Shprintzen RJ, Thorpy MJ. Endoscopic observations of obstructive sleep apnea in children with anomalous upper airways: predictive and therapeutic value. *Int J Pediatr Otorhinolaryngol* 11:135–146, 1986.

Stammberger H. Endoscopical diagnosis and treatment of paranasal sinus mycosis. In: *Recent Advances in E.N.T.—Endoscopy*. Ceuterick, Belgium: Scientific Society for Medical Information, 1985, pp 245–252.

Stammberger H. An endoscopic study of tubal function and the diseased ethmoid sinus. *Arch Otorhinolaryngol* 243:254–259, 1986.

Straatman NJA, Buiter CT. Endoscopic surgery of the nasal fontanel—a new approach to recurrent sinusitis. *Arch Otolaryngol* 107:290–293, 1981.

Valentin A. Die cystoscopische Untersuchung des Nasenrachens oder Salpingoskopie. *Arch Laryngol Rhinol (Berlin)* 13:410–420, 1903.

Wigand ME, Steiner W, Jaumann MP. Endonasal sinus surgery with endoscopical control: from radical operation to rehabilitation of the mucosa. *Endoscopy* 10:255–260, 1978.

Yamashita K. Endonasal flexible fiberoptic endoscopy. *Rhinology* 21:233–237, 1983.

Yamashita K. Pneumatic endoscopy of the eustachian tube. *Endoscopy* 15:257–259, 1983.

Yamashita K. Endoscopy of eustachian tube. In: *Recent Advances in E.N.T.—Endoscopy*. Ceuterick, Belgium: Scientific Society for Medical Information, 1985, pp. 51–56.

Yanagisawa E. Endoscopic anatomy of the nasal cavity. *ENT J* 72:256, 1993.

Yanagisawa E. Endoscopic view of sphenoethmoidal recess and superior meatus. *ENT J* 72:331–332, 1993.

Yanagisawa E. Endoscopic view of sphenoid sinus cavity. *ENT J* 72:393–394, 1993.

Yanagisawa E. Endoscopic view of the inferior turbinate. *ENT J* 72:659–660, 1993.

Yanagisawa E. Endoscopic view of the middle turbinate. *ENT J* 72:725–727, 1993.

Yanagisawa E. Endoscopic view of the septal spur and ridge. *ENT J* 72:784, 1993.

Yanagisawa E. Endoscopic view of acute maxillary sinusitis. *ENT J* 73:146–147, 1994.

Yanagisawa E. The use of video in ENT endoscopy—its value in teaching. *ENT J* 73:754–763, 1994.

Yanagisawa E. The use of an adenoid punch in endoscopic intranasal surgery. *ENT J* 74:154–155, 1995.

Yanagisawa E. Endoscopic excision of an antral lesion via inferior meatal antrostomy. *ENT J* 74:321–322, 1995.

Yanagisawa E. Endoscopic excision of an antral lesion via middle meatal antrostomy. *ENT J* 74:520–522, 1995.

Yanagisawa E, Carlson RD. Videophotolaryngography using a new low cost video printer. *Ann Otol Rhinol Laryngol* 94:584–587, 1985.

Yanagisawa E, Citardi MJ. Clinical manifestation of unilateral choanal atresia. *ENT J* 73:360–362, 1994.

Yanagisawa E. Citardi MJ. Endoscopic view of malignant lymphoma of the nasopharynx. *ENT J* 73:514–416, 1994.

Yanagisawa E, Citardi MJ. Endoscopic view of a foreign body in the nose. *ENT J* 74:8–9, 1995.

Yanagisawa E, Citardi MJ. Endoscopic view of hidden superior meatal polyps contributing to anosmia. *ENT J* 74:74–75, 1995.

Yanagisawa E, Citardi MJ. Telescopic view of Woodruff's naso-nasopharyngeal plexus. *ENT J* 74:804–806, 1995.

Yanagisawa E, Citardi JC. Complications of canine fossa maxillary sinoscopy. *ENT J* 75:14–16, 1996.

Yanagisawa E, Hirokawa R, Yanagisawa K. Endoscopic view of nasopharyngeal carcinoma. *ENT J* 73:12–14, 1994.

Yanagisawa E, Latorre R. Choking spells following septorhinoplasty secondary to displaced nasal packing. *ENT J* 74:744–746, 1995.

Yanagisawa E, Salzer SJ, Hirokawa RH. Endoscopic view of antrochoanal polyp appearing as a large oropharyngeal mass. *ENT J* 73:714–715, 1994.

Yanagisawa E, Walker R. Instantaneous "video photography" with a low-cost black-and-white video printer: its value in otolaryngology and head and neck surgery. *Otolaryngol Head Neck Surg* 95:230–233, 1986.

Yanagisawa E, Walker R, Alberti P. Telescopic videorhinoscopy: a useful addition to the clinical practice of rhinology. *Laryngoscope* 96:1231–1235, 1986.

Yanagisawa E, Weaver EM. Anatomical variations of the middle turbinate. *ENT J* 75:194–197, 1996.

Yanagisawa E, Yamashita K. Fiberoptic nasopharyngolaryngoscopy. In: Lee KJ, Stewart CH, eds. *Ambulatory Surgery and Office Procedures in Head and Neck Surgery*. Orlando, FL: Grune & Stratton, 1986, pp 31–40.

Yanagisawa E, Yanagisawa K. Endoscopic view of ostium of nasolacrimal duct. *ENT J* 72:491–492, 1993.

Yanagisawa E, Yanagisawa K. Endoscopic view of maxillary sinus ostia. *ENT J* 72:518–519, 1993.

Yanagisawa E, Yanagisawa K. Endoscopic view of eustachian tube orifice. *ENT J* 72:598–599, 1993.

Yanagisawa E, Yanagisawa K. Endoscopic view of often unrecognized middle meatal polyps. *ENT J* 73:218–219, 1994.

Yanagisawa E, Yanagisawa K. Endoscopic view of antro-middle meatal polyp occluding the natural ostium of the maxillary sinus. *ENT J* 73:300–301, 1994.

Yanagisawa E, Yanagisawa K. Endoscopic view of exposed vital structures following sphenoethmoidectomy. *ENT J* 73:810–811, 1994.

Yanagisawa E, Yanagisawa K. Endoscopic view of Thornwaldt cyst of the nasopharynx. *ENT J* 73:884–885, 1994.

Yanagisawa E, Yanagisawa K. Endoscopic view of sphenoid sinus mucocele. *ENT J* 74:220–221, 1995.

Yanagisawa E, Yanagisawa K. Intranasal crusting following endoscopic surgery. *Ent J* 74:392–394, 1995.

Yanagisawa E, Yanagisawa K, Fortgang P. Endoscopic excision of a large benign antral lesion via a modified ("mini") Caldwell–Luc procedure. *ENT J* 74:620–621, 1995.

Yanagisawa E, Yanagisawa K, Yanagisawa R. Newer concepts in endoscopic imaging of the larynx. *Proceedings of the International Society for Optical Engineering* ("Lasers in Otolaryngology, Dermatology, and Tissue Welding") 1876:89–93, 1993.

Zaufal E. Zur endoskopischen Untersuchung der Rachenmundung der Tuba enface und des Tubenkands. *Arch Ohrenheilkd* 79:410–411, 1909.

LARYNX

Alberti PW. Still photography of the larynx—an overview. *Can J Otolaryngol* 4:759–765, 1975.

Albrecht R. Zur Photographie des Kehlkopfes. *HNO* 5:196–199, 1956.

Andrea M, Dias O. *Rigid and Contact Endoscopy in Microlaryngeal Surgery—Technique and Atlas of Clinical Cases*. New York: Lippincott-Raven, 1995.

Andrea M, Dias O, Santos A. Contact endoscopy during microlaryngeal surgery—a new technique for endoscopic examination of the larynx. *Ann Otol Rhinol Laryngol* 104:333–335, 1995.

Andrews AH. Laryngeal telescope. *Trans Am Acad Opthalmol Otolaryngol* 66:268, 1962.

Andrews AH Jr, Gould WJ. Laryngeal and nasopharyngeal indirect telescope. *Ann Otol Rhinol Laryngol* 86:627, 1977.

Benjamin B. Technique of laryngeal photography. *Ann Otol Rhinol Laryngol* 93 (Suppl 109):1984.

Benjamin B. *Diagnostic Laryngology—Adults and Children*. Philadelphia: Saunders, 1990.

Benjamin B. Art and science of laryngeal photography (Eighteenth Daniel C. Baker Jr Memorial Lecture). *Ann Otol Rhinol Laryngol* 102:271–282, 1993.

Berci G. *Endoscopy*. New York, Appleton-Century-Crofts, 1976.

Berci G. Analysis of new optical systems in bronchoesophagology. *Ann Otol Rhinol Laryngol* 87:451–60, 1978.

Berci G, Calcaterra T, Ward PH. Advances in endoscopic techniques for examination of the larynx and nasopharynx. *Can J Otolaryngol* 4:786–792, 1975.

Berci G, Caldwell FH. A device to facilitate photography during indirect laryngoscopy. *Med Biol Illus* 13:169–176, 1963.

Brewer DW, Gould LV, Casper J. Fiber-optic video study of the post-laryngectomized voice. *Laryngoscope* 85:666–670, 1975.

Brewer DW, McCall G. Visible laryngeal changes during voice therapy—fiber optic study. *Ann Otol Rhinol Laryngol* 83:423–427, 1974.

D'Agostino MA, Jiang JJ, Hanson D. Endoscopic photography: solving the difficulties of practical application. *Laryngoscope* 104:1045–1047, 1994.

Davidson TM, Bone RC, Nahum AM. Flexible fiberoptic laryngobronchoscopy. *Laryngoscope* 84:1876–1882, 1974.

Dellon AL, Hall CA, Chretien PB. Fiberoptic endoscopy in the head and neck region. *Plast Reconstr Surg* 55:466–471, 1975.

Ferguson GB, Crowder WJ. A simple method of laryngeal and other cavity photography. *Arch Otolaryngol* 92:201–203, 1970.

French TR. On photographing the larynx. *Trans Am Laryngol* 4:32–35, 1882.

French TR. On a perfected method of photographing the larynx. *NY Med J* 4:655–656, 1884.

Garcia M. Observations on the human voice. *Proc R Soc Lond* 7:399–420, 1855.

Gould WJ. The Gould laryngoscope. *Trans Am Acad Opthalmol Otolaryngol* 77:139–141, 1973.

Gould WJ, Kojima H, Lamblase A. A technique for stroboscopic examination of the vocal folds using fiberoptics. *Arch Otolaryngol* 105:285, 1979.

Hahn C, Kitzing P. Indirect endoscopic photography of the larynx—a comparison between two newly constructed laryngoscopes. *J Audiovisual Media Med* 1:121–130, 1978.

Hirano M. Phonosurgery, basic and clinical investigations. *Otologia (Fukuoka)* 21 (Suppl 1):239–440, 1975.

Hirano M. *Clinical Examination of Voice (Disorders of Human Communication, vol 5)*. New York: Springer-Verlag, 1981.

Holinger PH. Photography of the larynx, trachea, bronchi and esophagus. *Trans Am Acad Ophthalmol Otolaryngol* 46:153–156, 1942.

Holinger PH, Brubaker JD, Brubaker JE. Open tube, proximal illumination mirror and direct laryngeal photography. *Can J Otolaryngol* 4:781–785, 1975.

Holinger PH, Tardy ME. Photography in otorhinolaryngology and bronchoesophagology. In: English GM, ed. *Otolaryngology*, vol 5. Philadelphia: Lippincott, 1986, Chapter 22.

Inoue T. Examination of child larynx by flexible fiberoptic laryngoscope. *Int J Pediatr Otorhinolaryngol* 5:317–323, 1983.

Jako GJ. Laryngoscope for microscopic observations, surgery and photography. *Arch Otolaryngol* 91:196–199, 1970.

Jako GJ, Strong S. Laryngeal photography. *Arch Otolaryngol* 96:268–271, 1972.

Kantor E, Berci G, Partlow E, et al. A completely new approach to microlaryngeal surgery. *Laryngoscope* 101:678–679, 1991.

Kleinsasser O. Entwicklung und Methoden der Kehlkopffotografie (mit Beschreibung eines neuen einfachen Fotolaryngoskopes), *HNO* 11:171–176, 1963.

Kleinsasser O. *Microlaryngoscopy and Endolaryngeal Microsurgery*. Philadelphia: Saunders, 1968.

Kleinsasser O. *Tumors of the Larynx and Hypopharynx*. New York: Thieme, 1988, pp 124–130.

Konrad HR, Hopla DM, Bussen J, Griswold FC. Use of videotape in diagnosis and treatment of cancer of larynx. *Ann Otol Rhinol Otolaryngol* 90:398–400, 1981.

Mambrino L, Yanagisawa E, Yanagisawa K, et al. Endoscopic ENT photography—a comparison of pictures by standard color films and newer color video printers. *Laryngoscope* 101:1229–1232, 1991.

Muller-Hermann F, Pedersen P. Modern endoscopic and microscopic photography in otolaryngology. *Ann Otol Rhinol Laryngol* 93:399, 1984.

Olofsson J, Ohlsson T. Techniques in microlaryngoscopic photography. *Can J Otolaryngol* 4:770–780, 1975.

Parnes SM, Lavorato AS, Myers EN. Study of spastic dysphonia using videofiberoptic laryngoscopy. *Ann Otol Rhinol Laryngol* 1978, 87:322–326.

Rosnagle R, Smith HW. Hand-held fundus camera for endoscopic photography. *Trans Am Acad Ophthalmol Otolaryngol* 76:1024–1025, 1972.

Saito S, Isogai Y, Fukuda H, et al. A newly developed curved laryngotelescope. *J Jpn Bronchoesphagol Soc* 32:328–331, 1981.

Sawashima M, Hirose H. New laryngoscopic technique by use of fiber optics. *J Acoust Soc Am* 43:168–169, 1968.

Selkin SG. Flexible fiberoptics for laryngeal photography. *Laryngoscope* 93:657–658, 1983.

Selkin SG. The otolaryngologist and flexible fiberoptics—photographic considerations. *J Otolaryngol* 12:223–227, 1983.

Silberman HD, Wilf H, Tucker JA. Flexible fiberoptic nasopharyngolaryngoscope. *Ann Otol Rhinol laryngol* 85:640–645, 1976.

Steiner W, Jaumann MP. Moderne Otorhinolaryngologische Endoskopie beim Kind. *Padiatr Prax* 20:429–435, 1978.

Stone JL, Peterson RL, Wolf JE. Digital imaging techniques in dermatology. *J Am Acad Dermatol* 23:913–917, 1990.

Strong MS. Laryngeal photography. *Can J Otolaryngol* 4:766–769, 1975.

Stuckrad H, Lakatos I. "Uber ein neues Lupeniaryngoskop (Epipharyngoskop). *Laryngol Rhinol Otol* 54:336–340, 1975.

Tsuiki Y. *Laryngeal Examination*. Tokyo, Kanehara Shuppan, 1956.

Tardy ME, Tenta LT. Laryngeal photography and television. *Otolaryngol Clin North Am* 3:483–492, 1970.

Tobin HA. Office fiberoptic laryngeal photography. *Otolaryngol Head Neck Surg* 88:172–173, 1980.

Ward PH, Berci G, Calcaterra TC. Advances in endoscopic examination of the respiratory system. *Ann Otol Rhinol Laryngol* 83:754–760, 1974.

Williams GT, Farquharson IM, Anthony J. Fiberoptic laryngoscopy in the assessment of laryngeal disorders. *J Laryngol Otol* 1975; 89:299–316.

Yamashita K. Endonasal flexible fiberoptic endoscopy. *Rhinology* 21:233–237, 1983.

Yamashita K. *Diagnostic and Therapeutic ENT Endoscopy*. Tokyo, Medical View, 1988.

Yamashita K, Mertens J, Rudert H. Die flexible Fiberendoskopie in der HNO-Heildunde. *HNO* 32:378–384, 1984.

Yamashita K, Oku T, Tanaka H, et al. VTR endoscopy. *J Otolaryngol Jpn* 80:1208–1209, 1977.

Yanagisawa E. Office telescopic photography of the larynx. *Ann Otol Rhinol laryngol* 91:354–358, 1982.

Yanagisawa E. Videolaryngoscopy using a low cost home video system color camera. *J Biol Photogr* 52:9–14, 1984.

Yanagisawa E. Videolaryngoscopy. In: Lee KJ, Stewart CH, eds. *Ambulatory Surgery and Office Procedures in Head and Neck Surgery*. Orlando, FL: Grune & Stratton, 1986, Chapter 6.

Yanagisawa E. Documentation. In: Ferlito A, ed. *Neoplasms of the Larynx*. Edinburgh, Churchill Livingston, 1993. Chapter 21.

Yanagisawa E. The use of video in ENT endoscopy—its value in teaching. *ENT J* 73:754–763, 1994.

Yanagisawa E, Carlson RD. Videophotolaryngography using a new low cost video printer. *Ann Otol Rhinol Laryngol* 94:584–587, 1985.

Yanagisawa E, Carlson RD. Physical diagnosis of the hypopharynx and the larynx with and without imaging. In: Lee KJ, ed. *Textbook of Otolaryngology and Head and Neck*. New York: Elsevier, 1989, Chapter 37.

Yanagisawa E, Carlson RD, Strothers G. Videography of the larynx—fiberscope or telescope? In: Clement Par, ed. *Recent Advances in ENT—Endoscopy*. Brussels, Scientific Society for Medical Information, 1985, pp 175–183.

Yanagisawa E, Casuccio JR, Suzuki M. Video laryngoscopy using a rigid telescope and a video home system color camera—a useful office procedure. *Ann Otol Laryngol* 90:346–350, 1981.

Yanagisawa E, Driscoll B. Laryngeal photography and videography. In: Rubin JS, et al, eds. *Diagnosis and Treatment of Voice Disorders*. New York: Igaku-Shoin, 1995.

Yanagisawa E, Eibling DE, Suzuki M. A simple method of laryngeal photography through the operating microscope—"macrolens technique." *Ann Otol Rhinol Laryngol* 89:547–550, 1980.

Yanagisawa E, Estill J, Mambrino L, et al. Supraglottic contributions to pitch raising. *Ann Otol Rhinol Laryngol* 100:19–30, 1991.

Yanagisawa E, Horowitz JB, Yanagisawa K, et al. Comparison of new telescopic video microlaryngoscopic and standard microlaryngoscopic techniques. *Ann Otol Rhinol Laryngol* 101:51–60, 1992.

Yanagisawa E, Kmucha ST, Estill J. Role of the soft palate in laryngeal functions and selected voice qualities: Simultaneous velolaryngeal videoendoscopy. *Ann Otol Rhinol Laryngol* 99:18–28, 1990.

Yanagisawa E, Owens TW, Strothers G, et al. Videolaryngoscopy—a comparison of fiberscopic and telescopic documentation. *Ann Otol Rhinol Laryngol* 92:430–436, 1983.

Yanagisawa K, Shi J, Yanagisawa E. Color photography of video images of otolaryngological structures using a 35 mm SLR camera. *Laryngoscope* 97:992–993, 1987.

Yanagisawa E, Yamashita K. Fiberoptic nasopharyngolaryngoscopy. In: Lee KJ, Stewart CH, eds. *Ambulatory Surgery and Office Procedures in Head and Neck Surgery*. Orlando, FL: Grune & Stratton 1986, pp 31–40.

Yanagisawa E, Yanagisawa R. Laryngeal photography. *Otolaryngol Clin North Am* 24:999–1022, 1991.

Yoshida Y, Hirano M, Nakajima T. A video-tape recording system for laryngo-stroboscopy. *J Jpn Bronchoespophagol Soc* 30:1–5, 1979.

STROBOSCOPIC VIDEOLARYNGOSCOPY

Bell Telephone Laboratories. *High Speed Motion Pictures of the Vocal Cords.* New York Bureau of Publication, 1937.

Bless DM. Assessment of laryngeal function. In: Ford CN, Bless DM, eds. *Phonosurgery: assessment and surgical management of voice disorders.* New York: Raven Press, 1991, pp 95–122.

Bless DM, Hirano M, Feder RJ. Videostroboscopic evaluation of the larynx. *Ear Nose Throat J* 66:289–296, 1987.

Hirano M. *Clinical Examination of Voice.* New York; Springer-Verlag, 1981.

Hirano M. Yoshida Y, Yoshida T, Tateishi O. Strobofiberscopic video recording of vocal fold vibration. *Ann Otol Rhinol Laryngol* 94:588–590, 1985.

Kallen LA. Laryngostroboscopy in the practice of otolaryngology. *Arch Otolaryngol* 16:791–807, 1932.

Kanell MP. Synchronized videostroboscopy and electroglottography. *J Voice* 1:68–75, 1987.

Kitzing P. Stroboscopy—a pertinent laryngological examination. *J Otolaryngol* 14:151–7, 1985.

Mahieu HF, Dikkers FG. Indirect microlaryngostroboscopic surgery. *Arch Otolaryngol Head Neck Surg* 118:21–24, 1992.

Moore DM, Berke GS, Hanson DG, Ward PH. Videostroboscopy of the canine larynx: the effects of asymmetric laryngeal tension. *Laryngoscope* 97:543–53, 1987.

Morrison MD. A clinical voice laboratory: videotape and stroboscopic instrumentation. *Otolaryngol Head Neck Surg* 92:487–488, 1984.

Oertel MJ. Das Laryngo-strobskop und die laryngostroboskopische Untersuchung. *Arch Laryngol Rhinol (Berlin)* 3:1–16, 1985.

Perlman HB. Laryngeal stroboscopy. *Ann Otol Rhinol Laryngol* 54:159–165, 1945.

Powell LS. The laryngostroboscope. *Arch Otolaryngol* 19:708–710, 1934.

Saito S, Fukuda H, Kitahara S, Kokawa N. Stroboscopic observation of vocal fold vibration with fiberoptics. *Folia Phoniatr (Basel)* 30:241–244, 1978.

Sataloff RT, Spiegel JR, Carroll LM, Schiebel BR, Darby KS, Rulnick R. Strobovideolaryngoscopy in professional voice users: results and clinical value. *J Voice* 1:359–364, 1988.

Sawashima M, Hirose H. New laryngoscopic technique by use of fiberoptics. *J Acoust Soc Am* 43:168–169, 1968.

Selkin SG. Flexible fiberscopics for laryngeal photography. *Laryngoscope* 93:657, 1983.

Sercarz JA, Berke GS, Ming Y, Gerratt BR, Natividad M. Videostroboscopy of human vocal fold paralysis. *Ann Otol Rhinol Laryngol* 101:567–577, 1992.

Steiner W, Jaumann MP. Moderne otorhinolaryngologische Endoskopie beimn Kind. *Padiatr Prax* 20;429–435, 1978.

Timcke R, von Leden H, Moore P. Laryngeal vibrations: measurements of the glottic wave. Part I. The normal vibratory cycle. *Arch Otolaryngol* 68:1–19, 1958.

Timcke R, von Leden H, Moore P. Laryngeal vibrations: measurements of the glottic wave. Part II. Physiologic vibrations. *Arch Otolaryngol* 69:438–444, 1959.

Von Leden H. The electronic synchron-stroboscope. Its value for the practicing laryngologist. *Ann Otol Rhinol Laryngol* 70:881–893, 1961.

Von Leden H, Moore P, Timcke R. Laryngeal vibrations: measurements of the glottic wave. part III. The pathologic larynx. *Arch Otolaryngol* 71:16–35, 1960.

Wendler J. Stroboscopy. *J Voice* 6:149–154, 1992.

Yamashita K. *Diagnostic and Therapeutic ENT Endoscopy.* Tokyo, Japan, Medical View Co., 1988.

Yanagisawa E, Godley F, Muta H. Selection of video cameras for stroboscopic videolaryngoscopy. *Ann Otol Rhinol Laryngol* 96:578–585, 1987.

Yanagisawa E, Owens TW, Strothers G, Honda K. Videolaryngoscopy—a comparison of fiberscopic and telescopic documentation. *Ann Otol Rhinol Laryngol* 92:430–436, 1983.

Yanagisawa E, Yanagisawa R. Laryngeal photography. *Otolaryngol Clin North Am* 24:999–1022, 1991.

Yanagisawa E, Yanagisawa K. Stroboscopic videolaryngoscopy—a comparison of fiberscopic and telescopic documentation. *Ann Otol Rhinol Laryngol* 102:255–265, 1993.

Yoshida Y, Hirano M. Yoshida T, Tateishi O. Strobofiberscopic colour video recording of vocal fold vibration. *J Laryngol Otol* 99:795–800, 1985.

INDEX

Italic numbers refer to figures.

A

Abducens palsy, caused by nasopharyngeal carcinoma, *100*
Adenoid
  examination of, 93
  hypertrophied, 94
    before swallowing, *94*
    on swallowing, *94*
  transnasal microscopic mirror examination of, *93*
  transnasal telescopic examination of, *93*
  transoral telescopic examination of, *93*
Adenoiditis, torus tubarius in, *94*
Adhesive otitis media, adhesive, 35
Allergic rhinitis, 58
Alphabet, saying, with exam, simultaneous velolaryngeal videoendoscopy, *162*
Angiofibroma, nasopharyngeal, 99, *99*
Antrochoanal polyp, 96, *96*
Antrostomy
  meatal
    inferior, *84*
    middle, 72, *84*
      transnasal telescopic view, *72*
Aryepiglottic fold cyst, *135*
Arytenoid contact ulcers, larynx, 138
Arytenoid granuloma, *138*
Aspergillosis, maxillary sinus, 80

B

Bilobed tonsil, *109*
Breathing examination, simultaneous velolaryngeal videoendoscopy, 162
  nasal, *162*
  oral, *162*
Bullous myringitis, 30

C

Camera
  for simultaneous velolaryngeal videoendoscopy, *161*
  video, for examination, 9–12, *11*
Carcinoma
  epiglottic squamous cell, *143*
  larynx, 142
    verrucous, *142*
  nasopharyngeal, 100, *100*
    abducens palsy, caused by, *100*
    serous otitis media caused by, *100*
  supraglottic squamous cell, 143, *143*
  tonsil, squamous cell, 110, *110*
  transglottic squamous cell, *142*, *143*
  vallecular squamous cell, *143*
Carotid artery
  internal, *75*, *85*
    pterygoid recess and, *75*
  pharyngeal, anomalous, *111*
CEMS, see Microlaryngeal surgery, contact endoscopy
Cerumen, 24, *24*
  impacted, *24*
  large, *24*
Choanal atresia, 65, *66*
  postoperative, *66*
  unilateral, 66, *66*
  with sinusitis, *66*
Choanal polyp, 97, *97*
Cholesteatoma, 33
  keratosis obturans, *29*
  middle ear, *33*
    videoendoscopy, *178*
  multiple, *32*
  posterior superior canal wall, *29*
  postoperative, *29*
    posterior canal wall, *29*
Cocaine rhinitis, 62
Computer, 14–15, 148
Concha bullosa, right, medially bent, *47*
Contact endoscopy in microlaryngeal surgery, 168–173
Coughing, examination, simultaneous velolaryngeal videoendoscopy, *163*
Cryptic chronic tonsillitis, *109*
Cyst
  aryepiglottic fold, *135*
  epidermoid, 134
  epiglottic, 135, *135*, *136*
  maxillary sinus, 81
  mucous retention, 134
  saccular, 134
  Thornwaldt, nasopharynx, 98, *98*
  vallecular, 136, *136*
  vocal fold, 134, 155
    on abduction, *155*
    composite of glottic cycles, *155*
    microphotographic representation of, *155*

D

Deformity of middle ear, congenital, 40
  anomalies of middle ear, *40*
  aural atresia, *40*
  cholesteatoma of middle ear, *40*
Deviated nasal septum, *59*
Documentation, 13–15
  endoscopic, in otorhinolaryngology, historical background, 3–6
  transfer of video images, to print, slides, 13–15, *14*

185

E

Ear
  external, *see* External ear
  middle, *see* Middle ear
Ear canal, infections of, 26
  furuncle, *26*
  otitis externa
    acute circumscribed, *26*
    acute diffuse, *26*
    necrotizing, *26*
Endoscopes, 7–9, *8*
  contact, 168, 172
  in CEMS, 168, 172
  in simultaneous velolaryngeal video endoscopy, 161
Endoscopy, in otorhinolaryngology
  history of, 3–6, *5*
  laryngology, 6
  otology, 3–5
  overview, 3–6
  rhinology, 6
Enhancer, video, 12
Epidermoid cyst, true vocal fold, 134
Epiglottic cyst, 135, *135, 136*
Epiglottic squamous cell carcinoma, *143*
Epiglottis, unfolding, simultaneous velolaryngeal videoendoscopy, *166–167*
Epiglottitis, acute, *125*
Epistaxis, 61
  anterior, *61*
  ethmoidal, anterior, *61*
Equipment, 7–12, *11*
  endoscopes, 7–9, *8*
  light sources, 12
  video cameras, 9–12, *11*
  video enhancer, 12
  video monitors, 12
  video recorders, 12
Ethmoidectomy cavity, postoperative, *64*, 85
Ethmoid sinus, ostium, 69, *74*
  posterior, *52*
Ethmoidal artery, posterior, 85
Eustachian tube, 90, 91
  orifice
    left, *91*
    right, *91*
    transnasal view, *90*
  Rosenmüller's fossa, *92*
  torus tubarius, *92*
Exostoses, 23
  advanced obstructive, *23*
  asymptomatic, *23*
  multiple, *23*
External ear
  disorders of, 23–30
  cerumen, 24, *24*
    impacted, *24*
    large, *24*
  cholesteatoma of ear canal, 29
    canal wall, posterior, *29*
    keratosis obturans, *29*
    postoperative, *29*
      canal wall, posterior, *29*
  ear canal, infections of, 26
    furuncle, *26*
    otitis externa
      acute
        circumscribed, *26*
        diffuse, *26*
      necrotizing, *26*
  otomycosis, *27*
  exostoses, 23
    advanced obstructive, *23*
    asymptomatic, *23*
    multiple, *23*
  foreign bodies, 25
    construction debris, *25*
    insect, live, *25*
    pebbles, multiple, *25*
  hairs, 27
    contacting tympanic membrane, *27*
  trauma of ear canal, 28
    bleeding from floor of ear canal, *28*
    fracture of anterior canal wall, *28*
    hematoma, *28*
  endoscopy, 19–40
    techniques, 22
      pneumatic video-otoscopy, *22*
      video-otoscopy, *22*

F

Facial nerve, dehiscent, middle ear, videoendoscopy, *178*
Fiberscopic
  vs. telescopic optical distortion, comparison, 151
  vs. telescopic strobovideolaryngoscopy, 149
Fiberscopic laryngoscopy, simultaneous velolaryngeal videoendoscopy, *161*
Fiberscopic strobovideolaryngoscopy, *149*
Fontanelle
  anterior, 48, 78
  posterior, 48
Foreign body
  in ear, 25
  in nose, *60*
Frontal recess, *50*, 73
Frontal sinus
  recess, *50*, 73, *73*
  sinusitis, 79, *79*
Fungus ball, sinus, *80*

G

Glomus tumor, middle ear, *178*
Glossoepiglottic fold, stroboscopy of larynx, *151*
Glottis
 arytenoid, 138
 anterior views of, 122
 intraoperative diagnostic telescopic view, 122, 123
 lateral view, 123
 squamous cell carcinoma, *142*
 telescopic view, *122, 123*
 transoral telescopic view, *121*
Granuloma
 larynx, 133, *133*
  bilateral, *133*
 middle ear, 33
 nasal septal, 62
 vocal fold, Teflon, *133*

H

Hairs in ear, 27
Hemorrhage
 laryngeal, *128*
 submucosal, larynx, 128
 vocal fold, *128*
Hiatus semilunaris
 inferior, 49, *50*, 69
 superior, *50*, 73
Historical background, endoscopy in otorhinolaryngology, 3–6

I

Incus, traumatic dislocation of, *28*
Infraorbital nerve, middle meatal sinoscopy, *72*
Inverting papilloma, 63

K

Kirchner's ridge, *144*
Kissing tonsils, *106*

L

Laryngeal nerve paralysis, *140*
Laryngectomy
 partial, postoperative findings, *144*
 postoperative findings, 144, *144*
Laryngitis
 acute, 125, *125*
 chronic, 126, *126*
  radiation-induced, *126*
 reflux, chronic, *126*
 sicca, *126*
Laryngocele, internal, *134*
Laryngology, 6
Larynx
 carcinoma, 142

cyst, 134–136, 155
disorders of, 125–144
effort closure of, simultaneous velolaryngeal videoendoscopy, 163
endoscopy, 114–145
 anatomy, 115–116, 121–124
 arytenoid contact ulcers, 138
 axial section, through glottis, *121*
 carcinoma of larynx, 142
 coronal section, *121*
 cyst, 134–136, 155
 disorders of larynx, 125–144
 epiglottic cyst, 135
 glottis, 121
  anterior views of, 122
  lateral view of, 123
 granulomas, 133, 138
 laryngectomy, total, postoperative findings, 144
 laryngitis
  acute, 125
  chronic, 126
 lingual tonsil hypertrophy, 137
 office techniques, *117*
 operating room diagnostic techniques, *119*
 papillomatosis, 141
 Reinke's edema, 127
 strictures, 139
 subglottis, 124
 submucosal hemorrhage, 128
 sulcus vocalis, laryngeal strictures and, 139
 supraglottic squamous cell carcinoma, 143
 techniques, 117–120
 vallecular cyst, 136
 vocal fold
  nodules, 129
  polyp, 130
   extra large, 132
   large, 131
  true, paralysis, 140
microlaryngeal surgery, 168–173; see also Microlaryngeal surgery
papillomatosis, *141*
simultaneous velolaryngeal videoendoscopy, *158–167*
stroboscopy, 145–157
 cyst, vocal fold, 155
 fiberscopic
  vs. telescopic optical distortion, comparison of, 151
  vs. telescopic strobovideolaryngoscopy, comparison of, 149
 glottic closure patterns, strobovideolaryngoscopy, 152
 leukoplakia, vocal fold, 156
 nodules, vocal fold, 153

Larynx (*contd.*)
    papilloma, vocal fold, 157
    polyp, vocal fold, 154
    techniques, 148–151
    vocal fold
        anatomy, 146–147
        true, disorders of, 152–157
    transoral telescopic view, *121*
    verrucous carcinoma, *142*
Laughing, examination, simultaneous velolaryngeal videoendoscopy, *163*
Light sources, 12
Lingual tonsil, hypertrophy, 137, *137*
Lingual tonsillitis, acute, *137*
Lymphoma, nasopharyngeal, 101, *101*
    MRI, *101*

M

Maxillary sinoscopy, 68
    middle meatal antrostomy, *72*, 84
    natural ostium, *68*, 70–71, 76–78
Maxillary sinus
    aspergillosis, *80*
    cyst, 81, *81*
    drainage, recirculation of, *77*
    ostium, *71*
        accessory, 49, 51, *51*, 68, *68*, 71, 76, 78
            nasal telescopic view, *68*
        natural, 68, 70,71, 76–78
    polyp, 82, *82*, 96
Maxillary sinusitis
    acute, *76*
        treated, *76*
    chronic, 77, *77, 78*
        ostium disease and, 78
Meatus, nasal
    middle, 49, 50, 69
        antrostomy, *64*
        polyp
            antro-middle, *56*
            inferior, 57, *57*
            middle, 55, *55*, 56, *56*
            superior, 57, *57*
    superior, *52*, 69
Microlaryngeal surgery
    contact endoscopy, 168–173, *170, 172*
    laryngeal papilloma, contact endoscopy, *173*
    overview, 169–170
    rigid endoscopy, 168–173, *169, 171*
    true vocal fold histology, normal, *173*
Middle ear
    atelectasis, 35
    cholesteatoma, *33*
        multiple, *32*
    deformity of middle ear, congenital, 40
        anomalies of middle ear, *40*
        aural atresia, *40*
        cholesteatoma of middle ear, *40*
    disorders of, 30–40
    otitis media
        acute, 30
            bullous myringitis, *30*
            with pressure equalizing tube, *32*
            suppurative stage, *30*
        adhesive, *35*
            advanced, *35*
        chronic, 33
            with cholesteatoma, *33*
            with granuloma, *33*
        mucoid, *31*
        serous, 31
            with air-fluid level, *31*
    postoperative changes, 37
        fenestration cavity, *37*
        malleus head ossiculoplasty, tympanoplasty with, *37*
        myringostapediopexy, *37*
        stapedectomy, *37*
        tympanoplasty
            with malleus head ossiculoplasty, *37*
            type III, *37*
    pressure equalizing tube, 32, *32*
    scarred tympanic membrane, 35, *35*
    trauma, 38
        fracture dislocation of incus, *38*
        hemotympanum, *38*
        incudomallear joint, traumatic dislocation of, *38*
        incudostapedial joint separation, *38*
        incus, fracture dislocation of, *38*
        traumatic dislocation of incudomallear joint, *38*
    tumor of, primary, 39
        glomus jugulare tumor, *39*
        glomus tympanicum tumor, *39*
    tympanic membrane
        attenuated segment, *35*
        perforation, 34
            anterior middle, *34*
            near-total, *34*
            posterior, *34*
    tympanosclerosis, 36, *36*
        with large tympanic membrane perforation, *36*
    videoendoscopy, 174–178
        cholesteatoma, *178*
        facial nerve, dehiscent, *178*
        glomus tumor, transmastoid telescopic view, *176*
        stapedial prosthesis, *178*
        techniques, 177
        transtympanic endoscopy, *177*
        transtympanic telescopic view, *175*

Monitor, video, 12
Mononucleosis, tonsillitis, infectious, *109*
Mucormycosis, sinus, *80*

N

Nasal anatomy, overview of, 42–43
Nasal cavity
   anatomical structures of, *42*
   congenital anomalies of, 65
   disorders of, 53–66
   endoscopic anatomy of, *43*
   inverting papilloma of, *63*
   postoperative findings, 64, 84
Nasal endoscopy, 41–66
   anatomy, 45–52
     overview of, 42–43
   cavity
     congenital anomalies, 65
     disorders of, 53–66
     postoperative findings, 64
     tumor of, 63
   choanal atresia, unilateral, 66
   epistaxis, 61
   foreign bodies, 60
   granulomatous disease, 62
   maxillary sinus ostium, accessory, 49, 51, 68, 71, 76, 78
   meatus
     middle, 49, 50
     polyp, 55, 56
       inferior, 57
       superior, 57
   nasolacrimal duct ostium, 46
   nasopharyngeal plexus, 46
   polyp, 54–57, 96, 97
   rhinitis, 58
   septum
     deviation, 59
     perforation, 60
   sinusitis, 53
   techniques, 44
   turbinate
     middle, variations of, 47
     superior, and meatus, 52
   uncinate process, variations of, 48
Nasal polyposis, diffuse, *54*
Nasal septum
   deviated, *59*
   granuloma of, *62*
   hemangioma of, *63*
   hypertrophy, posterior, 97, *97*
   spur, 59
Nasolacrimal duct ostium, 46, *46*
Nasopharyngeal plexus (Woodruff's plexus), 46, *46*

Nasopharyngitis, 95
   acute, *95*
   chronic, *95*
Nasopharyngoscopy
   techniques of, 89
   transnasal rigid, simultaneous velolaryngeal videoendoscopy, *161*
   transnasal telescopic, *89*
Nasopharynx, 86–101
   adenoids
     examination of, 93
     hypertrophied, 94
   anatomy
     endoscopic, 90–93
     overview of, 87–88
   angiofibroma, 99
   antrochoanal polyp, 96
   carcinoma, 100
   choanal polyp, 97
   disorders of, 94–101
   eustachian tube, 90
     pharyngeal ostium, transnasal telescopic views, 91
   lymphoma, 101
   nasal septal hypertrophy, posterior, 97
   nasopharyngitis, 95
   Thornwaldt cyst, 98
   transoral telescopic view, *88*, 92
   velopharyngeal port, 90

O

Optical factor, stroboscopy of larynx, *151*
Optic nerve, *75, 85*
Oropharynx, 102–113
   anatomy, 103–104
     endoscopic, 106–108
   carotid artery, pharyngeal, anomalous, *111*
   disorders of, 109–113
   foreign body, pharyngeal, *111*
   pharyngeal flap, *113*
     postoperative findings, 113
   pharyngoscopy, 105
   postoperative findings, 112
   soft palate defect, *111*
   tonsil
     bilobed, *109*
     hypertrophy, *106*
     kissing, *106*
     palatine, 106
       enlarged, *106*
       normal, *106*
     plug, *107*
     squamous cell carcinoma, 110
       left, *110*
       right, *110*

Oropharynx (*contd.*)
   tonsillar fossa, superior, 107, *107*
   tonsillectomy, postoperative findings, *112*
   tonsillitis, 109
     acute, *109*
     cryptotic chronic, *109*
     infectious mononucleosis, *109*
   transoral pharyngoscopic view, *105*
   transoral telescopic view, *103*, *104*
   uvula
     bifid, *108*
     long, *108*
     papilloma, *108*
     variations of, 108
     wide, *108*
   uvulopalatal web, *111*
   uvulopalatopharyngoplasty, postoperative findings, *112*
Osler-Weber-Rendu disease, *61*
Otitis externa, 26
   fungal, 27
Otitis media
   acute, 30
     bullous myringitis, *30*
     with pressure equalizing tube, *32*
     suppurative stage, *30*
   adhesive, *35*
     advanced, *35*
   chronic, 33
     with cholesteatoma, *33*
     with granuloma, *33*
   mucoid, *31*
   serous, 31
     with air-fluid level, *31*
     from nasopharyngeal carcinoma, *100*
Otology, 3–5
Otomycosis, 27
Otorhinolaryngology, endoscopy in, *see also* Larynx
   contact endoscopy, microlaryngeal surgery, 168–173
   documentation, 13–15
     historical background, 3–6
   equipment, 7–12
   external ear, 19–40; *see also* External ear
   historical background, 3–6
   laryngology, 6
   larynx, 114–144; *see also* Larynx
   middle ear, 174–180; *see also* Middle ear
   nasopharynx, 86–101; *see also* Nasopharynx
   nose, 41–66; *see also* Nasal endoscopy
   oropharynx, 102–113; *see also* Oropharynx
   otology, 3–5
   paranasal sinuses, 67–85; *see also* Paranasal sinuses
   rhinology, 6
   rigid endoscopy, microlaryngeal surgery, 168–173

   simultaneous velolaryngeal videoendoscopy, 158–167; *see also* Velolaryngeal videoendoscopy, simultaneous
   stroboscopic videolaryngoscopy, 145–157
   tympanic membrane, 19–40
   videoendoscopy, middle ear, 174–178
   videolaryngoscopy, 114–144
   videonasal endoscopy, 41–66
   videonasopharyngoscopy, 86–101
   videopharyngoscopy, 102–113
   videorhinoscopy, 41–66
   videosinoscopy, 67–85

P

Palate, soft, defect, *111*
Palatine tonsils, 106
   enlarged, with visible epiglottis, *106*
   normal, *106*
Papilloma, of nasal septum, *63*
Papillomatosis, laryngeal, 141, *141*, 174
Paranasal sinuses, 67–85
   anatomy, 68–69
     endoscopic, 71–75
     overview of, 68–69
   antrostomy window, meatus, middle, 72
   disorders of, 76–85
   endoscopic anatomy, 71–75
   ethmoid sinus ostium, 69, *74*
   frontal sinus
     recess, 50, 73
     sinusitis, 79
   maxillary sinus
     accessory ostium, 49, 51, 68, 71, 76, 78
     cyst, 81
     natural ostium, 68, 70, 71, 76–78
     ostium, 49, 51, 68,70, 71, 76–78
     polyp, 82, 96
     sinusitis, chronic, 77, 78
   acute, 76
   meatus, nasal
     middle, 49, 50, 69, *69*
     superior, 52, *69*
   mycotic infections, 80
   postoperative findings
     ethmoidectomy, 64, 85
     nasal cavity, 84
     sphenoethmoidectomy, 85
   retrobullar recess, *73*
   sinoscopy, 70
   sphenoethmoidal recess, 74
   sphenoid sinus
     cavity, endoscopic view, 75
     ostium, *74*
     pyocele, 83

Pharyngeal carotid artery, anomalous, *111*
Pharyngeal flap, *113*
  postoperative findings, 113
Pharyngeal foreign body, *111*
Pharyngeal ostium, transnasal telescopic view, 91
Pharyngoscopy
  techniques of, 105
  transoral, *105*
Phonation
  in examination, simultaneous velolaryngeal videoendoscopy, 162
  larynx, ninety-degree view, *115*
Polyp
  antrochoanal, 96, *96*
  choanal, 97, *97*
  meatal, nasal
    antro-middle, *56*
    inferior, 57, *57*
    middle, 55, 56, *56*
    superior, 57, *57*
  nasal, 54, *54*, *55*
  vocal fold, *128*, 154
    on adduction, *154*
    glottic cycles, *154*
    microphotographic representation of, *154*
Postadenoidectomy, scarring of nasopharynx, patulous eustachian tube, 95
Postcricoid edema, transoral telescopic exam, 125
Posterior ethmoidal artery, 85
Postlaryngectomy swallow, *144*
Pressure equalizing tube, middle ear, 32, *32*
Printer, 14–15
Pseudodiverticulum, *144*
Pterygoid recess, internal carotid artery and, *75*
Pus
  in middle nasal meatus, *53*
  from superior nasal meatus, *53*

R
Recorder, video, 12
Reinke's edema, 127, *127*
  bilateral, *127*
    advanced, *127*
    unilateral, *127*
REMS, *see* Microlaryngeal surgery, rigid endoscopy
Rhinitis, 58
  cocaine, *62*
Rhinitis sicca, *58*
Rosenmüller's fossa, *92*

S
Sarcoidosis, nasal, *62*
Scarring, tympanic membrane, 35, *35*

Septum
  deviation, 59
  perforation, *60*
    nasal, *60*
      foreign bodies, 60
  spur
    nasal, *59*
    posterior, *59*
Simultaneous velolaryngeal videoendoscopy, *see* Velolaryngeal videoendoscopy, simultaneous
Sinoscopy
  maxillary, via canine fossa, *70*
  techniques, 70
Sinus
  ethmoid, ostium, 69, *74*
    posterior, *52*
  frontal
    recess, 73, *73*
      suprabullar recess, *73*
    sinusitis, 79, *79*
  fungus ball, *80*
  maxillary
    accessory ostium, nasal telescopic view, *68*
    aspergillosis, *80*
    chronic, sinusitis, 77
      natural, accessory ostium disease, 78
    cyst, 81, *81*
    drainage, recirculation of, *77*
    ostium, *71*
      accessory, 49, 51, *51*, 68, *68*, 71, 76, 78
      natural, 68, 70, 71, 76, 77, 78
        accessory, 68
    polyp, 82, *82*, 92
  meatus, nasal
    middle, *69*
    and ostium ethmoid and sphenoid sinuses, 69
    superior, *69*
  mycotic infections, 80
  paranasal, 67–85
    anatomy, 68–69
      endoscopic, 71–75
      overview, 68–69
    antrostomy window, middle meatus, 72
    disorders of, 76–85
    endoscopic anatomy, 71–75
  postoperative findings
    nasal cavity, 84
    sphenoethmoidectomy, 85
  retrobullar recess, *73*
  sinoscopy techniques, 70
  sphenoethmoidal recess, 74
  sphenoid sinus
    cavity
      endoscopic view, 75

Sinus (contd.)
    postoperative
        internal carotid artery, 75, *85*
        optic nerve, 75, *85*
    ostium, *52*, 69, *69*, *74*
    postoperative, internal carotid artery, *85*
    pyocele, 83, *83*
Sinusitis, 53
  frontal sinus, 79, *79*
  maxillary sinus
    acute, *76*
      treated, *76*
    chronic, 77, *77*, *78*
      with natural, accessory ostium disease, *78*
Siren
  high-frequency range, simultaneous velolaryngeal videoendoscopy, *164–165*
  lowest-frequency range, simultaneous velolaryngeal videoendoscopy, *164–165*
  low-frequency range, simultaneous velolaryngeal videoendoscopy, *164–165*
  middle-frequency range, simultaneous velolaryngeal videoendoscopy, *164–165*
  simultaneous velolaryngeal videoendoscopy, 164–165
Soft palate
  defect, *111*
  relaxing, simultaneous velolaryngeal videoendoscopy, *166–167*
  simultaneous velolaryngeal videoendoscopy, *166–167*
Sphenoethmoidal recess, *52*, *69*, 74
  and sphenoid sinus ostium, *74*
Sphenoethmoidectomy findings, postoperative, 85, *85*
Sphenoidotomy opening, *75*
Sphenoid sinus
  cavity
    endoscopic view, 75, *85*
    internal carotid artery, 75, *85*
    postoperative, optic nerve, *85*
  ostium, *52*, 69, *69*, *74*
  pyocele, 83, *83*
Sphenoid sinusotomy, *84*
Squamous cell carcinoma
  epiglottic, *143*
  supraglottic, 143, *143*
  tonsil, 110, *110*
  transglottic, *142*, *143*
  vallecular, *143*
'Stapedial prosthesis, middle ear, videoendoscopy, *180*
Straining, in examination, simultaneous velolaryngeal videoendoscopy, *163*
Strobovideolaryngoscopy, 145–157
  fiberscopic, *149*
  glottic closure patterns, 152
    anterior and posterior gaps, *152*
    complete closure, *152*
    hourglass closure, *152*
    incomplete closure, *152*
    pseudo-hourglass closure, *152*
    spindle-shaped closure, *152*
  techniques, 148–151
  telescopic, *150*
    vs. fiberscopic, 149
Subglottis, 124
  stricture, *139*
  translaryngoscopic telescopic view, *124*
  transnasal fiberscopic view, *124*
  transoral telescopic view, *124*
  transtracheotomy telescopic view, *124*
Sulcus vergeture, *139*
Sulcus vocalis, *139*
  laryngeal strictures, 139
Suprabullar recess, paranasal sinus, *73*
Supraglottic squamous cell carcinoma, 143, *143*
Supraglottic stricture, *139*
Supraglottitis, *125*
  acute, *125*
Swallowing, simultaneous velolaryngeal videoendoscopy, 166–167
Synechiae, postoperative, *64*

T

Telangiectasias, laryngeal, *128*
Telescopic optical distortion, vs. fiberscopic, comparison, 151
Telescopic strobovideolaryngoscopy, vs. fiberscopic, 149
Thornwaldt cyst, nasopharynx, 98, *98*
Tonsil
  bilobed, *109*
  hypertrophy, *106*
    lingual, 137, *137*
  kissing, *106*
  palatine, 106
    enlarged, with visible epiglottis, *106*
    normal, *106*
  plug, *107*
  squamous cell carcinoma, 110, *110*
Tonsillar fossa, superior, 107, *107*
Tonsillectomy, postoperative findings, *112*
Tonsillitis, 109
  acute, *109*
  cryptic chronic, *109*
  follicular, lingual, *137*
  infectious mononucleosis, *109*
Torus tubarius, *92*
Transfer, of video images, to print, slide, 13–15, *14*
Transglottic squamous cell carcinoma, *142*, *143*
Trauma, of ear canal, 28
  bleeding from floor of ear canal, *28*
  fracture of anterior canal wall, *28*
  hematoma, *28*

Index

Tumor
  middle ear
    glomus, videoendoscopy, *176*
    primary, 39
      glomus jugulare tumor, *39*
      glomus tympanicum tumor, *39*
  nasal cavity, 63
Turbinate
  with anterior polypoid mucosa, *47*
  inferior, 45
    atrophic, after total laryngectomy, *45*
    decongested, *45*
    deformed, *65*
    hypertrophied, *45*
    posterior end of, *45*
  L-shaped, *47*
    with marked horizontal lamella, *47*
  medially displaced, with uncinate process, basal lamella, *47*
  middle, *69*
    right, *47*
      medially bent, *47*
      sagittally clefted, *47*
      variations of, *47*
  superior, and meatus, 52
  triangular, *47*
Tympanic membrane, 19–40
  anatomy
    overview, 20–21
    right tympanic membrane, normal, *20, 21*
  attenuated segment, *35*
  disorders of, 23–30
  perforation, 34
    anterior middle tympanic membrane perforation, *34*
    near-total tympanic membrane perforation, *34*
    posterior half tympanic membrane perforation, *34*
    posterior superior tympanic membrane perforation, *34*
Tympanoplasty, 37
Tympanosclerosis, 36, *36*

U

Ulcers
  arytenoid, 138
Uncinate process, 48
  medially bent, *48, 65*
    anteriorly, *48*
  unusually shaped, *48*
  variations of, 48
Uvula
  bifid, *108*
  long, *108*
  papilloma, *108*
  variations of, *108*
  wide, *108*

Uvulopalatal web, *111*
Uvulopalatopharyngoplasty, postoperative findings, *112*

V

Vallecular cyst, 136, *136*
Vallecular squamous cell carcinoma, *143*
Velolaryngeal videoendoscopy, simultaneous, 158–167
  anatomy, 159–160
  breathing, 162
  closed velopharyngeal port, *159*
  examination, 162–167
  larynx, effort closure of, 163
  open velopharyngeal port, *160*
  phonating, 162
  siren, 164–165
  swallowing, 166–167
  techniques, 161
  whistling, 162
Velopharyngeal port, 90
  closed, velolaryngeal videoendoscopy, simultaneous, *159*
  open, larynx elevated, simultaneous velolaryngeal videoendoscopy, *166–167*
Velum palatini, 158–167; see also Velolaryngeal videoendoscopy, simultaneous
Video camera, with endoscopy, 9–12, *11*, 148
Videoendoscopy, middle ear, 174–178; see also Middle ear, videoendoscopy
Video enhancer, 12
Video images, transfer of, to print, slides, 13–15, *14*
Videolaryngoscopy, 114–145
Video monitor, 12
Video nasal endoscopy, see Nasal endoscopy
Videonasopharyngoscopy, 86–101
Videopharyngoscopy, 102–113
Video printer, 14–15
Video recorder, 12
Videorhinoscopy, see Nasal endoscopy
Video-otoscopy, 19–40
Video-to-print transfer, 14–15
Video-to-slide transfer, 13–14
Vocal fold
  anatomy, overview, 146–147
  coronal section, *146*
  cyst, 155
    on abduction, *155*
  epidermoid cyst, *134*
  granulomas, *133*
  hemorrhage, *128*
  leukoplakia, 156
    on abduction, *156*
    on adduction, *156*
    composite of glottic cycles, *156*
    microphotographic representation of, *156*
  mucous retention cyst, *134*

Vocal fold (*contd.*)
  nodules, 129, *129*, 153, *153*
    on abduction, *153*
    on adduction, *153*
    stroboscopic composite, glottic cycle, *153*
  papilloma, *141*, 157, 179
    on abduction, *157*
    on adduction, *157*
    composite of glottic cycles, *157*
    microphotographic representation of, *157*
  paralysis, 140
  polyp, *128*, 130–132, *130–132*, 154
    on adduction, *154*
    excision, *132*
    glottic cycles, *154*
    microphotographic representation of, *154*
    pedunculated, *130*
  saccular cyst, anterior, *134*
  true
    disorders of, 152–157
    telescopic strobovideolaryngoscopic view, *147*
Vocal process, contact ulcer, *138*

W

Whistling, in examination, simultaneous velolaryngeal videoendoscopy, *162*
Woodruff's plexus, *46*